Essentials of
Respiratory Disease

R. B. COLE, MA, MD (Cantab.), FRCP (Lond.)

Consultant Physician,
North Staffordshire Hospital Centre,
formerly Senior Lecturer, Department of Medicine,
Queen's University of Belfast

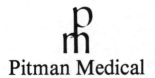

Pitman Medical

First published 1971
Reprinted 1973
Second edition 1975

Pitman Medical Publishing Co Ltd
42 Camden Road, Tunbridge Wells,
Kent TN1 2QD

Associated Companies

UNITED KINGDOM
Pitman Publishing Ltd, London
Focal Press Ltd, London

USA
Pitman Publishing Corporation, New York
Fearon Publishers Inc, California

AUSTRALIA
Pitman Publishing Pty Ltd, Melbourne

CANADA
Pitman Publishing, Toronto
Copp Clark Publishing, Toronto

EAST AFRICA
Sir Isaac Pitman and Sons Ltd, Nairobi

SOUTH AFRICA
Pitman Publishing Co SA (Pty) Ltd, Johannesburg

ISBN 0 272 79366 3
Cat. No. 21 0442 81

Printed in Great Britain by
The Whitefriars Press Ltd, London and Tonbridge

£5·00

ESSENTIALS OF RESPIRATORY DISEASE

To Sister & The
Chest Dept.

With very best wishes ___

Ashley Grossman
MRCP (Part I !)

August 1977

To Janie

Preface

Many of the commonest problems in clinical medicine are due to respiratory illnesses and I have always felt that a thorough understanding of the manifestations of pulmonary disease is an invaluable asset to the general physician, particularly in a field of medicine in which a knowledge of physiological principles plays so large a part in the logic of diagnosis and management. In this book I have tried to bring together the techniques of bedside diagnosis, the essential concepts of pulmonary physiology and the clinical characteristics of the commoner respiratory diseases, in the hope of providing a practical guide to clinical problems that may be useful to senior medical students and to doctors in their early postgraduate years.

In writing this book I have been constantly encouraged by Professor John Vallance-Owen, for whose interest and advice I am sincerely grateful. I also acknowledge with gratitude the valuable advice of those who were good enough to find time to read the manuscript, including my father, Dr Leslie Cole, and my friends and colleagues, Professor Peter Elmes, Dr Ross McHardy, Dr Ian Green, and Dr Leslie Capel.

My warmest thanks are due to Miss Anne Wilkie and to Mrs Joan Beattie who undertook the tedious task of typing the manuscript, and to Mr J. A. Robin and the staff of the Photographic Department, Belfast City Hospital, for their expert assistance with the diagrams. I am also grateful to Butterworth and Co Ltd for permission to reproduce certain material previously published in *Medical Progress* 1969/70.

R.B.C.
Belfast, 1970

Preface to the Second Edition

The preparation of a new edition of this book has given me a welcome opportunity to correct certain inaccuracies and ambiguities and to revise the text in the light of recent advances in the diagnosis and management of respiratory disorders. The reviewers of the first edition made many constructive comments which I have endeavoured to incorporate into this edition; few changes have seemed necessary in the first two sections of the book dealing with clinical methods and physiological principles but some rearrangements and additions have been made to the third section concerned with the commoner varieties of respiratory disease, including a chapter dealing with lung disorders induced by drugs. I have, however, tried to avoid excessive expansion of the text, for this remains a basic textbook designed for medical students and doctors in training rather than a reference book for specialists.

I would like to thank again all those whose help is acknowledged in the preface to the first edition, particularly Professor Peter Elmes who has once more given me invaluable advice. I am greatly indebted to Miss Diane Stirling for her able help in producing this revised book.

R.B.C
Belfast, 1975

Contents

PART I
Clinical Methods

1

The History

Throughout his interview with the patient the clinician's aim is to accumulate accurate clinical data which must be assessed mentally, tested by further questions, and stored in the mind in terms of a differential diagnosis. Besides listening to the patient it is important at this stage to observe every detail of his behaviour and appearance, noting all abnormalities and directing questions that may reveal their cause. In effect, during the interview a clinician must be a highly efficient and versatile computer, using his humanity and sympathy and his powers of observation as the vital means for obtaining the information needed to reach a correct diagnosis.

That the patient should be encouraged to give his own account of the symptoms is a well-tried maxim, and some patience may be needed before a general outline of the illness is revealed. Nevertheless, the main points that must be clearly understood at the end of this early stage of the interview provide a framework upon which the differential diagnosis must be built by direct questions. These main points are as follows:

1. The major symptoms and their duration.
2. The precise time and mode of onset of the first symptom.
3. The sequence and mode of onset of further symptoms.
4. The progress of the illness and of individual symptoms.

Once these points have been clearly established the clinician must turn to detailed probing of the patient by direct questions, designed not only to enlarge on the descriptions already obtained but also to acquire circumstantial evidence for one or other of the possible diagnoses that have been suggested by the patient's account. An example of this type of question might be, with regard to a primary complaint of haemoptysis, an enquiry into recent swelling or pain of a leg which might have seemed too slight or apparently too irrelevant to have been recounted by the patient but which, if present, would point to a possible diagnosis of pulmonary embolism.

It should be clear that these direct questions will cut across any

3

formal division of present, past or family history or systems of questioning that we all learn as junior students. Nevertheless, some such useful system should be deeply ingrained in the mind of the clinician so that once he has fully enlightened himself as to the patient's present illness he may survey the data he has already obtained and seek for unsuspected relevant information by formal questions about the patient's past history, his family, his occupation and social background that may lead to a modification or enlargement of the mental diagnosis he has already established.

By the time history-taking is completed the doctor should have a clear idea of the abnormal clinical signs he is likely to find on detailed examination of the patient, which will enable him to confirm or reject the various diagnoses that have already been suggested during the interview. However, he must bring to bear the same critical accuracy in clinical examination as in history-taking, remembering that new data may be revealed which will alter his earlier conclusions or raise new possibilities.

Symptoms of Respiratory Disease

These principles of the science of history-taking are applicable in all fields of medicine, but among diseases of the respiratory system certain symptoms are so common that more detailed consideration of their incidence and significance is necessary here. They are shortness of breath, cough, sputum, haemoptysis, and chest pain.

SHORTNESS OF BREATH

The sensation of shortness of breath, or dyspnoea, is a subjective one although the complaint may be supported by objective signs such as laboured or rapid breathing and evidence of hypoxia or hypercapnia. The sense organs and nervous pathways that convey the sensation are elusive, but it has been suggested that dyspnoea consists of an unpleasant awareness of inappropriate effort in performing the normal act of breathing (*see* page 68). This excessive effort may be demanded by neurochemical stimuli such as hypercapnia, or may be due to abnormal stiffness of the lungs as occurs in diffuse pulmonary fibrosis, or to weakness of the respiratory muscles as in myasthenia gravis.

Dyspnoea may present either as a complaint of persistent or progressive intolerance of exercise or as an acute attack, often paroxysmal. A complaint of reduced *exercise tolerance* should be defined precisely by questioning the patient's ability to walk on the flat or up an incline, to climb stairs and to perform activities such as carrying burdens, doing housework and gardening. These details should be recorded so that comparisons may subsequently be made,

particularly with regard to the effectiveness of treatment. The length of the history and the progress of the symptoms may give some guide to the nature of the underlying pathology, but exertional dyspnoea is a symptom of many conditions, not only diseases of the cardiac and respiratory systems but also of hyperthyroidism, obesity, anaemia, and anxiety. It is therefore an indication for enquiry into further symptoms which may reveal its cause, such as cough, wheeze, chest pain, palpitation and dependent oedema.

The mode of onset of dyspnoea may be more informative in diagnosis. Severe dyspnoea of sudden onset in a previously normal person suggests either *spontaneous pneumothorax,* which is often associated with pain or tightness in the chest, or *massive pulmonary embolism.* Recurrent paroxysms of dyspnoea suggest *bronchial asthma,* especially when precipitated by emotion, exposure to a known antigen, by exercise or by breathing cold air. Evidence of other forms of hypersensitivity and of a family history should also be sought. Bronchial asthma may present in an otherwise normal person or against a background of permanent exertional dyspnoea caused by recurrent attacks and by bronchial infection. The distinction between the dyspnoeic attacks of the middle-aged asthmatic and those of the chronic bronchitic is often difficult since both are liable to have chronic exertional dyspnoea with recurrent exacerbations due to bronchial infection.

Acute attacks of dyspnoea occurring when the patient is recumbent at night indicate impaired cardiac output, due usually to left ventricular failure or to severe mitral stenosis. The history of *paroxysmal nocturnal dyspnoea* is characteristic: the patient wakes from sleep with an intense feeling of suffocation, getting relief after a few minutes by sitting on the side of the bed or by standing at the window. Often he admits that this occurs when he slips down from his pillows during sleep, and enquiry into the number of pillows used by the patient may reveal his intolerance of the horizontal position, a condition known as *orthopnoea.* It is due to a reduction in the influence of gravity upon the peripheral circulation, causing increased pulmonary venous engorgement at a time when the pulmonary circulation is already overfilled because of left ventricular failure or mitral stenosis. Orthopnoea also occurs in patients with severe airways obstruction, but in this case it is due to the impaired ventilation that results from limitation of diaphragmatic movement when they are lying down.

Wheezing is due to bronchial narrowing, either by secretions or bronchospasm, and tends to be most marked during expiration, when slight bronchoconstriction occurs physiologically. It is therefore a characteristic symptom in asthma, bronchitis, and pulmonary oedema

and is often associated with coughing as the patient attempts to clear obstructing mucus. Wheeze in a localised area, unaffected by coughing, may indicate partial obstruction of a bronchus due to a neoplasm or an inhaled foreign body.

A complaint of dyspnoea is an indication for further interrogation of the patient with regard to other symptoms of respiratory or cardiac disease, his past history of respiratory infection, a family history of asthma, his occupational background, and his smoking habits. In examination, the clinician must be alert for evidence of cardiac arrhythmias, cardiac failure, and mitral stenosis, for signs of pneumothorax or pleural effusion, and of infection or neoplasm in the airways and lung parenchyma, for evidence of diffuse pulmonary fibrosis, for skeletal abnormalities of the thorax, and for neuromuscular disorders.

COUGH, SPUTUM, AND HAEMOPTYSIS

Cough is due to irritation of the mucous membrane anywhere in the respiratory tract between the pharynx and the small bronchi. To the clinician, cough is most commonly an indication of infection of the airways or lung parenchyma, when inflammation and excessive mucus production act as irritant stimuli. Other important causes of cough are inhaled foreign bodies, most often occurring in children, pulmonary oedema, and irritation of the mucous membrane by bronchial tumours arising either within or outside the bronchi, or by enlarged lymph nodes encroaching upon the airway from the mediastinum.

An unproductive cough denotes airway irritation without telling much about the underlying cause; only rarely does the character of the cough itself provide information about the underlying pathology, as does, for example, the long, inspiratory 'whoop' of whooping cough or the 'bovine' cough which characterises adductor paralysis of a vocal cord due to interruption of the fibres of the recurrent laryngeal nerve by tumour or by aortic aneurysm. In general, the diagnosis of the cause of cough depends not on an analysis of the cough itself, on its painfulness, its paroxysmal nature, its precipitating factors, but upon associated symptoms and signs. Common examples are the history of nasal discharge and sore throat, which usually precede the cough of acute pharyngitis or laryngitis; and the association of haemoptysis with cough in a smoker, which arouses the suspicion of bronchial carcinoma.

The most informative coincidental feature of cough is the character of the material coughed up. Occasionally, the cough is actually dry, either because there is no excessive mucus production or because the

mucus is too viscid or the patient too weak to expectorate it. This type of dry cough is characteristic of the early stages of acute bronchitis and pneumococcal pneumonia, and during an acute attack of bronchial asthma. More commonly the patient protests that his cough is dry when in fact he swallows his sputum; in such a case a sputum specimen must be obtained by personal encouragement, if necessary with the help of postural drainage.

The patient's description of the *sputum* must be confirmed by inspection. Large quantities of sputum in excess of 50 ml in 24 hours suggests three possible diagnoses: if it is purulent, either chronic bronchitis or bronchiectasis is likely and the possibility of underlying cystic fibrosis should be borne in mind; in chronic bronchitis the sputum may be quite copious even when it is not purulent, but excessive quantities of thin watery sputum should raise the suspicion of alveolar cell carcinoma. Although it is commonly supposed that bronchiectasis is characterised by a large sputum volume it must be remembered that localised bronchiectasis, particularly in the well-drained upper lobes, may occur without much sputum.

The sputum may be black if it contains smoke or carbon particles, and green, yellow, or khaki if it contains pus. An excessive number of eosinophils in the sputum may give it a lemon-yellow appearance. The observation of pus is an indication for bacteriological examination, to determine the infecting organism and its sensitivities. Specimens sent for bacteriological examination should be freshly taken and contain obvious pus. Mucoid sputum is white, grey or 'clear', and is characteristic of quiescent chronic bronchitis, diffuse fibrosing alveolitis and bronchial asthma. During acute attacks of asthma the sputum is more than usually viscid and difficult to expectorate, becoming 'looser' and sometimes frothy when the attack begins to subside. Bronchial casts are often found in such sputum following an acute asthmatic attack.

The coughing up of blood-stained sputum, or *haemoptysis*, is an indication for thorough investigation to exclude serious underlying disease. If the sputum is 'rusty' in appearance due to admixture of haemoglobin breakdown products, pneumococcal pneumonia is strongly suggested. Pink frothy sputum occurs in pulmonary oedema because of the exudation of red cells with oedema fluid into the airways. Otherwise, the appearance of the sputum varies only as to the relative proportions of blood and mucus, from 'frank blood' to blood-staining or streaking. The quantity of blood produced and the frequency of the haemoptysis do not give a reliable guide to the underlying cause, but the relationship of the haemoptysis to other symptoms and signs may be of prime importance, as for example the coincidence of haemoptysis and pleuritic pain ten days after an

abdominal operation, indicating the diagnosis of deep venous thrombosis and pulmonary embolism.

The commoner causes of haemoptysis which should always be considered, and excluded by thorough investigation, are:

1. Bronchial tumour, either carcinoma or carcinoid.
2. Pulmonary infarction.
3. Pulmonary tuberculosis.
4. Acute pneumonia.
5. Bronchiectasis.
6. Lung abscess.
7. Mitral stenosis.
8. Pulmonary oedema.
9. Chronic bronchitis.
10. Trauma, particularly lung contusion.
11. Abnormalities of blood coagulation.

CHEST PAIN

Chest pain should be analysed in a fashion similar to that of pain elsewhere in the body, by enquiry into its: 1, mode of onset; 2, character; 3, site; 4, area of radiation; 5, duration; 6, intensity; 7, precipitating or aggravating factors; and 8, means of relief. The most characteristic pain of lung disease is that due to inflammation of the pleura. Typical pleurisy may come on gradually or abruptly, is sharp or knife-like in character, and usually occurs at the site of inflammation, although diaphragmatic pleurisy is often referred to the point of the shoulder, and pleurisy in the lower thorax may be referred to the back or abdomen. The pain is continuous and severe, but is characteristically sharply aggravated by movement, coughing or deep breathing, so that the patient adopts a pattern of rapid, shallow respiration and tends to avoid unnecessary movement. The commonest causes of pleuritic pain are pulmonary infection or infarction, but many other conditions may present with, or be complicated by pleurisy, including primary and secondary malignant tumours, tuberculosis, spontaneous pneumothorax, and rheumatoid arthritis. The development of pleural effusion is usually accompanied by some relief of pain, due probably to limitation of lung movement by the fluid and to separation of the inflamed pleural surfaces.

Retrosternal pain accompanies acute tracheitis and bronchitis, usually aggravated by coughing, and relieved when the patient begins to bring up sputum. A rather vague, indefinite aching pain often occurs in bronchial carcinoma situated in the hilar region, poorly localised but sometimes referred to the neck, back or abdomen. This pain is most troublesome at night and is relieved by activity or occupation.

In assessing the cause of chest pain the clinician must give due consideration to alternative possibilities such as myocardial ischaemia, aneurysm of the aorta, oesophageal obstruction or reflux, subdiaphragmatic disease, Bornholm disease and affections of the intercostal muscles, herpes zoster, and diseases of the spinal cord, vertebral column and ribs.

Significance of Previous Illness and Family History

Enquiry into the past history may reveal that the present illness is either a recrudescence or a complication of a previous one. Similarly, the health of other members of the patient's family may have a direct bearing on his present illness. Since patients do not usually give a complete answer to questions such as, 'Have you ever had any serious illness in the past?', or 'Do you come from a healthy family?', specific questions must be put which are designed to throw light on the background of the present complaint. A past history of the following diseases may be relevant:

1. *Asthma.* This disorder is well-recognised by the patient who can often give a good account of spasmodic attacks going back to childhood. The opportunity should be taken to enquire about other allergies such as hay fever and skin disorders, and also about the incidence of asthma in other members of the patient's family.

2. *Bronchitis.* Recurrent illnesses with cough and purulent sputum are the customary precursors of chronic bronchitis, respiratory failure and cor pulmonale. Often such illnesses have been present since childhood when a severe attack of measles or whooping cough with secondary pulmonary infection may have initiated pulmonary damage.

3. *Pneumonia and Pleurisy.* These illnesses are often symptomatic of underlying lung disease, e.g. chronic bronchitis and emphysema. A history of recurrent attacks can sometimes be obtained in pulmonary thromboembolic disease, due to repeated episodes of pulmonary infarction. In the middle-aged a short history of recurrent pneumonia that fails to clear up satisfactorily is one of the commonest presenting features of bronchial carcinoma.

4. *Tuberculosis.* Previous tuberculosis infection may have caused lung damage which is responsible for bronchiectasis and pulmonary fibrosis. Recrudescence of quiescent pulmonary tuberculosis should also be considered.

5. *Cystic Fibrosis.* Enquiry into the childhood and family history of patients who present with symptoms and signs of bronchiectasis may rarely reveal a chronic respiratory history throughout early life, and similar illness or early death among one or more of the patient's siblings.

6. *Surgical operations,* especially those on the thorax or abdomen, radiotherapy, motor accidents, and any illness that imposes a period of prolonged bed rest may be responsible for pulmonary damage from fibrosis, infection, or pulmonary embolism.

Occupational and Environmental History

Occupational exposure to dust or antigenic material by inhalation is a common cause of lung disease, especially pulmonary fibrosis. The clinician should be careful to enquire not only into the patient's present occupation but into all other occupations in which he has been engaged throughout his working life. The actual nature of the work should be enquired into, with specific reference to the type of dust and the duration of exposure. In reaching a clinical diagnosis the following occupational hazards should be borne in mind:

1. As a cause of pulmonary fibrosis:
   (a) The mining, quarrying or handling of coal, or of any rock containing silica.
   (b) Sand-blasting.   –
   (c) Foundry-work, particularly the freeing of sand from castings.
   (d) The manufacture of china or earthenware.
   (e) Stone-masonry.
   (f) Grinding, using a sandstone grinder.
   (g) Boiler-scaling.
   (h) The handling of asbestos.
   (i) The manufacture or use of beryllium.
   (j) Farmers or horticulturists who are liable to handle mouldy hay.
   (k) Mushroom growing.
   (l) Handling sugar-cane pulp (bagassosis).
   (m) Bird-fanciers, including chicken farmers and pigeon breeders.

2. As a cause of chronic obstructive airways disease:
   (a) Spinning or manipulation of cotton or flax (byssinosis).
   (b) Inhalation of cadmium fumes, e.g. among scrap-metal cutters.

3. As a cause of pulmonary malignant disease (carcinoma or mesothelioma):
   (a) Exposure to asbestos dust (e.g. workers in the building or ship-building industries).
   (b) Workers in the chromate industry.
   (c) Miners exposed to radioactive dust.

It should be remembered that exposure by proximity to a hazardous dust may occur among workers who do not actually handle the material themselves. This is particularly important with regard to asbestos, for example, among ship-yard workers.

Besides the milieu of his work the patient's environment includes the neighbourhood in which he lives and the personal surroundings of his home. Careful questions about home surroundings are relevant to a history suggestive of atopic asthma, since unsuspected antigens originating from household pets or furnishings may be identified as the stimulus for asthmatic attacks. Both lung cancer and chronic bronchitis are statistically more frequent among urban dwellers than among countrymen, but for both conditions this factor is far outweighed in importance by cigarette smoking. A history of pulmonary symptoms is incomplete without an enquiry into the past and present smoking habits of the patient.

2

External Signs of Lung Disease

Much may be learned by watching the patient as he talks about his illness. If he appears to be short of breath, his respiratory movements may indicate the type of pulmonary disability from which he is suffering, and signs such as cyanosis or digital clubbing may be readily recognisable at a distance. Awareness of such abnormalities as the clinical history unfolds should stimulate the clinician to consider how they may fit in with the possible diagnoses, and alert him to make a closer study when he comes to his clinical examination. The integration of symptoms and clinical observations should be a continuous mental process throughout the interview.

Respiratory Distress

A complaint of shortness of breath is often accompanied by suggestive signs that indicate both the degree of disability and its cause. The appearance of a patient as he walks into the room or alters his position in bed, his ability to undress himself, and even his ability to talk may indicate the severity of his breathlessness. The adoption of an upright posture in bed suggests that he may suffer from orthopnoea, and fixation of the thorax by rigid clamping of the hands to the sides of the bed is particularly suggestive of the respiratory distress seen in obstructive airways disease, especially severe asthma and advanced chronic bronchitis. Analysis of the rate, depth, and rhythm of breathing may give further diagnostic information.

RESPIRATORY RATE

The normal rate of breathing at rest is about 14 breaths per minute. Rapid breathing is seen in acute pulmonary infection, particularly pneumonia, in left ventricular failure, diffuse pulmonary fibrosis, thyrotoxicosis, and in anxiety states. Slow breathing results from narcotic overdose and head injury, and may occur in myxoedema coma, and in the hypoventilation syndrome of obesity.

DEPTH OF BREATHING

Shallow breathing occurs in diffuse pulmonary fibrosis, in which the patient adopts a rapid, shallow respiratory pattern to reduce the excessive effort of expanding 'stiff' lungs. It is also characteristic of pleurisy, to avoid the severe pain caused by deeper breaths. Deep breathing occurs in metabolic acidosis, for example, diabetic ketosis or renal failure, and also in severe salicylate poisoning, in some head injuries or subarachnoid haemorrhage, and in hepatic encephalopathy.

Hysterical overbreathing is rapid and deep, and may be accompanied by peripheral paraesthesiae and carpopedal spasm due to lowering of the serum ionised calcium from respiratory alkalosis. Suspicion of a psychological origin for undue breathlessness is indicated if the symptom occurs at rest, is poorly related to exercise, and fluctuates very rapidly. It is usually associated with difficulty on inspiration and occurs in hysterical or obsessional people, being precipitated by an expectation of consequent pain, or by bereavement, illness or resentment.

RHYTHM

The rhythm of breathing is characteristically altered in airways obstruction by prolongation of the expiratory phase. This is most marked in patients with chronic bronchitis and emphysema, and is often accompanied by a number of characteristic additional signs such as pursing of the lips, contraction of the accessory respiratory muscles and distension of the neck veins during expiration. Cheyne-Stokes respiration is characterised by periods of apnoea alternating with increasing and then decreasing hyperventilation, and occurs in patients with raised intracranial pressure, and also in heart failure. It is occasionally seen in elderly normal people during sleep.

Breathing may be noisy, usually because of wheezing due to bronchial narrowing in asthma or chronic bronchitis. Harsh, strident breathing is known as *stridor,* which is due to narrowing of the large airways, for example in laryngeal spasm or in tracheal compression due to enlarged malignant paratracheal lymph nodes.

Signs of Respiratory Failure

When respiratory function is seriously impaired carbon dioxide tension in the tissues and blood rises and oxygen tension falls, states which are known as hypercapnia and hypoxia respectively.

HYPERCAPNIA

Hypercapnia causes reversible deterioration in cerebral function and peripheral vasodilatation with the following clinical signs:

1. Drowsiness, intellectual impairment, disorientation progressing to coma.
2. Headache due to cerebral vasodilatation, occasionally associated with papilloedema.
3. Flapping tremor of the outstretched hands.
4. A pulse of large volume with warm sweaty extremities.

The mental confusion, sleeplessness and restlessness are often wrongly attributed to senile dementia and are aggravated by drugs that are reputed to act as respiratory stimulants. In hypercapnia the patient becomes abnormally tolerant of high levels of arterial carbon dioxide tension, the principal drive to respiration being hypoxia; if a gas mixture containing a high concentration of oxygen is administered, respiration diminishes and the hypercapnia is increased. Hypercapnia is always accompanied by hypoxia unless the patient is breathing a hyperoxic gas mixture, but hypoxia may occur in the absence of hypercapnia.

HYPOXIA

The chronic hypoxia of respiratory failure affects cerebral and cardiac function directly, causes vasoconstriction of the pulmonary vessels, and stimulates secondary polycythaemia. The clinical signs of chronic hypoxia, some of which are difficult to distinguish from those of hypercapnia, are:

1. Intellectual impairment, behaviour disturbances and increased neuromuscular irritability.
2. Cardiac arrhythmias, tachycardia, and peripheral vasodilatation.
3. Central cyanosis.
4. The plethoric appearance of secondary polycythaemia.

Cyanosis is a bluish discoloration of the skin or mucous membranes which is usually due to hypoxia. This causes a reduction in the oxyhaemoglobin saturation of arterial blood which is normally 95 to 98 per cent saturated with oxygen during air breathing. A fall in arterial oxyhaemoglobin saturation to less than 75 per cent causes clinical cyanosis, but because the degree of 'blueness' is directly related to the quantity of circulating reduced haemoglobin, a greater degree of desaturation is necessary to produce cyanosis in an anaemic patient whereas a patient with polycythaemia will appear cyanotic when only mildly desaturated. Methaemoglobinaemia and sulphaemoglobinaemia may rarely cause a somewhat similar colour change.

The term *peripheral cyanosis* means that cyanosis is limited to the extremities, for example the fingers, toes, nose, and ear lobes. It is due

to sluggish peripheral circulation with excessive reduction of oxy-haemoglobin in the capillary blood, and it occurs commonly in the cold, when there is peripheral circulatory failure, or in venous obstruction. *Central cyanosis* means that the cyanosis affects not only the periphery but also the warm, central areas of the body such as the mucous membranes of the mouth and lips. The distinction between peripheral and central cyanosis can be quickly made by inspecting the tongue and inside of the mouth.

Central cyanosis is due to inadequate oxygenation of arterial blood because of a disorder of pulmonary gas exchange. The commonest causes of central cyanosis are:

1. Diseases that upset the normal relationship between pulmonary ventilation and perfusion, e.g. chronic bronchitis and emphysema, asthma, bronchiectasis, pulmonary fibrosis, pulmonary emboli.

2. Conditions causing underventilation of the alveoli in the presence of structurally normal lungs, e.g. hypoventilation associated with obesity, narcotic overdose, neuromuscular disorders leading to paralysis of the respiratory muscles.

3. Diseases that cause mixed venous blood to bypass ventilated lung tissue, e.g. some congenital cardiac defects such as Fallot's tetralogy, intrapulmonary arteriovenous aneurysms, intrapulmonary lesions such as pneumonic consolidation and, occasionally, tumours.

Obstruction of the superior vena cava, usually because of mediastinal spread of bronchial carcinoma, causes cyanosis of the arms, face and neck, because of the sluggish venous return from these areas. It is really a 'peripheral' cause of cyanosis but the tongue and mucous membrane of the mouth and lips are also cyanosed because they lie within the region drained by the superior vena cava (*see* page 33).

Secondary Polycythaemia. A common accompaniment of cyanosis is secondary polycythaemia due either to chronic hypoxia or to methaemoglobinaemia and is suggested by plethoric facies and the deep purplish-red colour of the mucous membranes. It should be distinguished from polycythaemia rubra vera by the evidence for chronic respiratory or cardiac disease, the absence of splenic enlargement and of generalised pruritus, and the normal white cell and platelet counts. Secondary polycythaemia with normal pulmonary function may occur in patients with primary alveolar hypoventilation, and in association with an abnormal haemoglobin with a high affinity for oxygen which leads to relative tissue hypoxia and consequently stimulates polycythaemia. Measurement of arterial oxygen tension and the oxygen affinity of haemoglobin is necessary in doubtful cases.

Methaemoglobinaemia and Sulphaemoglobinaemia. The observation of lavender-hued cyanosis in the absence of dyspnoea or
of other evidence of respiratory or cardiac disease should arouse
suspicion of sulph- or methaemoglobinaemia. These compounds are
derived from normal haemoglobin but do not take part in oxygen
transport, so that in severe cases symptoms of acute hypoxia may be
present, characterised by headache, dizziness, exertional dyspnoea,
mental confusion and even coma.

Methaemoglobin is present in normal red cells, but in a concentration of less than 1 per cent. This low concentration is maintained by
the activity of intracellular enzymes, which reduce methaemoglobin as
soon as it is formed by the auto-oxidation of haemoglobin. Excessive
accumulation of methaemoglobin usually occurs because the
methaemoglobin-reducing system is swamped by excessive auto-
oxidation of haemoglobin (*toxic methaemoglobinaemia*), but rarely
because either the enzyme system is genetically defective, or because
the haemoglobin is genetically abnormal and resistant to reduction
(*congenital methaemoglobinaemia*). Toxic methaemoglobinaemia is
most commonly caused by excessive ingestion of analgesics
containing phenacetin, but a large number of other substances may
also be responsible, including nitrites and nitrates, sulphonamide
derivatives, and analine and its derivatives.

Sulphaemoglobin is often present at the same time as
methaemoglobin, especially in constipated people, due, it is thought,
to absorption of sulphur from hydrogen sulphide formed in the bowel.
It causes cyanosis similar to that of methaemoglobinaemia. Both
sulphaemoglobinaemia and methaemoglobinaemia are treated by
removal of the causative agent. The chemical change to sulphaemoglobin is irreversible, so that it persists until the red cells are
destroyed; methaemoglobin, on the other hand, may be rapidly re-
converted to haemoglobin by intravenous injection of methylene blue.

Digital Clubbing

Digital clubbing is a peculiar change in the shape of the tips of the
fingers and toes which is clinically associated with a number of
different diseases. The earliest sign is loss of the angle between the nail
and the dorsum of the terminal phalanx, associated with a shiny
appearance of the skin at the base of the nail and a feeling of
'sponginess' of the nail root on gentle pressure. As the condition
progresses the tissue at the root of the nail becomes heaped up and the
curvature of the nail becomes more pronounced, until finally the soft
tissue of the whole of the tip of the digit becomes swollen, producing
the classical drum-stick appearance.

Recognition of these changes should lead to a careful search for the

underlying disease, giving particular attention to the following six groups of conditions which include those most commonly associated with digital clubbing in the United Kingdom.

1. *Intrathoracic Tumours:*
Bronchial carcinoma, particularly peripheral tumours
Mesothelioma of the pleura
Tumours of the mediastinum, including thymoma, aneurysm of the aorta, Hodgkin's disease and neurofibroma

2. *Mixed Venous-to-arterial Shunts:*
Intracardiac shunt, e.g. in cyanotic congenital cardiac lesions
Pulmonary arteriovenous aneurysm

3. *Chronic Pulmonary Diseases:*
Bronchiectasis
Diffuse pulmonary fibrosis
Chronic bronchitis and chronic pulmonary tuberculosis (probably only when associated with bronchiectasis)
Empyema and lung abscess

4. *Chronic Hepatic Fibrosis:*
Biliary cirrhosis
Portal cirrhosis

5. *Chronic Diarrhoea:*
Ulcerative colitis
Crohn's disease
Coeliac disease

6. *Subacute Bacterial Endocarditis*

Clubbing occurs rarely in a number of other miscellaneous diseases, and is also occasionally seen as a familial condition in the absence of any underlying disorder. The pathogenesis of clubbing is not known. Inspection of the above list of associated diseases (which is by no means exhaustive) shows that arterial desaturation occurs in a number of them, and in such cases correction of the cause of the desaturation nearly always leads to regression of the clubbing. Nonetheless, many patients with clubbing are not cyanosed or hypoxaemic, nor does arterial desaturation always lead to clubbing. Morphological and radiological studies of clubbed fingers indicate that the digital vasculature is abnormally profuse and physiological investigations suggest that finger blood flow may be excessively high, although both these views have been contested. One theory of clubbing is that the altered shape of the nail bed and finger tip is due

to hypertrophy of the muscular arteriovenous anastomoses which are particularly numerous in those areas, but no adequate hypothesis has been offered to explain the connection between these vascular changes and the diverse disease patterns with which clubbing is associated. Both humoral and neurological stimuli have been suggested.

Clubbing is so distinctive that it is not easily confused with any other abnormality of the fingers. A rare condition, known as 'pseudo-clubbing', may cause confusion; it occurs in hyperparathyroidism when excessive bone resorption results in virtual disappearance of the terminal phalanges with telescoping of the soft tissues and a resulting 'drum-stick' appearance of the fingers. The curvature of the nails is not abnormally pronounced, however, and the shortening of the finger is readily apparent, the condition being confirmed radiologically.

Hypertrophic Pulmonary Osteoarthropathy

This rare condition should be differentiated from other causes of acute arthritis of the wrists and ankles. It occurs in association with certain forms of pulmonary disease, particularly peripherally-located bronchial carcinoma and pleural fibromata. It is characterised by painful swelling of the wrists and ankles, the pain being of an intolerable burning character. The skin around the affected joints is warm, thickened and somewhat oedematous, and the face may also have a coarse, furrowed appearance. Digital clubbing is usually, but not always, associated, and gynaecomastia is present in about 7 per cent of the cases. The bone changes consist of a proliferative periostitis with lymphocyte and plasma cell infiltration of the periosteum, the subperiosteal new bone formation being readily apparent in radiographs of the distal ends of the forearm and leg. A somewhat similar condition, known as thyroid achropachy, occurs rarely in patients treated for thyrotoxicosis; it is associated with digital clubbing and pretibial myxoedema, but differs from hypertrophic pulmonary osteoarthropathy in that the periosteal new bone formation affects the metacarpals, metatarsals, and digits rather than the long bones.

The cause of hypertrophic pulmonary osteoarthropathy is unknown, although it has been suggested that it is due to the action of a humoral substance similar to growth hormone, which is secreted by the pulmonary tumour. The joint pain is quickly relieved by excision of the lung lesion, and the clubbing and periosteal changes regress gradually. It has been observed that the symptoms of pulmonary osteoarthropathy subside rapidly following cervical vagotomy on the side of the pulmonary lesion, but experimental attempts to define a neurological or neurohumoral mechanism for the condition have been unproductive.

3

Examination of the Chest

Examination of the chest should be undertaken with the patient sitting in a comfortable position, preferably leaning back against the pillows at an angle of about 45°. To avoid undue disturbance the front of the chest should first be fully examined before the patient is asked to lean forward to allow examination of the back. It is convenient at this stage to look for superficial signs of disease in the upper half of the body.

External Appearance

The Patient's Build. Wasting and weight loss occur not only in advanced pulmonary malignant disease and in pulmonary tuberculosis but also in other forms of longstanding disease causing diffuse pulmonary fibrosis or chronic bronchitis and emphysema. In the latter case a cachetic appearance seems to be associated with preponderant emphysematous changes rather than chronic bronchitis. Gross obesity is occasionally associated with alveolar hypoventilation and even respiratory failure. Excessive somnolence in such patients may be attributable to carbon dioxide retention, the usual accompaniments of this syndrome being cyanosis with secondary polycythaemia.

The skin may present evidence of certain common respiratory diseases, particularly bronchial carcinoma. Pigmentation of the skin folds, nipples, and exposed areas may be an indication of Addison's disease due to metastases to the adrenal glands, and further search should be made for the typical bluish-black blotches of pigmentation on the inside of the lips and cheeks. It may also occur in Cushing's syndrome secondary to oat-cell carcinoma of the bronchus. Metastatic skin nodules are evidence of widespread dissemination of bronchial cancer, and occasionally acanthosis nigricans and dermatomyositis may herald the development of this disease (page 239). Pulmonary sarcoidosis may be associated with cutaneous sarcoid lesions (page 206) or with erythema nodosum, and the latter may occasionally be a feature of pulmonary tuberculosis. Diffuse

19

pulmonary fibrosis due to systemic sclerosis may be associated with the typical skin changes of the disease: pinched facial features and hard, tethered skin over the chest, and particularly over the backs of the hands and fingers (page 254).

The breasts should be examined for carcinoma. Gynaecomastia in the male may be associated with hypertrophic pulmonary osteo-arthropathy as a rare manifestation of bronchial carcinoma.

The Lymph Nodes. Swelling of the neck or in the axillae may be observed. Palpation of the lymph nodes in the axillae should be carried out with the patient's arm supported and relaxed, the medial, posterior and lateral walls and apex of the axilla being explored gently but systematically. The infraclavicular nodes may be examined from the front but the nodes in the supraclavicular fossae, posterior triangle of the neck and the cervical chain are best examined from behind with the patient's head slightly flexed and the sternomastoids relaxed. The size, mobility, hardness and tenderness of the enlarged nodes should be noted. Enlargement of cervical nodes, particularly on the right side, may be the only indication of dissemination of bronchial carcinoma, but tuberculosis, sarcoidosis or one of the reticuloses may also have to be considered. Examination of the cervical lymph nodes also offers a convenient opportunity to palpate the thyroid gland.

The Shape of the Thorax. Gross distortion of the thoracic cage due to longstanding kyphoscoliosis may restrict lung expansion and so impair ventilation that respiratory failure results. An angular kyphosis sometimes results from collapse of a vertebra, usually because of spinal tuberculosis but occasionally because of injury or vertebral metastases.

In generalised emphysema the chest becomes 'barrel-shaped', due to an increase in antero-posterior diameter relative to the transverse diameter. This change results from longstanding over-inflation of the lungs, but is also sometimes seen in old people with relatively normal lungs, suggesting that age as well as hyperinflation is responsible for the change of shape. Pectus excavatum, a developmental defect in which the whole sternum and the costal cartilages may be depressed, can occasionally cause impairment of ventilatory function, displacement of the heart and abnormal cardiac murmurs.

Localised areas of flattening of the chest wall indicate underlying lung damage, usually fibrosis or longstanding pulmonary collapse. Local swelling may be due to metastatic malignant deposits in a rib or to direct extension of a pleural or pulmonary tumour into the thoracic wall.

Abnormal respiratory movements occur when breathing is obstructed or in severe chest injury. The commonest abnormal movement is the contraction of the accessory muscles of respiration in

patients with asthma or chronic bronchitis and emphysema. During inspiration the trapezius, scalene and sternomastoid muscles may be seen and felt to contract, and excavation of the suprasternal and supraclavicular fossae becomes apparent with paradoxical inward movement of the lower intercostal muscles due to the excessive negative intrathoracic pressure. In expiration the patient attempts to overcome airways obstruction by clasping the sides of the bed or the bed table, thus fixing the scapulae and allowing contraction of the latissimus dorsi to assist in expelling the air from his chest.

A 'flail' chest is produced by severe injury which results in multiple rib fractures or disruption of the costochondral junction of several ribs. Respiration causes paradoxical movement of the injured part of the chest wall which bulges inwards during inspiration and outwards during expiration, with the result that ventilation of the underlying lung also assumes a paradoxical pattern. Asynchrony of ventilation between the normal and abnormal sides leads to the shunting of air from one lung to the other with consequent hypoventilation and respiratory failure in severe cases.

Surface Anatomy of the Thorax

Whereas the diagnosis of generalised respiratory diseases such as chronic bronchitis or diffuse pulmonary fibrosis depends largely upon correct interpretation of the patient's history and of the external signs of lung disease described above, the diagnosis of localised lung lesions such as pneumonic consolidation or pleural effusion requires an understanding of the anatomical landmarks of the thoracic contents so that the examiner has a mental picture of what lies beneath his fingers or his stethoscope.

The area of the chest wall that overlies the lung varies according to the depth of inspiration, but the accompanying diagrams illustrate the lung margins as they apply in a normal individual during quiet breathing. The essential landmarks are the sternal angle anteriorly, which marks the level of the second rib, the seventh cervical spine posteriorly which may be identified as the uppermost prominent projection at the junction of the neck and thorax, and the mid-axillary line which may be projected vertically downwards from the apex of the axilla when the patient stands relaxed with the arms hanging at the sides.

Bearing these landmarks in mind, the oblique fissure can be traced as an imaginary line over the chest wall from the second thoracic spine posteriorly (two below the prominent seventh cervical spine) to the sixth costochondral junction anteriorly (Figs 3.1 and 3.2). On the right side the horizontal fissure may be traced from the fourth

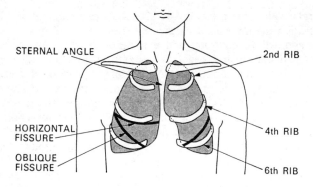

Fig. 3.1   Surface anatomy of the lobes and fissures: anterior view

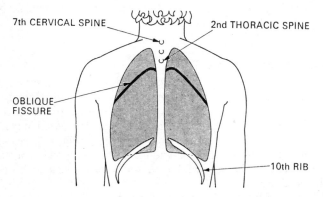

Fig. 3.2   Surface anatomy of the lobes and fissures: posterior view

intercostal space at the right sternal margin laterally to the mid-axillary line close to where it cuts the line of the oblique fissure (Fig. 3.3). These lines mark the contiguous margins of the various lung lobes and are useful in defining interlobar effusions and collapse or consolidation of single lobes of the lungs.

The anterior surface of the heart is not normally covered by lung tissue, and that area is consequently dull to percussion (Fig. 3.1). In quiet breathing the dull percussion note that indicates the upper margin of the normal liver is perceived at the level of the eighth rib in the mix-axillary line (Fig. 3.3).

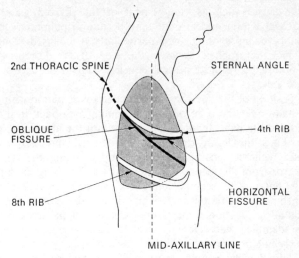

Fig. 3.3 Surface anatomy of the lobes and fissures: right lateral view

Chest Expansion

Asymmetry of chest expansion suggests that pulmonary disease is present on the side that moves less, for example, unilateral pleural effusion or pneumothorax. Inequality of movement between the two sides of the chest may be best appreciated by viewing the patient from directly in front while he takes one or two deep breaths. Any gross abnormality can be appreciated by palpation, the two hands being spread out against the chest wall at corresponding sites on either side of the mid-line. The palmar surfaces of the hands and fingers should be 'anchored' to the chest wall by firm pressure, the tips of the thumbs being brought together in the mid line at the end of expiration. The comparative degree of movement of the two hands and of the thumbs away from each other during deep inspiration is an indication of the symmetry of movement of the chest. This procedure is easily mis-interpreted and greater reliance should be placed on simple inspection of chest expansion.

Mediastinal Displacement

Shift of the mediastinum can be recognised by palpation of the trachea and the apex beat. The position of the trachea is estimated by placing the tip of a finger in the suprasternal notch and pushing it gently backwards: lateral displacement of the trachea is indicated if the finger tip tends to slip to one or other side. This may be due

to local causes such as enlargement of the thyroid gland or of paratracheal lymph nodes; or it may be due to pulmonary disease. Pulmonary collapse or fibrosis, particularly if localised to the lung apex, pull the trachea towards the side of the lesion, whereas pneumothorax or a large pleural effusion tend to displace it to the opposite side.

The position of the apex beat is identified by palpation with the flat of the hand over the praecordium, beginning well back in the axilla and moving the hand forward by stages until the apical pulsation is felt. A finger tip of the right hand is then held precisely over the pulsation while its position is defined by counting the rib spaces downwards from the second left intercostal space using the fingers of the left hand. The second intercostal space is identified by its relationship to the sternal angle which lies at the level of the second costochondral junction. Lateral displacement of the apex beat may then be identified with reference to the mid-clavicular line: this is an imaginary line drawn perpendicularly downwards from the mid point of the left clavicle, a point most easily defined as lying half way between the suprasternal notch and the tip of the acromion. The apex beat normally lies medial to this line in the fifth intercostal space.

Displacement of the apex beat is often due to cardiac enlargement but may be due to mediastinal shift, usually because of extensive fibrosis or pulmonary collapse which tends to draw the heart towards the side of the lesion. Pneumothorax and pleural effusion have the opposite effect. Failure to locate the apex beat may be due to a number of causes:

1. A fat or muscular chest wall.
2. Left-sided pneumothorax or pulmonary hyperinflation.
3. Large left-sided pleural effusion.
4. Large pericardial effusion.
5. Dextrocardia.

The Percussion Note
Percussion of the chest conveys to the ear a sound that varies in quality according to the density of the underlying tissue. Four types of sound can be distinguished: hyperresonant, resonant (or normal), impaired resonance, and dull. (The addition of 'tympanitic' at one end of this scale and 'stony dull' at the other does not increase diagnostic precision.) Dullness is a quality distinctive enough to be easily recognised but the other abnormal types of percussion note can be clearly appreciated only by comparison with the normal. It is therefore essential to percuss the chest in a systematic way, directly comparing the percussion note on one side with that obtained at the

corresponding site on the opposite side. The apices may be compared by percussing the clavicles directly; thereafter the chest should be examined from above downwards, both anteriorly, posteriorly, and in the axillae by alternate percussion on either side. Where a difference in percussion note is observed between the two sides ancillary evidence (such as unilateral reduction in chest expansion or local increase in vocal resonance) may help to decide whether the percussion note is hyperresonant on one side or impaired on the other.

The normal resonant percussion note can be appreciated over the whole lung, the margin between resonance and dullness being readily recognised at the left border of the heart and at the upper margin of the liver. The level of the diaphragm posteriorly may be identified (normally the upper margin of the tenth rib), and equality of diaphragmatic movement between the two sides may be recognised by percussing the margin between resonance and dullness at maximal inspiration and expiration ('tidal percussion'). Paralysis of the diaphragm due to a phrenic nerve lesion or a subdiaphragmatic abnormality such as hepatic enlargement or subphrenic abscess may cause this margin to be elevated.

Hyperresonance has a low-pitched, hollow quality due to diminution in density of the underlying tissue, and is usually due to a large cavity or emphysematous bulla closely underlying the percussing finger, or to pneumothorax. It also occurs in generalised hyperinflation of the lungs due to spasmodic asthma or to widespread emphysema, but in these conditions it is difficult to recognise with certainty because no comparison is possible with the percussion note of normal lung. Consequently the diagnosis of hyperinflation or emphysema is best confirmed by finding loss of the normal area of cardiac dullness and downward displacement of the upper margin of hepatic dullness, often associated with a barrel-shaped chest and wheezy breath sounds.

An impaired percussion note may be observed over areas of local pulmonary fibrosis, pulmonary collapse, consolidation, and sometimes as an indication of pleural thickening in the absence of underlying parenchymatous disease. A dull note indicates the presence of pleural fluid, and the extent of the effusion should be mapped out by percussing the dividing line between resonant and dull. Elevation of the diaphragm may simulate pleural effusion.

The Breath Sounds

The sound of normal breathing heard through a stethoscope is due to the noise of air passing through the larynx, and it varies both in loudness and in rhythm according to the distance of the stethoscope from the larynx where the sound originates. Two varieties of normal

breath sounds may be distinguished: vesicular breathing and 'tracheal' breathing.

Vesicular breathing is a gentle rustling noise that is audible all over the periphery of the lungs. It has a characteristic rhythm, being loudest during inspiration and dying away rapidly during the early part of expiration. Over the trachea, and to some extent over the manubrium sterni and the areas immediately adjacent to it, the rhythm is different: both inspiration and expiration are of approximately equal loudness and the expiratory sound is continued for the greater part of expiration; in addition the inspiratory sound cuts off fairly abruptly at the height of inspiration and there is a momentary silent pause before the expiratory sound begins.

Bronchial breathing indicates the presence of underlying lung disease, and in most respects it simulates the 'tracheal' type of breathing but is heard in regions of the lung distant from the trachea. It has the following characteristics:

1. It has a blowing quality.
2. The inspiratory sound is loud.
3. There is a pause between the inspiratory and expiratory sounds.
4. The expiratory sound is loud and prolonged.

Bronchial breathing results when pathological changes in the lung cause increased conduction of sound from the large airways to the periphery. It has a high-pitched quality when it is due to pulmonary consolidation or collapse and is usually of lower pitch when due to local lung fibrosis. It is also occasionally heard at the upper margin of a pleural effusion. When it has a particularly hollow, blowing quality similar to that obtained by blowing across the mouth of a bottle it is termed 'amphoric' breathing and denotes a large superficial cavity opening into a patent bronchus. Both bronchial and amphoric breathing are frequently accompanied by changes in the voice sounds.

Diminished breath sounds indicate that there is some barrier to the conduction of the noise of breathing to the chest wall. This may be due to acute obstruction of a major bronchus or because of pleural thickening. It is also characteristic of pleural effusion and pneumothorax, presumably because the sound waves conducted from the airways are reflected back at the interface between collapsed lung and air or fluid. General reduction in intensity of the breath sounds is commonly due to emphysema.

The Voice Sounds

Vocal fremitus is the term given to the vibration felt by a hand placed flat on the chest wall when the patient speaks. It is due to the conduction of sound from the larynx via the airways and lung

parenchyma to the chest wall, being increased by the presence of consolidation or collapse of lung tissue and decreased by intervening
pleural effusion, pleural thickening or pneumothorax. Vocal fremitus
should be compared on the two sides of the chest by alternately
placing the palm of the hand firmly against the chest at corresponding
positions on either side, asking the patient to repeat 'ninety-nine' or
'one-one-one'. Changes in vocal fremitus are a crude reflection of
disturbances in sound conduction which may be more easily
appreciated on auscultation.

Vocal resonance is the auscultatory equivalent of vocal fremitus,
the sound of the voice being increased on auscultation over consolidation, cavitation, collapse or local fibrosis and diminished by pleural
effusion, pleural thickening or pneumothorax. Over consolidation and
areas of longstanding collapse the sound of the voice may assume a
nasal quality that is sometimes exaggerated enough to be described as
'bleating' (*aegophony*). Increases in conduction of the spoken voice
are usually accompanied by exaggeration of the whispered voice; the
term '*whispering pectoriloquy*' is given to the peculiar quality of the
patient's whisper which sounds magnified, as if it were direct into the
ear of the auscultator, a marked contrast to the almost inaudible
sound of whispering that is heard on auscultation over normal lungs.

Bronchial breathing is a characteristic clinical sign in pulmonary
consolidation, collapse and local fibrosis, and when a large cavity lies
directly between the stethoscope and a patent bronchus. From the
above paragraph it will be noted that increased vocal resonance,
aegophony and whispering pectoriloquy are signs commonly
associated with these conditions, and they should be sought to
confirm a diagnosis of bronchial breathing.

Adventitial Sounds

Crepitations (or râles) are fine crackling noises heard mainly during
inspiration. They occur in disease affecting the alveoli or terminal
airways, often but not necessarily only when there is an excessive
amount of exudate or transudate in these regions. It has been
suggested that during expiration the small peripheral airways become
obstructed by fluid or by collapse of their walls and that the miniature
explosions which constitute crepitations are due to opening of these
obstructions and sudden equalisation of pressure between regions of
differing pressure, mainly during the expanding phase of respiration.
This concept explains the presence of crepitations in exudative
conditions such as pneumonia and bronchiectasis; in pulmonary
oedema, in which transudate not only floods the airways but also
augments the interstitial tension of the alveolar and bronchiolar walls,
increasing their tendency to collapse on expiration; and in diffuse

Table 3.1

Lung Pathology	Chest Expansion	Mediastinal Shift	Percussion Note	Breath Sounds	Voice Sounds	Added Sounds
Consolidation, e.g. due to lobar pneumonia	Slightly reduced on affected side	Nil	Impaired	Bronchial	Increased, Aegophony, Whispering pectoriloquy	Crepitations
Large cavity	Slightly reduced on affected side	Nil	Locally hyperresonant	Amphoric	Increased, Whispering pectoriloquy	Crepitations
Localised fibrosis, e.g. due to apical tuberculosis	Slightly reduced on affected side	To affected side	Impaired	Bronchial	Increased, Whispering pectoriloquy	Crepitations
Peripheral collapse, e.g. postoperative obstruction of small, peripheral bronchi	Slightly reduced on affected side	Nil	Impaired	Bronchial	Increased, Aegophony, Whispering pectoriloquy	Crepitations
Extensive collapse, e.g. of lung or lobe due to inhaled foreign body	Reduced on affected side	To affected side	Impaired	Diminished vesicular	Reduced	Nil
Pneumothorax	Reduced on affected side	To opposite side	Hyperresonant	Diminished vesicular	Reduced	Nil
Pleural effusion	Reduced on affected side	To opposite side	Dull	Diminished vesicular (Bronchial at air/fluid margin)	Reduced	Sometimes a pleural rub
Pleural thickening	Slightly reduced on affected side	Nil	Impaired	Diminished vesicular	Reduced	Sometimes a pleural rub
Generalised emphysema	Reduced overall	Nil	Hyperresonant	Diminished vesicular	Reduced	Wheezing

pulmonary fibrosis, in which the alveoli and small airways tend to collapse on expiration because of their inelasticity.

In chronic bronchitis and emphysema, crepitations originating from collapsed proximal airways are heard early in inspiration; in contrast, the crepitations characteristic of diffuse pulmonary fibrosis occur late in inspiration because they arise from distal airways.

Coarse crepitations are loud bubbling sounds heard during both inspiration and expiration. They are due to air bubbling through copious secretions in the large airways, and occur in bronchiectasis and bronchitis among patients who are too ill to expectorate these secretions effectively.

Rhonchi or wheezes are musical sounds of low or high pitch that may occur in inspiration or expiration. They are due to the passage of air through narrowed airways at high velocity, the pitch of the sound varying directly with the narrowness of the opening and with the velocity of air movement. Rhonchi occur whenever there is airway narrowing, commonly in chronic bronchitis or in bronchial asthma when the obstruction is due to secretions and bronchospasm. In such circumstances the rhonchi may be eliminated or altered in tone by coughing. Rhonchi are usually most prominent during the expiratory phase of respiration since a slight degree of physiological bronchoconstriction occurs during expiration, but inspiratory rhonchi occur in bronchi narrowed by secretions in asthma and bronchitis, or stiffened by inflammation, fibrosis or malignant infiltration. Inspiratory rhonchi are usually of lower pitch than their expiratory counterpart.

A *pleural friction rub* is due to sounds generated by friction between two inflamed pleural layers. It has a crackling quality frequently similar to and sometimes indistinguishable from the sound of crepitations. The diagnosis of pleural rub is aided by recognition of the sound during expiration as well as inspiration, by its localisation to a small area of the chest wall and by its occasional tendency to increase if the pressure of the stethoscope is increased. It may occur in any condition causing pleural inflammation, commonly pulmonary infarction, pneumonia and neoplastic infiltration. Separation of inflamed pleural surfaces by an effusion eliminates the friction rub.

Splash. The presence of air and fluid in the pleural space (hydropneumothorax) is indicated if a splash can be heard on auscultation when the thoracic cage is gently shaken. It should not be confused with the splashing of gastric contents.

Interpretation of Clinical Signs
The signs characteristic of the common local pulmonary lesions are shown in Table 3.1. Interpretation in any individual case may be

made difficult by the absence of one or more of the typical signs listed, or by the coincidence of more than one type of lesion. Analysis of the pulmonary signs must also depend upon careful consideration of the patient's history and of the clinical signs revealed by examination of the rest of the body, particularly of the cardiovascular system. The evidence of the chest radiograph may be conclusive, for extensive pulmonary abnormality may be present in spite of apparently normal physical signs.

4

Cardiovascular Aspects of Lung Disease

The major symptoms of lung disease such as dyspnoea, cough, and haemoptysis also occur commonly in diseases of the heart; in addition, disease of either system may cause secondary disease in the other. Examination of the respiratory system cannot therefore be considered complete without a thorough examination of the heart and peripheral circulation.

The Pulse

Attention should be paid to the rate, rhythm, volume, and character of the radial pulse, to the hardness of the vessel wall which is usually best observed in a larger vessel such as the brachial artery, and to the comparative volume of the opposite radial pulse.

Three observations are of particular relevance in pulmonary disease:

1. The finding of a large volume, *bounding pulse* associated with cyanosis and a history of chronic bronchitis and emphysema suggests carbon dioxide retention due to respiratory failure, when the associated signs of drowsiness, sweating, flapping tremor, and papilloedema should be looked for.

2. Diminution in the volume of the radial pulse during inspiration, known as *pulsus paradoxus,* is classically attributed to limitation of venous return to the right side of the heart due to constrictive pericarditis or restrictive cardiomyopathy, but also occurs in severe obstructive airways disease, presumably due to direct reduction in aortic and arterial blood pressure because of the extreme fall in intrathoracic pressure which occurs during inspiration. Pulsus paradoxus is also found in massive pulmonary embolism because the gross reduction in left ventricular filling which results from obstruction to pulmonary arterial blood flow is exaggerated by the increased capacity of the pulmonary venous bed during inspiration.

3. *Differences in volume* between opposite radial pulses should be confirmed by comparing the blood pressure in the two arms, values

31

differing by more than 10 mm Hg being considered significant. A number of factors may be responsible for diminution or obliteration of one radial pulse, including arteriosclerosis, arterial embolism or thrombosis, aneurysm of the aorta or subclavian artery, and coarctation of the aorta. An important pulmonary cause is an apical carcinoma of the lung (Pancoast tumour) which may be associated with lesions of the brachial plexus, Horner's syndrome and malignant invasion of the first rib.

The Jugular Venous Pressure

The jugular venous pressure is best observed with the patient reclining at an angle of 45°, his head supported by a pillow. The height of the column of blood distending the external or internal jugular veins above the sternal angle should be recorded. In normal subjects in this position the jugular veins appear completely collapsed, or slight venous pulsation may be seen behind the medial end of the clavicle. Confirmation that the central venous pressure is normal may be obtained by obstructing the jugular venous return by gentle pressure of a finger at the root of the neck, and observing the immediate collapse of the distended vein when the obstructing finger is removed. Incorrect conclusions may be drawn if the patient's head is not relaxed since contraction of the sternomastoid may obstruct the venous return of the external jugular vein.

The commonest respiratory cause of raised jugular venous pressure is congestive heart failure due to chronic lung disease, or 'cor pulmonale'. The associated clinical signs are oedema of the dependent parts of the body, a distended, tender liver and right ventricular enlargement due either to hypertrophy or dilatation. Right ventricular dilatation may eventually distort the tricuspid valve sufficiently to cause tricuspid incompetence, producing the characteristic systolic pulsation of the neck veins and liver, and the typical tricuspid pansystolic murmur.

Considerable *fluctuation of the jugular venous pressure* between inspiration and expiration occurs in severe airway obstruction (e.g. asthma or advanced chronic bronchitis) because of the violent swings in intrathoracic pressure. In such cases the jugular veins may become distended during expiration but collapse completely as soon as inspiration begins.

In congestive heart failure the distended jugular veins may be seen to pulsate in time with the cardiac cycle. A discussion on the interpretation of the jugular venous wave lies outside the scope of this book, but the *absence* of pulsation in distended jugular veins is of great significance and should be confirmed by firm pressure over the

liver to demonstrate the concurrent absence of hepato-jugular reflux. It indicates *obstruction to the superior vena cava,* most commonly by mediastinal spread of bronchial carcinoma although other upper mediastinal tumours may also be responsible. When partial superior vena caval obstruction is suspected delayed emptying of the neck veins may be demonstrated by asking the patient to bend forward, and observing abnormally slow drainage of blood from the jugular veins when he stands upright again. This observation may be an important indication for prompt radiotherapy.

The other signs of superior vena caval obstruction are plethora and cyanosis of the face, neck and arms, proptosis, distended thoracic wall veins which drain caudally, and sometimes pitting oedema of the backs of the hands and elbows.

Palpation of the Heart

Location of the apex beat is described in the previous chapter (page 24). If cardiac enlargement is suspected the *character of the apex beat* must be identified. Left ventricular hypertrophy produces a well-localised, strongly-pronounced thrust, whereas in right ventricular hypertrophy the actual apex beat is more difficult to define but the vigorous contractions of the right ventricle may be felt as a diffuse systolic impulse in the left parasternal area at the level of the fourth intercostal space. In mitral stenosis this type of right ventricular heave is characteristically associated with a pronounced systolic tap at the apex due to transmission of the shock wave set up by abrupt closure of the stiffened mitral valve cusps.

Systolic pulsation over the third intercostal space close to the sternum occurs in *pulmonary hypertension,* due to the pulsation of the pulmonary artery. In advanced pulmonary hypertension the pulmonary second sound, which is produced by closure of the pulmonary valve, becomes so accentuated that it may be felt with the flat of the hand as a sharp tap in the same area.

When palpating the praecordium attention should be paid to the presence of *thrills*. A thrill is the palpable vibration caused by turbulent blood flow and is the tactile counterpart of a loud murmur. It is always of pathological significance, and its timing in the cardiac cycle should be carefully assessed by comparison with the apex beat or with carotid pulsation. A systolic thrill may be felt: (1) at the base of the heart, due to either aortic or pulmonary stenosis; (2) at the left parasternal region in the fourth or fifth intercostal space, due either to tricuspid incompetence or to ventricular septal defect; and (3) at the apex, due to mitral incompetence. A diastolic thrill at the apex is due to mitral stenosis.

The Heart Sounds

Appreciation of the sounds heard on auscultation can be successful only if the observer concentrates strictly on the individual features of the cardiac cycle in turn. The first essential is correct identification of the first and second heart sounds, and this is facilitated by simultaneously palpating the carotid pulse which is felt immediately after the first heart sound is heard. The first sound is due to the closure of the mitral and tricuspid valves, and marks the beginning of systole; the second heart sound is caused by closure of the aortic and pulmonary valves, marking the beginning of diastole. In the normal, the first heart sound is the louder at the apex, the second sound being the louder on auscultation at the base of the heart.

SPLITTING

Slight splitting of the first heart sound can occasionally be appreciated but is of no clinical significance. Splitting of the second sound is normally heard in the pulmonary area on inspiration, due to slight delay in pulmonary valve closure. This occurs because increased negative intrathoracic pressure augments the venous return during inspiration, increasing right ventricular stroke volume and slightly prolonging right ventricular systole. Pathological splitting of the pulmonary second sound is indicated by appreciable splitting even during expiration ('fixed split') and is a sign of prolonged right ventricular contraction due either to right ventricular hypertrophy or to right bundle branch block, as occurs in atrial septal defect. When the first or aortic element of the second sound is delayed because of left bundle branch block or left ventricular hypertrophy it may occur *after* the pulmonary element of the second sound. Under these circumstances the splitting of the second sound will *narrow* on inspiration, a condition known as reversed or paradoxical splitting of the second sound.

INTENSITY

The intensity of the first heart sound depends on the rate of closure of the atrioventricular valves which varies according to the position of the valve cusps at the onset of ventricular systole. Three abnormalities occur:

1. The cusps are widely separated in mitral stenosis because the high left atrial pressure keeps them apart until the very end of diastole: as a result they come together sharply at the beginning of ventricular systole, causing a loud first heart sound in the mitral area, the shock of which may sometimes be palpable. A corollary of this observation is that mitral stenosis is unlikely to be severe if the first heart sound at the apex is not accentuated.

2. The cusps begin to float together at the end of diastole if ventricular systole is delayed, as occurs in partial atrioventricular block when the P-R interval is prolonged, for example, in acute rheumatism. As a result the first heart sound is abnormally soft in this condition.

3. The position of the atrioventricular cusps at the beginning of ventricular systole may vary because there is an inconstant time relationship between atrial and ventricular systole. This occurs in complete heart block and is characterised by irregular variation in intensity of the first heart sound.

The intensity of the second heart sound is accentuated by high pressure beyond the valve. In pulmonary hypertension a loud second sound is audible in the pulmonary area, where occasionally it may also be palpable. Systemic hypertension causes a loud second sound in the aortic area, sometimes so marked as to have a ringing quality. Diminution in the intensity of the second heart sound occurs in pulmonary and aortic stenosis. The sound is also often soft or absent in emphysema due to hyperinflation of the lungs.

THIRD HEART SOUND

The third heart sound occurs early in diastole at the phase of rapid ventricular filling. It is normal in children and young adults, but when heard in middle age or later it is a sign of ventricular overfilling in ventricular failure.

FOURTH HEART SOUND

The fourth (or atrial) heart sound occurs late in diastole, coinciding with rapid ventricular filling consequent upon atrial contraction. It is a sign of ventricular strain and does not occur in atrial fibrillation.

GALLOP RHYTHMS

A gallop (or triple) rhythm signifies ventricular failure and may be heard over either the right or left ventricle. It is caused either by a third heart sound (diastolic or protodiastolic gallop) or by a fourth heart sound (atrial or presystolic gallop), or by both (quadruple gallop). Quadruple gallop can be appreciated only when the heart rate is slow, since the third and fourth sounds become superimposed in the presence of tachycardia, producing a triple rhythm known as summation gallop.

EJECTION CLICK

An ejection click may be heard in the aortic or pulmonary area and is associated with postvalvular dilation of the aorta or the pulmonary artery. In the aortic area it may be associated with systemic hyperten-

sion, aortic stenosis, and aneurysm of the ascending aorta as occurs, for example, in Marfan's syndrome. In the pulmonary area it may be due to pulmonary stenosis with poststenotic dilation, to idiopathic dilation of the pulmonary artery, and to pulmonary hypertension.

OPENING SNAP

The opening snap of mitral stenosis is heard at the apex or just medial to it. It is a sharp sound heard early in diastole and followed immediately by the rumbling diastolic murmur of mitral stenosis. A similar sound may be heard over the tricuspid area in tricuspid stenosis.

Cardiac Murmurs

A detailed discussion of cardiac murmurs is beyond the scope of this book, apart from a consideration of those murmurs associated with cardiac lesions of special relevance to respiratory disease which are discussed in the next section. The following general principles are of value in assessing the significance of a murmur:

1. Decide whether the murmur is systolic or diastolic.
2. Enquire into the precise timing of the onset and termination of the murmur.
3. Discover its point of maximal intensity, and the direction, if any, in which it radiates.
4. Decide whether it is high, medium or low-pitched, blowing or harsh.
5. Decide whether it is soft or loud (Grade 1, soft, to Grade 4, very loud) and whether it is crescendo, decrescendo or constant.
6. Observe the effect on the murmur of respiration, change of position and exercise.
7. Consider its significance in relation to other clinical signs, such as abnormalities of the pulse and the jugular venous wave form, ventricular enlargement, the presence of a thrill and abnormalities of the heart sounds.

PERICARDIAL FRICTION

A pericardial rub may be difficult to distinguish from a cardiac murmur, but is suggested by the following characteristics: it usually has a harsh, creaking character, and occurs in diastole as well as in systole; and its intensity is said to be occasionally increased by firm pressure of the stethoscope over the praecordium.

Cardiac Conditions of Special Relevance in Lung Disease

In a discussion on the clinical aspects of respiratory disease two types of cardiovascular disorder are particularly relevant:

1. Those complicated by respiratory symptoms so that their presentation may be respiratory although their root cause is cardiac; and

2. Those that are respiratory in origin but present as a cardiac complication.

RECURRENT CHEST INFECTIONS CAUSED BY CARDIAC DISEASE

Recurrent chest infections such as bronchitis and bronchopneumonia occur commonly as complications of mitral stenosis, and of those congenital heart lesions that are characterised by increased pulmonary blood flow, i.e. atrial and ventricular septal defects and aortopulmonary shunts. It is necessary to bear these conditions in mind when examining a patient with symptoms of recurrent lung infection.

Mitral Stenosis. The haemodynamic effect of narrowing of the mitral valve is to limit left ventricular output, especially on exercise, and to dam back blood in the pulmonary vascular bed, causing pulmonary hypertension and right ventricular enlargement, ultimately leading to congestive cardiac failure. The pulse is typically of small volume and the heart is enlarged due to right ventricular hypertrophy, a tapping impulse being apparent at the apex. An apical diastolic thrill may be felt. The first heart sound is accentuated in the mitral area, and the pulmonary second sound may be increased if there is pulmonary hypertension. An opening snap is audible shortly after the second sound and is immediately followed by a low, rumbling mid-diastolic murmur which extends towards the first heart sound and may be continuous with a presystolic crescendo murmur which immediately precedes the first sound. These murmurs are heard at the apex or just medial to it and do not radiate widely, becoming more distinct when the patient turns on to his left side, and following exercise. The diagnosis of mitral stenosis cannot be confidently excluded unless these manoeuvres have been carried out.

Left-to-right Shunts. This group of congenital cardiac conditions includes atrial septal defect, ventricular septal defect, patent ductus arteriosus and aortopulmonary septal defect, all of which are characterised by a left-to-right shunt which results in increased pulmonary blood flow and ultimately to pulmonary hypertension if the shunt is large enough. The liability to recurrent chest infections is attributed to the pulmonary hyperaemia. In *atrial septal defect* the shunt is at atrial level so that both atria and the right ventricle are affected by the increased flow, the right ventricle becoming hypertrophied. Because right bundle branch block is a usual accompaniment of the condition the pulmonary second sound is

widely split and does not vary with respiration; this is attributed to the presence of the atrial septal defect which allows intrathoracic pressure changes to affect flow on both sides of the heart. Blood flow through the defect is silent but increased flow through the pulmonary valve causes a systolic murmur in the pulmonary area, and torrential flow through the tricuspid valve often causes a mid-diastolic murmur at the left sternal border, increased during inspiration. Because of the recirculation of blood through the pulmonary vascular bed the left ventricle is relatively under-filled and the peripheral pulse is small.

In *ventricular septal defect* the increased flow affects both ventricles, so that the apex beat may be left ventricular in type, but at the same time right ventricular pulsation is palpable at the left sternal border. A loud pan-systolic murmur is heard in the fourth intercostal space due to blood flow through the defect, accompanied by a thrill. Increased blood flow through the pulmonary and mitral valves may cause a soft mid-systolic murmur in the pulmonary area and a short mid-diastolic murmur at the apex.

In *patent ductus arteriosus* and aortopulmonary septal defect the physiological changes and clinical signs are closely similar; recirculation occurs from the aorta through the pulmonary circulation and the left side of the heart. The pulse is of collapsing quality because of the 'leak' of blood from the systemic circulation, and the left ventricle is hypertrophied. The cardinal sign is a continuous 'machinery' murmur caused by flow of blood through the ductus, usually best heard in the first or second intercostal spaces a little distance from the left sternal edge. A mid-diastolic murmur may be audible in the mitral area due to increased flow through the mitral valve.

Long-sustained pulmonary hypertension due to left-to-right shunts leads to right ventricular hypertrophy and a rise in pressures on the right side of the heart. When right-sided pressure exceeds that on the left the shunt reverses, causing central cyanosis, and the murmurs attributable to increased flow through the pulmonary and atrioventricular valves alter in character or disappear. This effect is known as the Eisenmenger syndrome (pulmonary hypertension with reversed shunt).

PULMONARY HYPERTENSION

Pulmonary hypertension occurs as a complication of many forms of longstanding lung disease, either because of obliteration of the pulmonary vasculature by multiple emboli or thrombosis, fibrosis or alveolar destruction, or because of the vasoconstrictive effect of chronic hypoxia, or from a combination of these effects. Pulmonary hypertension may eventually lead to right ventricular hypertrophy and dilation, congestive heart failure, and tricuspid incompetence.

Signs of Pulmonary Hypertension. In the present context pulmonary hypertension is accompanied by the history and signs of chronic lung disease. In patients with carbon dioxide retention the peripheral pulse is bounding and the extremities are warm, but when pulmonary vascular resistance is very high cardiac output diminishes and the pulse becomes small and rapid with cold, cyanosed extremities. A giant 'a' wave may be seen in the jugular pulse. Palpation of the praecordium reveals a right ventricular impulse at the left sternal margin and the shock of pulmonary valve closure may be palpable. The pulmonary second sound is accentuated and narrowly split, and a systolic ejection click may be heard in the pulmonary area, associated with pulmonary artery dilatation. A right ventricular gallop rhythm is occasionally audible. The development of functional pulmonary incompetence is indicated by a blowing, early diastolic murmur in the pulmonary area.

In the presence of pulmonary hyperinflation in chronic airways obstruction these signs are masked, praecordial pulsation being absent and the auscultatory signs distant and indistinct.

Sustained pulmonary hypertension ultimately causes *congestive cardiac failure* with a rise in central venous pressure producing jugular venous distension and engorgement of the liver. This often leads to a complaint of right-sided upper abdominal pain and sometimes of nausea and vomiting due to engorgement of the abdominal viscera. Pitting oedema is a more variable sign, tending to develop in the dependent areas such as the feet and sacrum but often extending to involve the legs, scrotum or vulva and lower abdominal wall.

Dilatation of the right ventricle leads to expansion of the atrioventricular valve ring and *tricuspid incompetence*. This is indicated by the appearance of an unusually large 'v' wave in the jugular pulse accompanied by simultaneous systolic pulsation of the distended liver. A blowing pan-systolic murmur is audible over the right ventricle, usually best heard at the left sternal margin and characteristically increased in intensity during inspiration.

5

The Chest X-ray

It may seem unorthodox to consider examination of the chest radiograph under the heading of clinical methods. Nevertheless, the plain chest film has proved to be so useful in the diagnosis of cardiorespiratory disease that it has become the chief accessory to the history and clinical examination. It is important to recognise that the clinical examination and the chest X-ray each offer different sorts of information, the contribution of the radiograph being mainly an anatomical one from which pathological conclusions are drawn by inference with the help of the clinical data. Many pulmonary lesions are primarily diagnosed by clinical means, for example, multiple pulmonary emboli or the syndrome of chronic bronchitis, while others, such as the hilar lymphadenopathy of sarcoidosis, may only be suspected on clinical grounds but be readily apparent on the chest radiograph.

The principles of examining the chest radiograph are similar to the principles of clinical examination: systematic inspection, careful assessment of any apparent deviations from the normal, a search for any associated abnormality, and a logical conclusion that is consistent with the clinical data.

The Plain Film

PRINCIPLES OF EXAMINATION

It is important that the chest radiograph should be examined systematically, attention being paid first to the technical quality of the film so that due allowance may be made for apparent abnormalities that are merely due to deviations from the standard technique. Thereafter, the different anatomical parts of the chest should be inspected in a sequential fashion, ending with a second look at those parts that are notoriously difficult to demonstrate radiologically: the lung apices, the hilar regions, the costophrenic angles, and the retrocardiac area.

Positioning. The standard chest radiograph is the postero-anterior (PA) view taken at full inspiration with the subject in the upright

position at a distance of six feet. A portable film is usually taken in the antero-posterior position and at shorter range so that the relationship between the mediastinal shadows and the shadows of the thoracic cage differ from the standard. To check whether the patient has been radiographed in a straight position the horizontal distance between the end of the clavicle and the lateral edge of the vertebral body opposite which it lies should be compared on either side (Fig. 5.1). At the same time, curvature of the spinal column should be noted since this, like postural variations, can lead to incorrect conclusions about the chest radiograph, particularly with regard to the mediastinal shadows.

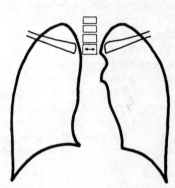

Fig. 5.1   Positioning
To judge whether the patient has been X-rayed in a straight position the distance between the ends of the clavicles and the vertebral body (marked with double arrow) should be compared on either side.

Translucency. Variations in the translucency or 'penetration' of the chest film sometimes make it difficult to assess whether the shadows visible in the lung fields differ from normal lung markings. As a guide to the correct degree of penetration it should be possible just to distinguish the outline of the vertebral bodies and ribs, but not the intervertebral disc spaces, through the heart shadow.

Sequence of Examination. Failures of observation will be less frequent if the chest radiograph is inspected systematically, a convenient sequence being the soft tissues and thoracic cage, the diaphragm, the mediastinum and the lung fields. Related abnormalities should be sought, since they may give insight into the pathology that underlies an observed lesion; for example, deviation of the trachea to the right, associated with elevation of the horizontal fissure and decreased density of the vascular shadows in the right lower zone, indicating a likely diagnosis of right upper lobe collapse.

SOFT TISSUES AND THORACIC CAGE

Certain extrathoracic tissues may cause a shadow that projects on to the lung fields and causes confusion unless its orign is recognised. In

general, such shadows are identifiable because they can be traced out beyond the lung fields. They include the scapulae, the muscles of the chest wall, particularly pectoralis major, the breast and nipple shadows. The breast shadows are liable to obscure the costophrenic angles in the obese, and *absence* of one breast shadow (as a result of mastectomy for malignant disease) may be relevant to other abnormal shadows in the chest X-ray due to metastases. The nipple shadows sometimes produce a localised opacity, apparently in the lung, but in cases of doubt the shadow can be identified by repeating the radiograph with a radio-opaque marker placed around the nipple.

The symmetry of the thoracic skeleton should be examined for evidence of spinal curvature and for differences in the pattern of the ribs on either side; local rib retraction may occur over an area of lung disease, and unilateral crowding of the ribs is seen in kyphoscoliosis. The bones should be examined for evidence of periostitis, seen as a thin, rather ragged line of new bone running parallel to the rib, and a sign of trauma or intrathoracic infection, classically actinomycosis. Fractures and erosions should be noted; the latter may be due to a primary rib tumour, invasion by pleural or pulmonary malignancy, secondary metastases, tuberculosis, oesteomyelitis, and pressure erosion from enlarged arteries. Notching of the ribs and scapulae due to the latter cause is a characteristic radiographic sign of coarctation of the aorta.

THE DIAPHRAGM

The dome of the diaphragm on the right side usually lies 1 to 2 cm higher than that on the left in all phases of respiration. Elevation of one dome of the diaphragm may be due to:

1. Excessive gas in the stomach.
2. Spinal curvature.
3. Phrenic nerve damage, resulting from trauma, malignant disease, lymph node enlargement or neuropathy.
4. Collapse of the middle or lower lobe of the lung on the affected side.
5. Basal pulmonary infection or infarction.
6. Subphrenic abscess.

The diaphragm is depressed and its curvature flattened in conditions characterised by hyperinflation of the lungs. Its movement may be assessed by fluoroscopy, immobility of one lobe being suggestive of paralysis or contiguous inflammation such as a subphrenic abscess.

THE MEDIASTINUM

Shift of the mediastinum to one or other side often results from

intrapulmonary disease and may provide important information about the underlying pathology, e.g. displacement of the mediastinum to the side opposite to a tension pneumothorax. In particular, movement of the trachea from the mid-line may be related to changes in the lung apices. The hilar region often reveals evidence of mediastinal tumours and abnormalities of the pulmonary vessels particularly relating to pulmonary hypertension. The lower half of the mediastinal shadow is mainly due to the heart which may be altered in size or shape by disease arising in the lungs, as well as to intrinsic lesions of the heart itself.

The *trachea* appears as a vertical translucent band overlying the spinous processes of the upper thoracic vertebrae. Its lower end is slightly inclined to the right. Collapse of an upper lobe causes the trachea to incline towards the affected side, whereas apical fibrosis usually results in more obvious kinking of the trachea towards the fibrosed area. The trachea may also be displaced by tumours of the upper mediastinum, recognisable by widening of the mediastinal shadow.

The *hilar shadows* are composed of the pulmonary vessels and hilar lymph nodes. The shadow of the left hilum normally lies 1 to 2 cm higher than on the right, but either may be displaced in association with an alteration in the pulmonary vascular pattern. Enlargement of the vascular shadows occurs in pulmonary hypertension and causes an increase in the horizontal distance between the main divisions of the pulmonary arteries on either side, a sign which constitutes useful radiographic evidence of raised pulmonary arterial pressure in chronic airways obstruction. Unilateral enlargement of the hilar shadow suggests carcinoma of the bronchus, but there are numerous other causes of widening of the middle part of the mediastinum which include sarcoidosis, Hodgkin's disease, lymphosarcoma, leukaemia, tuberculosis, malignant metastases, and aortic aneurysm.

The *heart shadow*. At its widest point the transverse diameter of the heart is normally less than half the maximum diameter of the thoracic cage. The main bulk of the heart shadow lies somewhat to the left of the mid-line, but the extent of this asymmetry depends partly on the build of the individual, patients of tall thin habitus having narrow centrally-placed flask-shaped hearts while those who are short and squat tend to have the heart in a more horizontal position with a prominent left border. Displacement of the cardiac shadow to one or other side is detected by observing its relationship to the shadow of the thoracic spine; it may be due to skeletal deformity such as kyphoscoliosis or pectus excavatum, or to disease of the lungs or pleura.

The borders of the heart shadow are formed on the right side by the superior vena cava in the upper half of the thorax, and by the right atrium in the lower half; on the left side the cardiac border consists of three prominences, the aortic knuckle above, the main pulmonary trunk in the middle, and the curving border of the left ventricle below (Fig. 5.2). The left atrial appendage lies just below the prominence caused by the pulmonary trunk and sometimes forms a small segment of the cardiac shadow at this site; in mitral stenosis it enlarges, causing the left cardiac shadow to be straighter and steeper than normal.

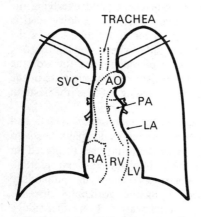

Fig. 5.2   The Mediastinal Shadow
Ao = aorta, LA = left atrium, LV = left ventricle,   PA = pulmonary   artery, RA = right atrium, RV = right ventricle, SVC = superior vena cava.

In the context of pulmonary disease it is important to recognise the changes in cardiac size and shape that characterise right-sided cardiac failure or cor pulmonale. Right ventricular enlargement increases the transverse diameter of the heart causing a prominence of the left border rather above the apex. The right atrium may be somewhat displaced to the right by the enlarged right ventricle, giving an impression of prominence of the right cardiac border which is often not very conspicuous. Associated enlargement of the main pulmonary artery and its major branches is due to pulmonary hypertension.

THE LUNG FIELDS

Systematic examination of the lung fields is aided by dividing the area into arbitrary zones: the upper zone is the area between the lung apex and a horizontal line at the level of the lower border of the 2nd costochondral junction; the middle zone lies between the lower margin of the upper zone and a horizontal line at the level of the lower border of the 4th costochondral junction; and the lower zone lies below the lower border of the middle zone.

The *boundaries of the lung* should be traced all round the thorax to

ensure there is no abnormal shadow that obscures or projects from the outlines of the thoracic cage, the mediastinal shadow, or the diaphragm. This inspection should lead to recognition of such abnormalities as a shadow in the costophrenic angles due to a small pleural effusion, loss of translucency in the cardiophrenic angles due to collapse of the lower lobes, impaired translucency along the lower lateral margins of the thoracic cage due to pleural thickening, apical shadowing, and the thin line of the visceral pleura slightly retracted from the inner surface of the thorax due to a small pneumothorax.

Opacity of normal structures may be increased by abnormalities lying in front or behind them; for example, increased opacity of one hilum due to a retrohilar tumour, or of the heart shadow because of left lower lobe collapse.

Movement of normal landmarks such as the mediastinum or the shadows of the interlobar fissures may indicate pulmonary fibrosis or collapse, and localised hyperinflation or emphysematous bullae.

Vascular Pattern. The pulmonary vessels normally spread outwards from the hilum in an evenly-spaced fan-shaped pattern and can be distinguished peripherally almost to the margins of the lungs. In areas where the lung is partially collapsed, however, the vessels appear crowded together and the translucency of the lung is correspondingly reduced; in contrast, areas of compensatory hyperinflation of lung tissue show a vascular pattern that is more spread out than normal, a factor that contributes to the increased translucency of the region. In emphysema, which is characterised pathologically by dilation of the air spaces with destruction of the alveolar septa, the overall translucency of the lungs is increased and the pulmonary vessels become so attenuated that the vascular pattern at the periphery of the lung fields is invisible. In contrast, when the pulmonary vascular bed becomes overfilled due to increased pulmonary blood flow or venous congestion the vascular shadows appear more prominent than usual; in severe congestion with pulmonary oedema an opaque fan-shaped shadow is seen on either side of the hilar region, and thin hair-like horizontal shadows are visible at the margins of the lungs in the costophrenic angles (Kerley's B lines), due to dilation of the lymphatics in the interlobular septa.

The Lobes and Fissures. The site of a radiological abnormality in the lung fields can be recognised more easily by determining its relationship to the interlobar fissures. In the PA view only the horizontal fissure can be seen, at the level of the anterior end of the right fourth rib. Both the oblique and horizontal fissures are visible in the lateral view, the oblique fissure running from the 4th or 5th thoracic vertebra downwards and forward through the hilum to the anterior costophrenic angle. The fissures normally appear as hair-line

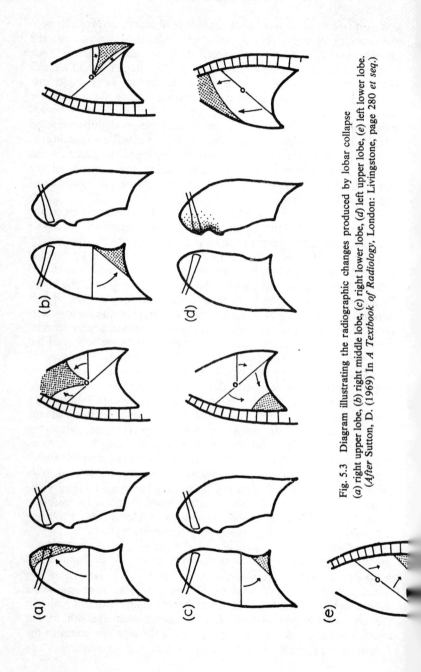

Fig. 5.3 Diagram illustrating the radiographic changes produced by lobar collapse (a) right upper lobe, (b) right middle lobe, (c) right lower lobe, (d) left upper lobe, (e) left lower lobe. (*After* Sutton, D. (1969) In *A Textbook of Radiology*, London: Livingstone, page 280 *et seq.*)

shadows but may be thicker and more prominent than usual if there is an increase in pleural fluid, most commonly due to heart failure. Loculation of an effusion within a fissure produces a characteristic eliptical opacity when seen in profile.

Complete consolidation of a lobe results in opacification of an area bounded by the margins of the lung and the interlobar fissures. In practice it is much commoner to find only a segment of the lobe affected, leading to a limited area of opacification with margins that are often poorly defined, the shadow commonly being most dense in the lowest, dependent part of the consolidated area.

If collapse occurs within a lobe, the fissure is drawn towards the collapsed area and some increase in the radio-opacity of the shrunken area of lung may occur, depending upon the degree of collapse and the presence or absence of associated consolidation (Fig. 5.3). Increased translucency may be observed in the remainder of the affected lung due to compensatory hyperinflation and spreading of the vascular pattern.

THE LATERAL VIEW

Examination of the lateral projection of the chest should follow the same principles of systematic assessment described already. Because the two lungs are superimposed it is difficult to make out much detail in the lung fields or to distinguish the features of one lung from those of the other. The fissures can usually be recognised readily and their displacement may provide useful evidence of lobar collapse. The anatomical position of opacities seen in the PA view can usually be confirmed more precisely in the lateral view, and lesions invisible in the PA film because they lie behind the hilum or the heart often become identifiable in the lateral projection. Particular attention should therefore be paid to the retrocardiac and hilar areas, especially the posterior costophrenic angle which may contain a localised lesion or the triangular shadow of a small pleural effusion. Attention may be drawn to such an abnormality by observing that the opacity of the vertebral bodies in the lower thoracic spine is accentuated by the presence of an overlying lesion, in contrast to the normal appearance of the thoracic spine which becomes increasingly translucent from above downwards.

Other Radiological Techniques

TOMOGRAPHY

This technique enables radiographs of the lung to be taken at different depths so that a detailed picture of the region of lung under inspection may be built up, in a manner similar to the histological examination of a

tissue in serial sections. It is of particular value in demonstrating or excluding a pulmonary cavity, for demonstrating the lumen of the trachea or a major bronchus to exclude stenosis or an intraluminal tumour, and, in general, for showing the extent and nature of abnormal shadows in the lungs and in the other tissues of the thorax.

FLUOROSCOPY

Fluoroscopy is a technique that subjects the patient to a considerable dose of X-rays, many times larger than resulting from the simple radiograph. It should therefore be employed in carefully selected cases only. It is most useful in the assessment of abnormal movement of the heart or lungs; for example, immobility or paradoxical movement of the diaphragm, abnormal pulsation of the pulmonary vessels ('hilar dance') in conditions of increased pulmonary blood flow, or of the left atrium in mitral incompetence, and absence of cardiac pulsation in constrictive pericarditis.

BRONCHOGRAPHY

Instillation of radio-opaque material such as iodised oil into the lumen of the tracheobronchial tree provides a detailed silhouette of the bronchial anatomy in the chest radiograph. Bronchography is most useful in demonstrating the presence or extent of bronchiectasis which is suspected on clinical grounds but cannot be seen in the plain chest film or on tomography, and it is a necessary preliminary investigation to the surgical treatment of localised bronchiectasis. It is also indicated in the investigation of haemoptysis unexplained by other investigations, including bronchoscopy, which might be due to a neoplasm or to bronchiectasis. Although relatively safe, it is unpleasant for the patient and should not be undertaken without a definitive objective in mind.

PULMONARY ANGIOGRAPHY

This technique is briefly described in Chapter 8 (page 95).

PART II

Pulmonary Physiology in Relation to Disease

6

Concepts of Pulmonary Physiology

INTRODUCTION

The lung has two essential functions: the maintenance of gas and blood flow to the alveoli, and the exchange of gases between the alveolar space and the blood. These functions are clearly interdependent, in that gas exchange cannot take place in the absence of an appropriate flow of gas and blood to the gas-exchanging region, but it is often useful to consider them separately when trying to define the physiological disturbance responsible for the clinical manifestations of lung disease.

The clinician may be required to approach the problem from either end: he may be presented with a clinical syndrome that represents impairment of gas exchange—for example, a patient with cyanosis or one showing the signs and symptoms of carbon dioxide retention—and he has to distinguish the defect of gas or blood transport that is responsible. Alternatively, the disease may be one that obviously disturbs the transport function of the lung—for example, airways obstruction or pulmonary embolisation—and the clinician must then be familiar with the consequent effect upon gas exchange.

A physiological approach to the problems of lung disease is presented in the following four chapters, beginning with a brief explanation of the current concepts of the various factors that control alveolar gas exchange and gas transport. In the next chapter the principles of the tests used to measure these aspects of lung function are described, while the following chapter is devoted mainly to the functional behaviour and investigation of the pulmonary circulation. In the final chapter of this section certain common clinical syndromes are described with particular reference to the physiological disturbances responsible for the clinical manifestations.

GAS EXCHANGE

The Alveolus

The lung is an organ primarily concerned in exchanging oxygen and carbon dioxide between the air and pulmonary capillary blood, and its functioning unit, analogous to the nephron of the kidney, is the alveolus. Each alveolus, of which there are approximately 300 million in the normal adult lung, is a minute air sac, about 250 microns in diameter, which is in continuity with the environmental air by a system of branching airways. The alveoli are packed together in a manner akin to the cells of a honeycomb, their walls consisting of a thin membrane of alveolar lining cells and fibrous tissue richly interspersed with pulmonary capillaries. The lumen of each alveolus opens widely into a terminal airway but there are also minute holes (the pores of Kohn) which perforate the alveolar walls and connect the lumens of adjacent alveoli.

The walls of the alveoli are the gas-exchanging surface of the lung, forming the interface between alveolar gas and pulmonary capillary blood. This surface, known as the alveolar-capillary membrane, has a total area of about 75 m^2 in the normal adult. The tissue layer of the membrane consists of a single alveolar lining cell, a thin basement membrane, and the endothelial cell of the capillary, and has a thickness of only 0·2 to 0·7 microns so that it causes little hindrance to the diffusion of gases between the alveolar space and the capillary blood.

The alveoli are lined with a surface film of lipoprotein, rich in lecithin, which reduces the surface tension and thereby prevents collapse of the alveoli. It is secreted by granular cells which lie in the alveolar epithelium. This surface activity ensures the stability of the alveoli over a wide range of size, for without it, smaller alveoli would tend to collapse on expiration and the larger ones to become over-inflated during inspiration. Moreover, in the absence of surfactant, abnormally high intra-alveolar surface tension would probably lead to transudation of fluid into the alveoli from the capillaries.

Gas Exchange in a Single Lung Unit

In a single alveolus, gas exchange is limited by its ventilation, by its diffusion characteristics and, in a particular way, by its blood flow. An understanding of these factors forms a useful introduction to the more complicated aspects of gas exchange in a lung consisting of multiple functioning units. For the sake of argument, the whole lung is considered as a single alveolar unit.

VENTILATION

The ventilation of the lung is the volume of gas inspired (or expired*) in unit time, e.g. 7·0 litres a minute in a normal adult breathing a tidal volume of 500 ml at a respiratory rate of 14 breaths a minute. However, this quantity of gas does not reach the alveoli because part of each breath merely fills the airways and takes no part in gas exchange; this is the *anatomical dead space,* amounting to about 150 ml. The *alveolar ventilation* in this example therefore consists of only $(500-150) \times 14 = 4,900$ ml/minute. The alveolar gas differs in composition from the inspired air because carbon dioxide is being continually added to it, and oxygen removed, by the blood perfusing the alveoli. Its composition therefore depends on a balance between ventilation and blood flow, hyperventilation causing a rise in alveolar oxygen tension and a fall in carbon dioxide tension whereas hypoventilation has the opposite effect. Alveolar hypoventilation occurs clinically when the respiratory centre is depressed by narcotic drugs or by intracranial disease or when the respiratory muscles are paralysed, but it is much more commonly due to disease of the lungs, when ventilation is restricted by narrowing of the airways or non-distensibility of the alveoli.

DIFFUSION IN THE AIRWAYS

The movement of gas molecules into and out of the alveoli—the process of 'alveolar ventilation'—is not solely due to the mass movement of gases brought about by the expansion and deflation of the lungs; it is also due to the diffusion of gas molecules within the airways and the alveoli. If we measure the total cross-sectional area of the air passages of the lung at various different points down the airways from the trachea to the alveoli we find that it remains relatively small down to the level of the respiratory bronchioles, and then suddenly increases enormously due to the branching out of myriads of alveolar ducts and alveoli (Fig. 6.1). The mass flow of gas, which is the major component of gas movement in the narrower portion of the airways, suddenly drops to zero as the airways widen out into the gas-exchanging zone of the lung, and the final millimetre or two of gas movement to and from the alveolar-capillary membrane is entirely due to molecular diffusion. One of the important adverse effects of airways obstruction on gas exchange is to impede the mass movement of the respiratory gases and, consequently, increase the distance over which gas molecules have to

---

* Strictly speaking, the expired and inspired gas volumes differ slightly because the volume of oxygen taken up is larger than the volume of carbon dioxide given off; in physiological estimations the expired volume is used as a measure of ventilation.

travel by molecular diffusion to and from the alveolar-capillary membrane.

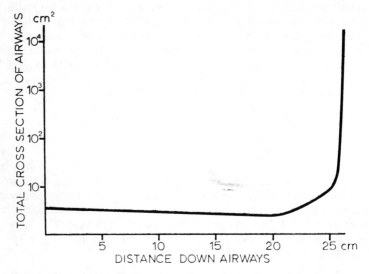

Fig. 6.1 Graph showing how the total cross-sectional area of the airways remains relatively small until the last few millimetres are reached, when it is increased enormously

DIFFUSION ACROSS THE ALVEOLAR-CAPILLARY MEMBRANE

The exchange of respiratory gases between the alveolar space and the capillaries is by diffusion, the gases flowing from a region of high partial pressure to one of low partial pressure. The blood that enters the alveolar capillary is mixed venous blood with a relatively high carbon dioxide tension and low oxygen tension, so that it takes up oxygen and gives off carbon dioxide to the alveolar gas. At rest, equilibration between alveolar gas and blood is virtually complete in about one third of the time available for gas exchange as the blood flows through the alveolar capillary, and even when the rate of blood flow is increased during maximal exercise the degree of equilibration is hardly affected. The efficiency of this diffusion mechanism is influenced by the oxygen pressure difference between alveolar gas and capillary blood, and therefore by the alveolar ventilation, because the partial pressure of oxygen in the alveolus depends upon its ventilation. If alveolar ventilation is adequate, oxygen diffuses readily from a high alveolar pressure to a low capillary pressure; this movement of oxygen is enhanced by the shape of the oxygen dissociation curve of haemoglobin, since, because the curve is so flat when the oxygen

tension is high, most of the oxygen will have crossed the gas : blood interface before the oxygen tension of the capillary blood has come close to that of the alveolar gas. If, on the other hand, alveolar oxygen tension is reduced by hypoventilation, the 'head of pressure' driving oxygen across the interface will be small, and the advantage of the shape of the oxygen dissociation curve will be lost because at low oxygen tensions the curve slopes steeply (Fig. 6.2).

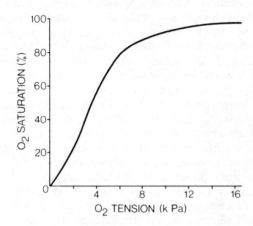

Fig. 6.2   The normal oxygen dissociation curve of haemoglobin

In a normal person, oxygen exchange is limited by diffusion only when he breathes an hypoxic gas mixture, either experimentally or when residing at a very high altitude. Under such conditions the resulting hypoxaemia is further enhanced by exercise because the increased rate of pulmonary blood flow diminishes the time available for oxygen uptake by blood as it passes through the alveolar capillaries. In diffuse pulmonary disease another critical factor may be the thickness of the alveolar-capillary membrane, although calculations suggest that the observed degree of thickening of the gas-blood barrier would be insufficient by itself to interfere significantly with the diffusion of oxygen. It seems most probable that in diseases characterised by diffuse thickening of the alveolar-capillary membrane any hypoxaemia is due to a combination of alveolar hypoventilation and uneven distribution of ventilation to perfusion (*see* next section) rather than to a tissue 'barrier' between the alveolus and the blood.

Carbon dioxide diffuses in the tissues much more readily than

oxygen, to such an extent that diffusion limitation across the alveolar-capillary membrane apparently has no effect on the exchange of carbon dioxide, even in disease.

BLOOD FLOW

In the context of this account of gas exchange in a lung consisting of a single functioning unit, blood flow affects gas exchange in only two ways. The first has been discussed in relation to diffusion, that in the special circumstances of alveolar hypoventilation or hypoxia, with or without associated thickening of the alveolar-capillary membrane, an increase in the rate of blood flow (e.g. by exercise) may be critical in determining the completeness of oxygen uptake by the blood.

Gas exchange is also affected when blood flow bypasses the lung altogether, i.e. when venous blood mixes with arterial blood without having perfused a ventilated part of the lung. The effect of such a *shunt* is to lower the oxygen tension and raise the carbon dioxide tension of arterial blood, the extent of these changes depending on the size of the shunt which in normal subjects amounts to about 1 to 2 per cent of the cardiac output. It is composed of the drainage of myocardial venous blood via the Thebesian veins and some slight contribution from direct communication between the pulmonary arteries and veins. In disease, however, large extrapulmonary shunts may occur between the right and left sides of the heart, e.g. in the tetralogy of Fallot, or within the lung as a result of congenital pulmonary arteriovenous anastamoses or, much more commonly, because of perfusion of unventilated areas of diseased lung.

Gas Exchange in Multiple Functioning Units

This description of pulmonary gas exchange has so far been simplified by considering the lung as a single alveolar unit. In fact, the lung consists of 300 million such units, each behaving *individually* according to the physiological principles described but each likely to vary slightly in its gas exchange according to the ventilation and blood flow it receives. The overall result of this variation in ventilation and perfusion is to impair the efficiency of gas exchange slightly even in the normal lung, while in disease this factor is the most important cause of respiratory insufficiency.

THE VENTILATION-PERFUSION RATIO $(\dot{V}A/\dot{Q})$

In a lung consisting of more than one 'compartment' (i.e. functioning unit or alveolus) the total ventilation and perfusion may be shared equally or unequally between the compartments. For example, taking representative normal values, a total alveolar ventilation of 4,850 ml might be matched by a total pulmonary blood flow of 5,000 ml, giving

an overall ventilation : perfusion ratio ($\dot{V}A/\dot{Q}$) of approximately 1. Total ventilation and perfusion might be distributed between the two compartments in various ways, including—

1. Both may be equally distributed between the two compartments (Fig. 6.3).
2. They may be unequally but similarly distributed between the compartments (Fig. 6.4).
3. They may be unequally and dissimilarly distributed between the compartments (Fig. 6.5).

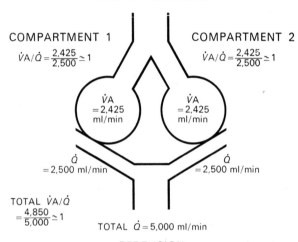

VENTILATION

TOTAL $\dot{V}A = 4,850$ ml/min

COMPARTMENT 1

$\dot{V}A/\dot{Q} = \dfrac{2,425}{2,500} \simeq 1$

COMPARTMENT 2

$\dot{V}A/\dot{Q} = \dfrac{2,425}{2,500} \simeq 1$

$\dot{V}A = 2,425$ ml/min

$\dot{V}A = 2,425$ ml/min

$\dot{Q} = 2,500$ ml/min

$\dot{Q} = 2,500$ ml/min

TOTAL $\dot{V}A/\dot{Q}$
$= \dfrac{4,850}{5,000} \simeq 1$

TOTAL $\dot{Q} = 5,000$ ml/min

PERFUSION

Fig. 6.3   Distribution of ventilation and perfusion

This is a nearly perfect situation in which both ventilation and perfusion are evenly distributed to all parts of the lung, and ventilation and perfusion are almost precisely matched.

In the first two examples the $\dot{V}A/\dot{Q}$ ratio is equal to 1 in both compartments even though there may be considerable variation in the distribution of ventilation and perfusion to different parts of the lung; the essential point is that variation in ventilation is accompanied by similar variation in perfusion. In the third example ventilation and perfusion are at variance in both compartments, each of which has a $\dot{V}A/\dot{Q}$ ratio widely different from 1 even though the total ventilation and perfusion of the lung remain unchanged. Clearly, $\dot{V}A/\dot{Q}$ ratios may vary from zero (perfused but unventilated alveoli) to infinity (ventilated but unperfused alveoli) although in the normal lung the

majority of $\dot{V}A/\dot{Q}$ ratios range from about 0·6 to 3·0 with an overall value of approximately 0·85. Variation in $\dot{V}A/\dot{Q}$ ratios has a profound effect on pulmonary gas exchange.

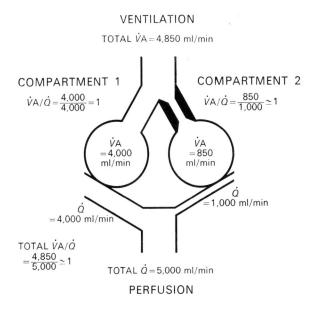

Fig. 6.4   Distribution of ventilation and perfusion

Although both ventilation and perfusion are unevenly distributed to different parts of the lung, in each part they are almost precisely matched. This example approximately represents the situation in the normal, healthy young adult.

THE EFFECT OF VARIATION IN $\dot{V}A/\dot{Q}$ RATIOS

The Alveolar-arterial Difference. To understand the significance of uneven distribution of ventilation and perfusion upon pulmonary gas exchange it is necessary to be acquainted with the concept of the alveolar-arterial gas tension difference. One way of judging the efficiency of the lung as a gas exchanger is to compare the tensions of oxygen and carbon dioxide in the arterial blood flowing out of the lungs with their tensions in the gas mixture expired from the alveoli; if the efficiency of the system is low, the alveolar tensions will differ widely from the arterial, whereas they will approximate closely to one another if the efficiency of gas exchange is high. In the first two examples given above (Figs. 6.3 and 6.4) the $\dot{V}A/\dot{Q}$ ratios of both

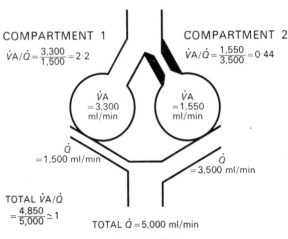

VENTILATION

TOTAL $\dot{V}A = 4,850$ ml/min

COMPARTMENT 1

$\dot{V}A/\dot{Q} = \dfrac{3,300}{1,500} = 2 \cdot 2$

COMPARTMENT 2

$\dot{V}A/\dot{Q} = \dfrac{1,550}{3,500} = 0 \cdot 44$

$\dot{V}A = 3,300$ ml/min

$\dot{V}A = 1,550$ ml/min

$\dot{Q} = 1,500$ ml/min

$\dot{Q} = 3,500$ ml/min

TOTAL $\dot{V}A/\dot{Q}$

$= \dfrac{4,850}{5,000} \simeq 1$

TOTAL $\dot{Q} = 5,000$ ml/min

PERFUSION

Fig. 6.5 Distribution of ventilation and perfusion

Both ventilation and perfusion are distributed unevenly to different parts of the lung, and their distribution does not match. This example represents the abnormality that occurs in various types of diffuse lung disease.

compartments are the same and therefore* the gas tensions in the blood and alveolar space of both compartments are the same (assuming no diffusion block). It follows that the gas tensions in the mixed alveolar gas and the mixed capillary blood leaving the lung are identical, i.e. the alveolar-arterial tension differences for oxygen and carbon dioxide equal zero. In the third example (Fig. 6.5) the $\dot{V}A/\dot{Q}$ ratios in each compartment differ widely and consequently the gas tensions in the alveolar gas and capillary blood leaving Compartment 1 are quite different from those in the gas and blood leaving Compartment 2. It can be calculated that the mixed alveolar gas from the two compartments has an O_2 tension of $14 \cdot 6$ kPa (110 mm Hg) and

* The logic of this statement may be questioned. Suffice it to say that, given certain reasonable assumptions about the composition of mixed venous blood and the shape of the haemoglobin dissociation curves for oxygen and carbon dioxide, only one set of values for oxygen, carbon dioxide and nitrogen tensions is possible for any given $\dot{V}A/\dot{Q}$ ratio. The physiological and mathematical explanations for this fact are beyond the scope of this book, but they are well described by West and by Rahn (*see* Bibliography).

a CO_2 tension of $4\cdot55\,kPa$ ($34\cdot2\,mm\,Hg$), while the mixed capillary blood leaving the lung has an O_2 tension of $11\cdot0\,kPa$ ($83\,mm\,Hg$) and a CO_2 tension of $5\cdot10\,kPa$ ($38\cdot4\,mm\,Hg$); the resulting alveolar-arterial difference for O_2 is therefore $3\cdot6\,kPa$ ($27\,mm\,Hg$) and the arterial-

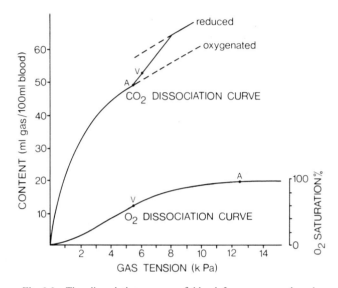

Fig. 6.6   The dissociation curves of blood for oxygen and carbon dioxide drawn on the same scale for comparison, assuming normal values of bicarbonate and haemoglobin concentration.

Since the amount of carbon dioxide that can be carried by blood depends on the degree of reduction of the haemoglobin, the 'physiological' carbon dioxide dissociation curve follows a course that lies between the curves for fully oxygenated and fully reduced haemoglobin. *A* and *V* mark the normal values for arterial and mixed venous blood respectively.

Note that the curve for carbon dioxide is steeper and straighter than that for oxygen, so that the increased ventilation effectively 'washes out' carbon dioxide from alveoli with high $\dot{V}A/\dot{Q}$ ratios and compensates for the reduced excretion of carbon dioxide from alveoli with low $\dot{V}A/\dot{Q}$ ratios. In contrast, hyperventilation of alveoli with high $\dot{V}A/\dot{Q}$ ratios does not have a similar compensatory effect for oxygen because it does not increase the oxygen *content* of the pulmonary capillary blood significantly.

(*After* Campbell, E. J. M., Dickinson, C. J. and Slater, J. D. H. (1963). In *Clinical Physiology*, 2nd Edn. Oxford: Blackwell, page 111.)

alveolar difference for CO_2 is $0\cdot55\,kPa$ ($4\cdot2\,mm\,Hg$). These values indicate the considerable effect that variation in VA/Q ratios can have upon the efficiency of gas exchange, compared with the zero alveolar-

arterial gas tension differences that occur when ventilation and perfusion are precisely matched. It should be remembered that impairment of gas exchange occurs in spite of the fact that equilibration between gas and blood in each compartment is perfect, and that any shunt or impairment of diffusion will reduce the efficiency of gas exchange still further.

It will be noticed that the alveolar-arterial tension difference for oxygen in the above example is much greater than that for carbon dioxide. This is partly because the difference between venous and arterial tensions is less for carbon dioxide than for oxygen, but it is also due to the difference between the shapes of the haemoglobin dissociation curves for the two gases (Fig. 6.6). The curve for carbon dioxide is almost straight over the physiological range, so that over-ventilation in Compartment 1 compensates for under-ventilation in Compartment 2; as a result, although rather less carbon dioxide is removed from the blood in Compartment 2, rather more is removed in Compartment 1. In the case of oxygen, however, there can be no significant compensation for diminished uptake in Compartment 2 because the blood in Compartment 1 is already fully saturated, i.e. lies on the flat part of the haemoglobin dissociation curve, so that a large increase in alveolar oxygen tension due to over-ventilation causes little increase in blood oxygen content.

Physiological Dead Space ('wasted ventilation') and Venous Admixture ('wasted blood flow'). It will be appreciated that the lung as a gas-exchanging organ must satisfy the metabolic needs of the body as a whole by supplying oxygen and removing carbon dioxide. Ideally, the lung would consist of one or more functional units with a single, common $\dot{V}A/\dot{Q}$ ratio exactly appropriate for the oxygen and carbon dioxide exchange of the whole organism. In other words, the ventilation and blood flow through the lung would be perfectly adjusted to exchange oxygen and carbon dioxide in precisely the quantities required by the metabolic needs. It has been shown that, in fact, the lung consists of many functioning units, each with a slightly different $\dot{V}A/\dot{Q}$ ratio, some over-ventilated in relation to their perfusion (high $\dot{V}A/\dot{Q}$ ratio, e.g. Compartment 1 in Fig. 6.5), others overperfused in relation to their ventilation (low $\dot{V}A/\dot{Q}$ ratio, e.g. Compartment 2 in Fig. 6.5), so that the required exchange of respiratory gases is only achieved at the expense of some waste of ventilation to the alveoli with high $\dot{V}A/\dot{Q}$ ratios, and some waste of blood flow to those with low $\dot{V}A/\dot{Q}$ ratios.

'Wasted ventilation' and 'wasted blood flow' can be quantitated and used as measures of uneven distribution of ventilation and perfusion. Both are made up of two components. Wasted ventilation consists of the anatomical dead space, plus the *alveolar dead space*, i.e. that

portion of the volume of inspired gas entering the alveoli with high $\dot{V}A/\dot{Q}$ ratios that is superfluous to the respiratory capacity of the perfusing blood. The classical name for wasted ventilation is *physiological dead space*, and it has a value of less than 30 per cent of the tidal volume in normal young adults. Wasted blood flow, otherwise known as *venous admixture*, consists of the blood flow that bypasses ventilated lung altogether, i.e. shunt, plus that portion of the blood flow perfusing alveoli with low $\dot{V}A/\dot{Q}$ ratios that exceeds the gas-exchanging potential of their ventilation.

CAUSES OF UNEVEN DISTRIBUTION OF VENTILATION AND PERFUSION

The organisation of the lung as a structure with 300 million functioning units allows a large volume of gas and blood to be brought into close proximity over an enormous area, and the efficiency of gas exchange depends to a great extent upon the precision with which the appropriate proportions of the total ventilation and the total blood flow are conveyed to each alveolus. Uneven distribution of ventilation and perfusion may arise either because ventilation is uneven but perfusion normally distributed as might occur in acute bronchial asthma, or because perfusion is uneven but ventilation normally distributed, as in multiple pulmonary embolisation. More commonly, both ventilation and perfusion are unevenly and dissimilarly distributed, e.g. in chronic bronchitis and emphysema or diffuse pulmonary fibrosis, but for simplicity we will describe the causes of uneven distribution of ventilation and perfusion separately.

Ventilation. A number of factors are responsible for the variations in ventilation to different parts of the lung which occur normally and in disease:

1. *The Effect of Gravity.* In the normal lung in the upright position ventilation is greatest at the lung base and diminishes towards the apex. This variation disappears in the supine position and is attributed to regional differences in intrapleural pressure due to the weight of the lung itself.

2. *Narrowing of the Airways.* Flow of gas into the lungs on inspiration depends upon a reduction in intrathoracic pressure produced by contraction of the respiratory muscles. For a given fall in pressure the volume of gas that enters an alveolus or group of alveoli within a finite time will depend on the calibre of the conducting airway and on the distensibility of the respiratory unit. If the conducting airway is narrowed the time required for gas to flow past the narrow portion in order to equalise pressures between the alveoli and the atmosphere will be longer than normal, and the ventilation of such

alveoli will vary with the duration of inspiration and, therefore, with the rate and rhythm of breathing. Such a unit is said to have a long *time constant,* and variation in time constants of different respiratory units leads to uneven distribution of ventilation of the type commonly seen in bronchial asthma or in chronic airways obstruction.

. 3. *Variation in distensibility* of different respiratory units leads to uneven ventilation because those units with stiff, inelastic walls expand to a smaller extent for a given intrathoracic pressure change than those which are easily distensible. This type of uneven ventilation is thought to be a major cause of impaired gas exchange in patients with diffuse fibrosis of the lungs.

4. *Dilatation of Terminal Airways.* In the normal lung the mass movement of gas as it is swept along the airways by inspiration carries individual gas molecules close to the alveolar-capillary membrane, so that the distance over which the molecules have to move by diffusion alone is small. If the terminal airways are dilated, for example by centrilobular emphysema, ventilation of the alveolar space diminishes because part of every inspired breath is used in filling the dilated airways. As a result, the distance respiratory gas molecules have to diffuse is increased and gas exchange becomes correspondingly impaired, attributable here to uneven ventilation *along* the lung unit.

Perfusion. The distribution of perfusion is affected by two major factors, namely variation in hydrostatic pressure in different parts of the lung, and obstructive changes in the pulmonary vascular bed.

1. *Variations in Hydrostatic Pressure.* Because the alveolar capillaries are collapsible tubes that are influenced by the pressure of gas in the alveoli which surround them as well as by the pressure of blood in the pulmonary arteries and veins, alveolar capillary blood flow depends on the relationship between these three variable pressures. In the upright resting normal subject, both arterial and venous pressure exceed alveolar pressure at the base of the lung where hydrostatic pressure is greatest, and flow is influenced by the arteriovenous pressure difference; at the apex alveolar pressure exceeds both arterial and venous pressure and there is no flow of blood; while in the intermediate zone, where alveolar pressure is less than arterial but greater than venous pressure, flow becomes independent of venous pressure. This variation in blood flow from top to bottom of the upright lung does not precisely match the similar variation in ventilation that has already been described, so that the overall effect of gravity in the normal lung is to cause high $\dot{V}A/\dot{Q}$ ratios at the upper end of the lung, and low ratios at the bottom.

The distribution of perfusion becomes more even in the supine

position and on exercise. This is also the case when pulmonary blood flow is increased by left-to-right intracardiac shunts, or when pulmonary vascular resistance is increased.

2. *Obstruction to the Pulmonary Vascular Bed.* This may be due either to multiple pulmonary embolisation, to obstructive vascular changes resulting from long-sustained pulmonary hypertension, to fibrotic or inflammatory lesions of the lung parenchyma causing obliteration of pulmonary capillaries, or to pulmonary vasoconstriction resulting from hypoxia. The latter mechanism may have a compensatory effect by reducing perfusion of poorly ventilated parts of the lung and, therefore, improving the relationship between ventilation and perfusion.

BREATHING

The primary physiological function of breathing is to provide adequate alveolar ventilation so that gas exchange is appropriately maintained throughout a wide range of physiological, environmental, and pathological states. The apparatus of breathing consists of the 'respiratory centre', the skeletal and muscular elements of the thoracic cage with the nerves which supply them, and the lungs themselves.

The Control of Breathing

The rhythmicity of breathing and the homeostatic ventilatory responses to change in blood gas levels and acid-base balance appear to be generated in nerve cells scattered in a limited area of the pons and the medulla, referred to as the 'respiratory centre'. Hypoxia causes an increase in breathing because low arterial oxygen tension directly stimulates peripheral chemoreceptors in the carotid and aortic bodies to send nerve impulses over the glossopharyngeal and vagus nerves respectively to the respiratory centre. Changes in arterial carbon dioxide tension or in arterial hydrogen ion concentration influence breathing chiefly by their action upon central chemoreceptors, an increase in either acting as a stimulus to ventilation. The chemoreceptors situated near the ventral and lateral surface of the medulla may be stimulated by changes in the hydrogen ion content of the cerebrospinal fluid (CSF), brought about by diffusion of molecular carbon dioxide into the fluid as a result of a rise in arterial carbon dioxide tension.

Although a rise in arterial carbon dioxide tension and a fall in arterial oxygen tension both act as a stimulus to breathing, the response to change in carbon dioxide tension is much the greater of the two. The respiratory centre appears to be 'set' to produce the appropriate ventilatory response when arterial carbon dioxide tension

varies outside a certain range, but changes in the 'setting' of the respiratory centre are brought about gradually by alterations in the level of CSF bicarbonate ion, which adjusts slowly to changes in plasma bicarbonate level. Thus, chronic hyperventilation induced by persistent hypoxia (e.g. in normal subjects at high altitude) leads to a lowering of the level of arterial carbon dioxide tension at which ventilation is stimulated. In contrast, in patients with carbon dioxide retention due to chronic bronchitis and emphysema the respiratory centre becomes relatively insensitive to carbon dioxide; the main stimulus to ventilation then results from hypoxaemia alone, and the inhalation of gas mixtures containing a high concentration of oxygen leads to depression of ventilation and a further rise in carbon dioxide tension. These changes in the setting of the respiratory centre revert to normal when the normal person returns to sea level or when the patient with chronic lung disease is effectively treated.

The respiratory centre is depressed by certain pharmacological agents, including barbiturates, anaesthetics, tranquillising agents, and morphine. The use of these drugs is therefore particularly hazardous in patients whose respiration is already jeopardised by chronic lung disease. Stimulation of the centre is caused by an increase in arterial hydrogen ion concentration and, therefore, by any cause of metabolic acidosis such as diabetic ketosis or renal failure. Ventilation is also increased by salicylate and amphetamine poisoning, although it is not clear whether the hyperventilation is due to direct stimulation of the respiratory centre. Hyperventilation, which is seen following certain brain injuries and in hepatic encephalopathy, may be due to interference with pyramidal or extrapyramidal inhibition of the supramedullary motor pathways and so represent an exaggerated motor response similar to the hyperreflexia and hypertonia seen in the limbs of such patients.

Mechanical Factors

THE THORACIC CAGE

Apart from any consideration of its higher control, breathing is a motor activity that depends on the integrity of the thoracic skeleton, the muscles that move it and the nerves that supply them. Any gross abnormality of these will lead to hypoventilation with or without impairment of ventilation/perfusion relationships, and hence to a deterioration in gas exchange.

The action of the respiratory muscles is to increase the volume of the thoracic cage chiefly in two dimensions; transversely, by the action of the scalene and intercostal muscles in elevating the ribs, and

in its longitudinal dimension by contraction of the diaphragm. Expansion of the chest produces a negative pressure in the pleural space, causing the lungs to expand and air to flow into them. Expiration, on the other hand, is normally a passive process brought about by the elastic recoil of the lungs, but in forced expiration or when there is abnormal resistance to the flow of gas in the airways due to bronchial disease the expulsion of air from the thorax is assisted by contraction of the intercostal and abdominal muscles and by the accessory muscles of respiration.

The diseases of the thoracic cage liable to lead to respiratory embarrassment include spinal deformities such as severe kypho-scoliosis, widespread indurative conditions of the skin such as scleroderma which restrict expansion of the thorax, severe deformities of the sternum such as pectus excavatum, and crush injuries of the chest in which multiple rib fractures prevent the proper movement of the thorax. Among the diseases of muscles that cause hypoventilation are myasthenia gravis, dermatomyositis, and muscular dystrophy, while respiratory failure is an important complication of diseases that involve the motor neurones supplying the respiratory muscles, such as poliomyelitis, polyneuritis, and disease or injury of the spinal cord. These various conditions and the way they affect respiration are dealt with more fully in Chapter 9.

PULMONARY COMPLIANCE

Pulmonary ventilation is accompanied by rhythmical changes in the volume of the lungs and thoracic cage. At any moment the volume of gas in the lungs depends on a balance between the expansile force of the respiratory muscles and thoracic cage, and the contracting force produced by the elastic recoil of the lungs. The effect of these two opposing forces is to produce a pressure in the pleural space—*the intrathoracic pressure*—which is negative relative to the pressure within the airways—*the intrapulmonary pressure*—and to the atmospheric pressure outside the chest. The relationship between in-trathoracic pressure and lung volume is used to gain an understanding of the distensibility of the lung in terms of volume change per unit of pressure change (1 kPa^{-1} or 1/cm H_2O), and is known as the *compliance* of the lung.

The concept of compliance is essentially that of a *static* relationship between volume and pressure, and it assumes that the measurement is made only when all flow of gas into or out of the lungs has ceased. Abnormalities of static compliance reflect changes in the elastic recoil of the lung, due either to abnormalities of the pulmonary elastic tissue or of the surface tension of the surface film that lines the alveoli. Static compliance may be high in emphysema, when loss of elastic tissue

renders the lung more distensible than normal, or low in pulmonary fibrosis when elastic tissue is increased.

AIRWAY RESISTANCE

Although the measurement of static compliance is useful in giving an indication of changes in the distensibility of the lung, it does not, by definition, give any information about the mechanical factors involved in the flow of gas into and out of the airways. For this purpose it is necessary to study the relationship between the pressure difference between the mouth and the alveoli, and the flow of gas into the lung. This is referred to as the *airway resistance*, measured in terms of pressure difference per unit of gas flow (kPa l^{-1}s or cm $H_2O/l/sec$).

Airway resistance is due to friction between molecules of the moving gas and between the gas molecules and the walls of the bronchi. During quiet breathing, airflow in the normal bronchi is streamlined (laminar), but because the bronchi have an irregular surface and branch frequently the flow of gas becomes turbulent during rapid breathing, requiring a greater pressure difference to produce a given rate of flow. The factors that increase airway resistance are narrowing and abnormal irregularity of the airways, as occur most strikingly in chronic bronchitis or bronchial asthma. In emphysematous patients the airways tend to collapse on expiration, causing a rise in airway resistance.

TISSUE RESISTANCE

One further factor influencing the flow of gas in the airways is the resistance of the tissues to displacement or distortion, known as the tissue or viscous resistance. These tissues include the lungs, thoracic cage, diaphragm and abdominal contents. Tissue resistance amounts to only 20 per cent of the total pulmonary resistance and is rarely a limiting factor to ventilation in disease.

THE WORK OF BREATHING

The total work of breathing is the sum of the mechanical work done in moving the lungs, the respiratory gases, the thorax, the diaphragm, and the chest wall during the breathing cycle. It can be measured only indirectly, but one of its components, the mechanical work done on the lungs, can be estimated relatively easily by making simultaneous measurements of volume change and the pressure exerted across the lungs. The mechanical work done on the lungs may be greatly increased in obstruction of the airways and in diffuse pulmonary fibrosis, and becomes disproportionately greater when ventilation is increased by exercise.

When the mechanical work of breathing increases, the oxygen

requirement of the respiratory muscles rises. During quiet breathing in normal subjects the oxygen consumption of the respiratory muscles amounts to only about 2 per cent of the total metabolic requirement, rising to as much as 20 per cent during strenuous exercise. In patients with an increased mechanical breathing load due to lung disease the oxygen cost of breathing may be so great that there is little oxygen available for other activity, and exercise tolerance may be limited by this factor alone.

Mechanical factors may be responsible for alterations in the pattern of breathing. In patients with reduced pulmonary compliance the work of breathing is increased by the excessive elastic recoil of the lungs and it appears to be more economical to breathe more shallowly, in order to minimise the elastic factor, but more rapidly, in order to maintain adequate alveolar ventilation.

Breathlessness

Breathlessness, or dyspnoea, is a subjective sensation that is a symptom of a wide range of cardiopulmonary disorders. It is also experienced by normal people during exercise or breath-holding and by patients suffering from neuroses without evidence of organic disease. The measurable physiological functions that characterise these various conditions differ widely from normality to gross disorder, but the symptom of dyspnoea is common to them all. No one has been able to produce a theory that satisfactorily explains all the manifestations of breathlessness, but some have speculated that it is really a composite term that includes a number of different but closely related sensations. It has been suggested that breathlessness is discomfort in breathing due to:

1. Increased work of ventilation, e.g. due to increased airway resistance in asthma or to reduced compliance in diffuse pulmonary fibrosis.

2. Feeling of need for increased ventilation, e.g. during breath-holding, or in paralysed patients maintained by artificial ventilation.

3. Increased awareness of ventilation, e.g. during exercise, in hyperventilation of organic cause and in psychogenic disease.

Because breathlessness is a manifestation of so many different disorders it has proved impossible to identify a single sensory end-organ or receptor and its afferent pathway. One interesting theory that could account for some of the observed characteristics of breathlessness is the concept of *'length-tension appropriateness'*, based on the idea that dyspnoea arises from an imbalance between the demand of the respiratory centre for ventilation and the actual ventilation produced. The train of events in such a system might be

that a 'demand' for increased ventilation from the respiratory centre, initiated perhaps by a change in blood gas tension, would stimulate the respiratory muscles to contract. The resulting contraction would normally be appropriate to satisfy the demand, but in the presence of an obstruction to airflow, for example, the same contraction would produce inadequate change in volume of the lungs. Information about muscle tension and change in shape of the thorax would be sensed by muscle spindles or joint receptors in the thoracic cage, or by stretch receptors in the lung, and relayed to centres of consciousness. The sensation of dyspnoea would result if previous experience indicated that the amount of volume increase of the lungs or thoracic cage was inappropriate for the amount of tension set up in the muscles by their contraction.

An extension of this idea is that if the output of the respiratory centre, or the 'demand message' for increased ventilation, is available for analysis by the centres of consciousness, the only additional information required to assess the appropriateness of the ventilatory response is some measure of expansion of the lungs or thorax, e.g. from stretch receptors or muscle spindles; awareness of a change in muscle tension becomes unnecessary.

7

Testing Pulmonary Function

In this chapter some of the simpler tests of pulmonary function are described in principle, to provide an understanding of their value in the assessment of lung disease. Details of the techniques have been deliberately excluded, but these can readily be found in the appropriate textbooks. In the final section of the chapter there is a short account of the ways in which pulmonary function tests are most commonly useful in clinical practice.

TESTS OF GAS EXCHANGE

The Blood Gases

OXYGEN

Oxygen is carried in the blood in two ways, either dissolved or combined with haemoglobin. The amount of dissolved oxygen is relatively small, being only $0 \cdot 0013$ mmol l^{-1} kPa^{-1} ($0 \cdot 003$ ml oxygen/ 100 ml blood/mm Hg) oxygen tension, and increases in direct relation to the tension of oxygen in the blood. The bulk of the oxygen is associated with haemoglobin, which has the capacity for combining with oxygen in the proportions of $1 \cdot 34$ ml ($0 \cdot 06$ mmol) of oxygen for every gram of haemoglobin. Assuming a normal haemoglobin level of 15 g/100 ml, 100 ml of blood when fully saturated contains $20 \cdot 1$ ml of oxygen in combination (9 mmol l^{-1}). The degree of saturation of the blood depends on its oxygen tension, but this relationship is a non-linear one depicted by the oxyhaemoglobin dissociation curve (Fig. 6.2, page 55).

The peculiar shape of this curve has three important effects on the oxygenation of arterial blood in disease:

1. A decrease in arterial oxygen tension from $13 \cdot 3$ to $10 \cdot 6$ kPa (100 to 80 mm Hg) due to pulmonary disease does not greatly alter the amount of oxygen in the blood.

2. If the disturbance of function is severe enough to cause a further fall in arterial oxygen tension, the resulting fall in arterial oxygen *content* is disproportionately greater.

3. Because the upper part of the curve is almost flat, increasing alveolar oxygen tension by hyperventilation in well-ventilated areas of the lung does not significantly increase the amount of oxygen in the blood leaving these areas, and cannot therefore compensate for the low oxygen content of blood leaving under-ventilated parts of the lung.

Measurement. The level of oxygen in arterial blood can be estimated either in terms of saturation (Sa_1O_2) or in terms of tension (Pa_1O_2). Measurements of saturation can be carried out by spectrophotometry with reasonable accuracy ($\pm 1\%$) on samples of blood obtained by arterial puncture, or with somewhat less accuracy ($\pm 3\%$) but with less disturbance to the patient by using an oximeter attached to an ear lobe. The usual arterial oxygen saturation lies between 95 and 98 per cent, increasing to 100 per cent when pure oxygen is breathed. Arterial oxygen tension can be derived from a measurement of saturation by means of the dissociation curve, but the method is imprecise for values above $10 \cdot 6$ kPa (80 mm Hg) because this part of the curve is relatively flat. Direct measurement of oxygen tension can be carried out accurately using a membrane-covered oxygen electrode, the value in normal subjects breathing air lying between $10 \cdot 6$ and $13 \cdot 3$ kPa (80 and 100 mm Hg). Methods are available for measuring arterial oxygen tension from capillary blood samples, with a reasonable degree of accuracy.

Value of Arterial Oxygen Estimations. In clinical medicine the commonest cause of arterial hypoxaemia is uneven distribution of ventilation and perfusion due to airways obstruction, and some idea of the severity of the functional defect can be obtained from arterial oxygen estimations. In practice measurement of both arterial oxygen and carbon dioxide tensions provide a useful guide to the management of patients in respiratory failure.

Measurement of saturation with an ear oximeter is a simple way of assessing the effect of exercise or hyperventilation on gas exchange. For example, hypoventilation in obese subjects may be detected by measuring the change in arterial oxygen saturation that occurs when they are encouraged to hyperventilate. Arterial oxygen tension is required in the estimation of the alveolar-arterial oxygen tension difference, and in the measurement of venous-to-arterial shunts.

CARBON DIOXIDE AND pH

Transport. Carbon dioxide is transported by the blood in three ways: in solution, as bicarbonate, and as carbamino compounds combined with protein, mainly haemoglobin. Carbon dioxide diffuses from the tissues into the plasma and then to the red cells where the following

reactions take place under the influence of the enzyme, *carbonic anhydrase*:

$$CO_2 + H_2O \rightleftharpoons H_2CO_3 \rightleftharpoons H^+ + HCO_3^-$$

The H^+ ions are buffered by haemoglobin, while the HCO_3^- ions diffuse back into the plasma, being replaced by Cl^- ions. Although most of the carbon dioxide is transported as HCO_3^- in plasma, the red cells play an important role because:

1. They contain the carbonic anhydrase necessary for accelerating the hydration of carbon dioxide to carbonic acid.

2. They contain haemoglobin necessary for buffering or donating H^+ ions in the above reaction.

3. Since reduced haemoglobin has a greater affinity for H^+ ions than oxyhaemoglobin, the removal of oxygen from haemoglobin in the tissues increases the tendency of the reaction to proceed to the right, and therefore facilitates the uptake of carbon dioxide.

4. The more haemoglobin is reduced in the tissues, the greater is its capacity for forming carbamino compounds.

The haemoglobin dissociation curve for carbon dioxide differs from that for oxygen because it is steeper and more nearly linear over the physiological range (Fig. 6.6, page 60). This means that hyperventilation of well-ventilated regions can remove carbon dioxide to compensate for an increase in blood carbon dioxide level due to underventilation in other parts of the lungs.

Measurement. Several methods are available for measuring arterial carbon dioxide tension (Pa,CO_2):

1. *Directly.* Using a membrane-covered glass electrode.

2. *The Interpolation Method of Astrup.* There is a linear relationship between pH and the logarithm of carbon dioxide tension. The line can be constructed by equilibrating a blood sample with two gas mixtures of known carbon dioxide concentration in turn, and measuring the pH at each level. Knowing the original pH of the blood sample, its original carbon dioxide tension can be determined. This technique can be adapted for very small capillary blood samples obtained by pricking a finger or ear lobe, but it is important that the site chosen for sampling should have a copious capillary blood flow, so that the values obtained are a true reflection of arterial carbon dioxide tension and pH.

3. *By calculation,* from knowledge of the pH and plasma bicarbonate. This method is based on the interrelationship between pH, plasma bicarbonate and plasma carbon dioxide tension according to the Henderson-Hasselbalch equation:

$$pH = pK' + \log \frac{(HCO_3^-)}{(CO_2)}$$

which can be alternatively written:

$$pH = 6 \cdot 1 + \log \frac{(HCO_3^-)}{0 \cdot 03 \, Pa,CO_2}*$$

4. *By the Rebreathing Method.* A sample of gas that has a carbon dioxide tension very close to that of mixed venous blood can be obtained by getting the patient to breathe in and out of a bag containing oxygen. After about 90 seconds the gas mixture in the bag reaches a carbon dioxide tension somewhat higher than that of mixed venous blood. The patient rests for a few minutes, then re-breathes again into the bag for 20 to 40 seconds, during which time equilibrium is reached between mixed venous blood, alveolar gas, and the gas in the bag. This is analysed to obtain the mixed venous carbon dioxide tension, from which arterial carbon dioxide tension is derived by subtracting $0 \cdot 8 \, kPa$ (6 mm Hg). The advantage of this method is that it avoids arterial or capillary blood sampling, but it is difficult to use in the severely ill patient who is apt to allow gas to leak around the mouth during re-breathing. The normal value for arterial carbon dioxide tension lies between $4 \cdot 7 - 6 \cdot 0 \, kPa$ (35 and 45 mm Hg).

The Interpretation of Acid-base Changes. The lungs play an important part in acid-base regulation, because alterations in ventilation can rapidly bring about changes in the rate of excretion of carbon dioxide, and hence in the levels of carbon dioxide, bicarbonate, and hydrogen ion in the blood. The role of the lungs in this respect complements that of the kidneys which control fluctuations in acid-base balance more slowly. In acid-base disturbances the regulatory functions of the lungs and kidneys are directed towards restoration of arterial pH to normal, but these compensatory mechanisms are not always completely effective. Interpretations of changes in the acid-base state cannot be unequivocal without knowledge of the plasma bicarbonate level as well as the pH and carbon dioxide tensions.

1. Metabolic Disturbances

The primary change in *metabolic acidosis* (e.g. accumulation of H^+ ion due to renal failure or diabetic ketosis, or loss of base due to chronic diarrhoea or biliary fistula) is a rise in H^+ ions and a fall in bicarbonate. The compensatory respiratory mechanism is hyperventilation, to produce a fall in H^+ ions and, incidentally, a fall in bicarbonate and carbon dioxide tension.

* If Pa,CO_2 is expressed in kPa the factor is $0 \cdot 225$.

ERD 6

The primary change in *metabolic alkalosis* (due to persistent vomiting, excessive ingestion of sodium bicarbonate, or in hypokalaemia) is a fall in H^+ ions and a rise in plasma bicarbonate. The compensatory respiratory mechanism, often slight, is hypoventilation to produce a rise in H^+ ions and, incidentally, a rise in bicarbonate.

2. Respiratory Disturbances

The primary change in *respiratory acidosis* (due to respiratory failure) is an increase in carbon dioxide tension with an increase in H^+ ion and in bicarbonate. The compensatory renal mechanism is excretion of H^+ ion and retention of bicarbonate.

The primary change in *respiratory alkalosis* (due to hyperventilation in conditions such as liver failure, salicylate poisoning and cerebral injury) is a reduction in carbon dioxide tension with a fall in H^+ ion and in bicarbonate. The compensatory renal mechanism is to excrete more bicarbonate and retain more H^+ ions.

Diffusion

The transfer of oxygen from the alveoli to the pulmonary capillary blood depends on three major factors. Firstly, oxygen exchange takes place only in areas where functioning alveoli and functioning capillaries are brought into close proximity; if airways are blocked, if the pulmonary vascular bed is occluded, or if the normal architecture of the lung is disrupted, the effective surface area for gas exchange becomes diminished and the transfer of oxygen is reduced. Secondly, oxygen transfer is affected by the distance the oxygen molecules must travel between the alveolar space and the haemoglobin molecules within the red cells of the pulmonary capillary blood. This pathway consists of the alveolar lining cell, the interstitial tissue of the alveolar wall, the endothelial cell of the capillary, the plasma, the red cell membrane and, finally, the chemical reaction of association between the oxygen molecule and haemoglobin. Each of these steps takes a finite time, and oxygen transfer is reduced if the time required for diffusion is increased, for example, by thickening of the alveolar wall due to fibrosis or oedema fluid. Thirdly, the diffusion of oxygen depends on the pressure difference for oxygen between the alveolar space and the pulmonary capillary blood; if the head of pressure in the alveolus is diminished because of hypoventilation the transfer of oxygen molecules may be limited.

Bearing these points in mind, it should be recognised that measured abnormalities in the diffusion of oxygen are not usually due to obstruction to diffusion at the alveolar-capillary

membrane—'alveolar-capillary block'—but to changes in the effective alveolar-capillary surface area, to uneven distribution of ventilation, or even to abnormalities in the number of red blood cells in the pulmonary capillaries and their haemoglobin content. Mainly for this reason there has been a recent change in terminology, from 'diffusing capacity' to the less specific term 'transfer factor'.

Measurement. The transfer factor for the lung (T_L)—or diffusing capacity (D_L)—is expressed in mmol min^{-1}kPa^{-1} (ml of gas/minute/mm Hg), according to the following equation:

$$T_L = \frac{\text{volume of gas taken up by the pulmonary capillaries/minute}}{\text{alveolar pressure of the gas—mean capillary pressure of the gas}}.$$

Although oxygen is the gas of physiological interest, measurement of the mean capillary pressure of oxygen is complicated, and probably based on false assumptions. For this reason carbon monoxide is used as the test gas because its rate of diffusion and its behaviour in associating with haemoglobin resemble those of oxygen. The advantage of using carbon monoxide is that its affinity for haemoglobin is so great that it is completely taken up by the red cells, and its partial pressure in capillary blood remains to all intents and purposes zero.

Two types of test are used in measuring transfer factor for carbon monoxide (T_L,CO); the *steady state* method, in which the subject breathes a gas mixture containing a low concentration of carbon monoxide for about a minute, after which the uptake of carbon monoxide and the alveolar tension are measured; and the *single breath* method, in which these values are calculated from the change in composition of a gas mixture containing carbon monoxide which is inspired and held in the lungs for about 10 seconds. The former method has the advantage that it can be used during exercise. The normal value for T_L,CO is in the region of 10 mmol min^{-1} kPa^{-1} (30 ml CO/min/mm Hg), but varies according to age and stature.

Interpretation. T_L,CO is reduced in diseases such as diffuse interstitial pulmonary fibrosis and pulmonary oedema, in which increased thickness of the alveolar walls leads to a disturbance of alveolar ventilation. It is also reduced when the surface area of the pulmonary capillary membrane is diminished by emphysema, loss of pulmonary tissue, and occlusion of the pulmonary vascular bed. It is increased in polycythaemia but reduced by severe anaemia, these changes being due to alterations in the amount of haemoglobin available to absorb carbon monoxide.

Uneven Distribution of $\dot{V}A/\dot{Q}$

ALVEOLAR-ARTERIAL GAS TENSION DIFFERENCES

As described in the previous chapter uneven distribution of ventilation and perfusion leads to an increase in the differences in partial pressures between alveolar gas and arterial blood. As far as oxygen is concerned a large alveolar-arterial tension difference merely suggests a defect in gas exchange without indicating its cause, since diffusion limitation and venous-to-arterial shunts also increase it. However, neither of these factors significantly affects the arterial-alveolar tension differences for carbon dioxide or nitrogen, and theoretically a useful picture of uneven $\dot{V}A/\dot{Q}$ ratios could be obtained by measuring the arterial-alveolar tension difference for carbon dioxide, which is only increased by the presence of over-ventilated but under-perfused alveoli (high $\dot{V}A/\dot{Q}$), while that for nitrogen is increased by alveoli with low $\dot{V}A/\dot{Q}$ ratios. In making such measurements the arterial value for carbon dioxide can be measured using a membrane-covered glass electrode, and that for nitrogen can be measured by gas chromatography or derived from the nitrogen tension of urine collected anaerobically; the major difficulty lies in obtaining a representative sample of alveolar gas, since end-tidal alveolar sampling or rapid analysis of gas concentrations in the expired breath gives a meaningful estimate of alveolar gas only if the distribution of ventilation and perfusion is relatively normal. The value of this method is therefore limited.

PHYSIOLOGICAL DEAD SPACE AND VENOUS ADMIXTURE

The concept of 'ideal' alveolar gas attempts to overcome these difficulties by the argument that since, in the steady state, gas exchange in the lung must represent the metabolic requirements of the body as a whole, there must exist an average ('ideal') value for alveolar gas that is appropriate to the overall respiratory exchange ratio. This ideal value for alveolar oxygen tension can be calculated using 'the alveolar air equation' if it is assumed that alveolar and arterial carbon dioxide tensions are equal, and on the same assumption values for physiological dead space ('wasted ventilation') and venous admixture ('wasted blood flow') can be obtained. These values can be estimated by simultaneous collections over a 3-minute period of expired gas and arterial blood from patients in a steady-state condition, and they give a useful assessment of uneven distribution of $\dot{V}A/\dot{Q}$.

REGIONAL DIFFERENCES IN THE DISTRIBUTION OF
VENTILATION AND PERFUSION

Such differences may be measured by external counting over the chest following the intravenous injection or inhalation of insoluble

radioactive gases such as ^{85}Kr or ^{133}Xe. After inhalation the distribution of ventilation can be assessed from the count rate in different parts of the lung, while after intravenous injection the count rate in different lung regions will depend on their blood flow since the insoluble gas diffuses into the alveolar space of perfused alveoli.

VENOUS-TO-ARTERIAL SHUNTS

The total shunt of mixed venous to arterial blood includes contributions from Thebesian veins and from pulmonary arterial blood which bypasses ventilated alveoli; for example, some normal blood flow at the lung bases in the upright posture, perfusion of areas of pulmonary consolidation or collapse, and occasionally pulmonary arteriovenous fistulae. When pure oxygen is breathed, shunt is the only factor to limit the uptake of oxygen by pulmonary capillary blood and therefore to cause an alveolar-arterial oxygen tension difference, provided that sufficient time is allowed for the inspired oxygen to diffuse into the most poorly ventilated alveoli. In practice, arterial blood samples are obtained after the patient has breathed pure oxygen for 15 or 20 minutes, and arterial oxygen and carbon dioxide tensions estimated. Assuming that all nitrogen has been washed out of the lungs and that arterial and alveolar carbon dioxide tensions are equal, alveolar oxygen tension can be calculated as atmospheric pressure minus water vapour pressure minus arterial carbon dioxide tension, and the alveolar-arterial oxygen tension difference estimated by subtraction. Shunt can be calculated using a 'shunt equation', the normal value being 1 to 2 per cent of the cardiac output.

TESTS OF VENTILATORY FUNCTION

Lung Volumes

The total volume of gas in the lungs is conventionally divided into several fractions that can be separately measured. The names of the various subdivisions are shown on the accompanying diagram (Fig. 7.1). Clearly, the measured amount of gas within each of these subdivisions will depend on the size and stature of the individual, but numerous surveys of normal people of different height, age, and sex have made it possible to define the range of normality for each measurement.

MEASUREMENT

The patient breathes in and out of a close-fitting oro-nasal mask which is connected by a wide-bore tube to a simple spirometer. During quiet breathing the *resting tidal volume* is recorded, the end-expiratory level being a useful reference point since it is relatively constant in any

individual because it represents a point of balance between the elastic recoil of the lungs and the expansile force of the thoracic cage and respiratory muscles. The volume of air enclosed in the lungs at this end-expiratory level is the *functional residual capacity* (FRC).

The volume inspired by maximal inspiration from the end-expiratory level or FRC is the *inspiratory capacity* (IC), and a maximal expiration from the height of inspiration expels the volume of gas known as the *vital capacity* (VC). The difference between end-tidal inspiration and maximal inspiration is the *inspiratory reserve volume* (IRV) and between end-tidal expiration (or FRC) and maximal expiration is the *expiratory reserve volume* (ERV).

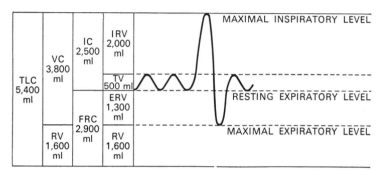

Fig. 7.1   The subdivisions of lung volume, giving normal values for a healthy adult of average stature

(Adapted from *The Lung: Clinical Physiology and Pulmonary Tests,* 2nd edition, by Julius Comroe, Jr. *et al.* Copyright 1962, Year Book Medical Publishers; by permission.)

The volume of gas remaining in the lungs at the end of a maximal expiration is the *residual volume* (RV). This cannot be measured directly by spirometry; instead, a dilution technique is used. Wearing a nose-clip, the patient is connected via a mouthpiece to a spirometer of known volume containing a helium gas mixture in known concentration. During the expiratory pause when his lung volume is at FRC a tap is turned so that he breathes in and out of the spirometer, the volume of which is kept constant by adding oxygen and removing carbon dioxide. The concentration of helium in the system is monitored, and recorded when equilibrium is reached. The volume of gas in the lungs and spirometer system, and hence the FRC, is calculated from knowing the initial volume of gas in the spirometer and the initial and final concentrations of helium. The residual volume is calculated by subtracting the ERV from FRC.

Total lung capacity (TLC) is calculated as the sum of RV + VC, or FRC + IC.

ABNORMALITIES OF LUNG VOLUME

A reduction in all the subdivisions of lung volume is characteristic of restrictive lung disease, i.e. those diseases in which lung expansion is limited by factors such as increased elastic recoil (diffuse pulmonary fibrosis), immobility of the thoracic cage (kyphoscoliosis) or weakness of the respiratory muscles (myasthenia gravis). Serial measurements of VC may be useful in judging the progress of such patients.

RV is normally less than 30 per cent of TLC, although increasing to 50 per cent in old age; an increase in RV at the expense of VC is characteristic of hyperinflation of the lungs, e.g. in bronchial asthma or in emphysema. In the latter condition FRC is often increased because elastic recoil is reduced and the resting position of the lungs is therefore at a more expanded level.

The *thoracic gas volume,* which can be measured with a body plethysmograph, is the volume of gas contained within the thorax, and normally equals TLC. When TLC is derived from measurements of FRC using the helium dilution technique the volume of gas in parts of the lung not in free connection with the airways is not included. In such circumstances the thoracic gas volume is larger than the measured TLC, a finding that suggests the presence of pulmonary bullae or areas of very poorly ventilated lung as occur in severe airway obstruction.

Airway Resistance

Precise estimation of the airway resistance depends on the simultaneous measurement of two variables, the rate of air flow at the mouth, and the pressure difference between the mouth (equal to atmospheric pressure) and the alveoli. The patient is seated in an air-tight box (the body plethysmograph); pressure is measured continuously in the box around the patient. As he inspires, the enlargement of the thorax lowers intrathoracic gas tension but increases the gas tension in the plethysmograph. At any point in the breathing cycle, therefore, the change in alveolar pressure is reflected by an equivalent change in the plethysmograph pressure, and the latter can easily be measured with a sensitive manometer. Air flow at the mouth during breathing is measured with a pneumotachograph. Normal values for airway resistance range from $0 \cdot 06 – 0 \cdot 24$ kPa l^{-1}s $(0 \cdot 6$ to $2 \cdot 4$ cm $H_2O/1/sec)$ in adults.

A more readily available method of evaluating airway resistance in the larger airways is by the use of a spirometer connected to a fast-

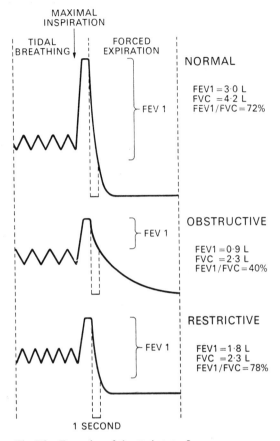

Fig. 7.2   Examples of the expiratory flow curve
Note that although the FEV1/FVC ratio for the restrictive pattern of lung disease is normal, the volume of the FEV1 is less than normal, due to the overall reduction in lung volumes.

moving recording system; the usual test is to ask the patient to breathe out as fast as possible following a maximal inspiration; three types of expiratory curve that may be obtained are shown in Fig. 7.2. From the expiratory flow curve the volume of gas expelled within a stated time can be measured, the usual measurement being the *forced expired volume in one second* (FEV1), i.e. the volume of gas expelled in one second beginning at the peak of a maximal inspiration. The

mean of three consecutive measurements should be recorded. In addition, the total volume of gas expired during the forced expiration should be measured; this is the *forced vital capacity* (FVC) which is equal to VC in normal subjects but may be less than VC in patients with airways obstruction because of '*air-trapping*', i.e. the retention of inspired gas in poorly ventilated areas of the lung. This occurs because the tendency of the airways to collapse is greatest in obstructive airway disease when transpulmonary pressure is increased by forceful expiration.

The FEV1 is reduced in obstructive airway disease because of increased airway resistance, and in restrictive lung disease because all lung volumes are diminished. Its size also depends upon the height and age of the subject. For these reasons the FEV1/FVC ratio is often used as it is independent of variations in lung volumes due to age or stature or restrictive lung disease, and gives a good indication of abnormality of airway resistance. Measurement of FEV1 before and after the inhalation of an isoprenaline aerosol gives an indication of the extent to which the airway obstruction can be reversed by bronchodilators.

A handy way of estimating changes in airway resistance is by the use of the peak expiratory flow meter which measures the *peak expiratory flow rate* (PEFR), i.e. the maximum flow over 10 msec at the beginning of expiration. The meter is easy to use and is particularly valuable in the serial assessment of airway obstruction.

The *maximal voluntary ventilation* (MVV) is the volume of gas expired per minute when the patient breathes as rapidly and as deeply as he can. The gas is usually collected over a period of 15 sec when the patient is ventilating maximally, the measured volume being multiplied by four and expressed in 1/min. This test is tiring and requires considerable co-operation from the patient, but it is useful whenever a repetitive test of muscle function is required, for example in myasthenia gravis.

Elastic Properties of the Lung

Of the simple tests already described, measurement of VC is the one most directly affected by changes in the compliance of the lungs or thoracic cage. It tends to be reduced in all forms of lung disease in which compliance is diminished, and serial measurements of VC are therefore of value in following the progress of such patients. It is not, however, a specific test for changes in compliance, and for this purpose the compliance itself must be measured.

Measurement of *pulmonary static compliance* depends on the measurement of transpulmonary pressure at a series of different end-inspiratory lung volumes. Transpulmonary pressure is strictly the

difference between mouth pressure (atmospheric pressure) and intra-pleural pressure, but a satisfactory approximation to the latter can be obtained by measuring intraoesophageal pressure by means of a small balloon in the oesophagus. The patient inspires a measured volume of gas from a spirometer and then pauses with the glottis open while oesophageal pressure is measured, the procedure being repeated several times at different lung volumes to obtain a pressure-volume curve, from which pulmonary compliance is estimated. The normal value is about 2 1 kPa^{-1} (0·2 l/cm H_2O), but varies according to sex, age and stature. It also varies according to the initial degree of pulmonary distension at which the measurement is made and, therefore, with FRC. For this reason measurements of compliance are most usefully recorded as *specific compliance,* i.e. in terms of com-pliance/FRC ratio expressed as l/cm H_2O per litre of FRC.

Static compliance is reduced in pulmonary fibrosis, pulmonary collapse, consolidation, pulmonary congestion or oedema, and hyaline membrane disease. It is increased in emphysema.

Dynamic Compliance. It is also possible to estimate pulmonary compliance during continuous breathing by measuring the transpulmonary pressure at the two lung volumes represented by the end-inspiratory and end-expiratory levels, when gas flow is momentarily at a standstill. Provided that gas flow *is* at a standstill at the instant that the pressure measurement is made, the value for dynamic compliance is similar to that for static compliance, as is usually the case in normal subjects breathing at normal respiratory rates. With rapid breathing, however, or in patients with narrowing of the airways the filling of terminal lung units may not be completed during the short end-inspiratory or end-expiratory pause so that the value for dynamic compliance turns out to be less than that for static compliance. A discrepancy of this nature indicates an abnormality of airway resistance rather than of the elastic properties of the lung, and may be an early sign of chronic airway obstruction.

Distribution of Ventilation

The evenness of distribution of inspired gas to the alveoli is an important factor in the efficiency of gas exchange. At best, uneven distribution implies wasted ventilatory effort to achieve adequate ventilation of the whole lung because minute volume must increase to compensate for a certain amount of ineffective ventilation; at the worst, it leads to hypoxaemia and carbon dioxide retention because of the resulting unequal distribution of ventilation with respect to blood flow.

Two methods of testing distribution of ventilation are available, both requiring rapid analysis of the gas expired at the mouth. The first

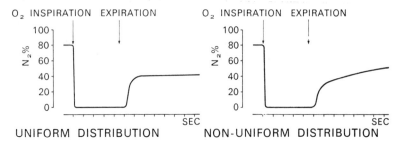

Fig. 7.3 The single breath test for distribution of inspired gas

Nitrogen concentration is measured by rapid analysis at the mouth of the expired gas. When a breath of pure oxygen is inspired the nitrogen concentration at the mouth falls to zero; during expiration it initially remains at zero but begins to rise as oxygen mixed with nitrogen from the gas-exchanging zone of the lung is expired, the latter part of the curve (the alveolar 'plateau') representing nitrogen from the alveoli. If the inspired oxygen is evenly distributed to all alveoli the concentration of alveolar nitrogen will be nearly uniform throughout the latter part of the expirate and the alveolar plateau will be nearly horizontal. If, on the other hand, the inspired oxygen is unevenly distributed, the end-inspired nitrogen concentration will vary in different parts of the lungs; this will lead to a steeply sloping alveolar plateau since the better-ventilated parts of the lungs which received the greater share of inspired oxygen will tend to empty earliest, while the poorly ventilated parts will empty last. Conventionally, the slope of the alveolar plateau is measured between the points that represent 750 and 1,250 ml of expired gas.

is a *multiple breath method,* depending on the principle that the time required for an inhaled gas to reach the same concentration in all parts of the lung will be longer if distribution is uneven than if it is even. If the patient breathes in and out of a spirometer containing a helium gas mixture the concentration of helium in the system will gradually fall until equilibrium is achieved in all parts of the lung; the rate of change of helium concentration is therefore an indication of the evenness of distribution in the lung. Alternatively, the patient breathes 100 per cent oxygen while the nitrogen concentration of the expired gas is analysed; the nitrogen in the alveoli is gradually replaced by oxygen so that the concentration of nitrogen in the expirate falls, the time taken for it to reach an arbitrary low level (usually 2·5%) being an indication of the evenness of distribution of the inspired oxygen.

The second method depends on rapid analysis of the gas concentration in a *single breath.* Poorly ventilated alveoli have a relatively high concentration of carbon dioxide and nitrogen, and tend to empty late in expiration. The concentration of carbon dioxide in an expired breath is low at the beginning of the expiration (because this portion

consists of dead space gas, i.e. air that contains virtually no carbon dioxide), then increases rapidly as the alveoli begin to empty, and finally increases more slowly as the alveoli make their major contribution to the expirate. The slope of the latter part of the expired carbon dioxide curve is nearly flat if all alveoli are equally ventilated, but rises steeply if there is a significant contribution from poorly ventilated alveoli, the steepness of the slope being a measure of the unevenness of alveolar ventilation. On the same principle, the concentration of nitrogen in the expired gas at the mouth may be analysed following a single breath of oxygen. The first part of the expirate contains no nitrogen; then in the second part the concentration of nitrogen rises sharply; and in the final part of the expirate the slope of the 'alveolar plateau' for nitrogen indicates the evenness with which the nitrogen in different alveoli has been diluted by the inhaled oxygen (Fig. 7.3).

The most marked disturbance of distribution of ventilation is seen in chronic bronchitis and emphysema. Distribution is also adversely affected by age, in local or diffuse fibrosis of the lungs, in diseases of the thoracic wall and the respiratory muscles and in hypoventilation syndromes.

Airway Closure

There is considerable interest in methods of testing function that will identify the changes of chronic bronchitis and emphysema at an early stage before permanent lung damage has occurred. An abnormality of dynamic compliance is thought to reflect early changes in small airways but the method is too complicated for routine use in large surveys, and at present the most useful simple technique is probably the forced expiratory spirogram from which the FEV1, FVC and maximum mid-expiratory flow rate can be measured.

Closing volume is a measurement designed to detect collapse of small airways occurring towards the end of maximal expiration. A bolus of a marker gas such as helium or argon is introduced at the mouth at the end of full expiration; the subject then takes a slow maximal inspiration which has the effect of distributing the marker gas preferentially to the upper zones of the lungs. During the subsequent slow expiration, marker gas concentration and expired gas volume are monitored, and expiration of the upper zone gas is indicated by a sudden increase in the concentration of marker gas towards the end of expiration; this is taken as a sign that airway closure has occurred in the lower zones. The volume of gas remaining in the lungs at this point is called the closing volume, and is usually expressed as a percentage of the vital capacity.

In normal young subjects the closing volume is less than 15 per cent

of vital capacity, but increases with age. It is greater in smokers than non-smokers but the range of normal values is wide, and present evidence suggests that the test is not sufficiently specific to distinguish the early bronchitic from the normal subject.

PRACTICAL ASSESSMENT OF LUNG FUNCTION

In ordinary clinical practice pulmonary function tests may be used in one of two ways: to obtain a quantitative assessment of a functional disability that is readily recognisable on clinical grounds; or, less frequently, as an aid to the diagnosis of pulmonary disease.

Quantitative Assessment

MEDICAL TREATMENT

It is often useful to follow the progress of patients with chronic lung disease such as bronchial asthma or chronic airways obstruction by making base-line observations on the state of their pulmonary function when they are first seen, followed by a serial record of those aspects of function that most accurately reflect the physiological abnormality being treated. The choice of pulmonary function tests will vary according to the functional pathology of the underlying disease; three examples of this type of management are briefly described:

1. In *bronchial asthma* the use of corticosteroids is occasionally indicated because of the severe, persistent nature of the disease; on the other hand, it is obligatory to keep the dose of corticosteroid to a minimum effective level because of the important side-effects. One method of achieving this result has been proposed as follows: in a control period lasting about a week the patient is maintained on a dose of 20 mg prednisolone daily, and the FEV is measured daily. The prednisolone is then replaced with placebo tablets, and further daily measurements of FEV recorded to determine the duration of action of the prednisolone. In this way it is possible to decide whether adequate control of bronchospasm can be obtained with intermittent (e.g. twice or thrice weekly) doses of prednisolone, or whether daily dosage is necessary.

2. In *sarcoidosis* and in other diseases characterised by diffuse pulmonary fibrosis, it is sometimes necessary to decide whether corticosteroid therapy is effective in retarding the progress of the disease. In such conditions the lung volumes, especially VC, and transfer factor (T_L,CO) are characteristically diminished. Having obtained a base-line record of these measurements, corticosteroid

therapy may be begun; further measurements made at three and six months will show the effect of therapy on the progress of the disease, and indicate whether there is a place for continued steroid treatment.

3. In *respiratory failure* due to airways obstruction the patient is affected by hypoxia and by carbon dioxide retention. Correction of the hypoxia by giving inspired gas mixtures containing an increased concentration of oxygen is liable to cause hypoventilation and further carbon dioxide retention. To avoid dangerous hypercapnia it is necessary to measure the arterial carbon dioxide tension before oxygen therapy is started, and to make repeated measurements thereafter at intervals of 1 to 2 hours, lowering the concentration of the inspired oxygen mixture if the arterial carbon dioxide measurements indicate that excessive carbon dioxide retention is occurring.

SURGICAL TREATMENT

It is often difficult to decide whether a patient with chronic lung disease is fit to have an elective surgical operation; for example, pros-tatectomy in an elderly bronchitic. The danger lies mainly in the development of postoperative respiratory failure precipitated by infection, pulmonary collapse and alveolar hypoventilation. In such cases it is important to know the patient's level of activity prior to his illness, and to test his exercise tolerance by a simple procedure such as walking him up a flight of stairs. It is not possible to lay down strict criteria in deciding the suitability of a patient for operation, but a combination of the following factors would tend to contra-indicate major surgery:

1. Inability to perform a simple exercise test, such as climbing a flight of stairs, without undue breathlessness.
2. FEV1 less than 40 per cent of the predicted value for age and height.
3. Arterial carbon dioxide tension more than 6·6 kPa (50 mm Hg).
4. RV/TLC ratio of more than 50 per cent.

If the operation is necessary in spite of severe lung disease it is important that careful pre-operative preparation should be carried out, using physiotherapy, antibiotics, and bronchodilators to ob-tain maximum pulmonary function. Following operation, serial measurements of arterial oxygen and carbon dioxide tensions may be useful indications of impending respiratory failure.

DISABILITY CLAIMS

In assessing pulmonary disability attributed to occupational hazards a

comprehensive appraisal of pulmonary function must be available, to be used in conjunction with the clinical and radiological findings.

Diagnosis

RESPIRATORY FAILURE

Respiratory failure often develops insidiously and may be recognised by the unwary only when the patient's condition has deteriorated sufficiently to make corrective measures difficult to carry out. Changes in the arterial blood gas tension are the critical measurements in diagnosing respiratory failure, and where there is doubt concerning a patient's respiratory capacity serial measurements of arterial carbon dioxide tension should be performed.

Progressive weakness of the respiratory muscles in neuromuscular disorders leads gradually to respiratory incapacity and failure of gas exchange. Apart from the measurements of blood gas tension mentioned above, it is helpful to make serial tests of ventilatory function; in particular, vital capacity and maximal voluntary ventilation are diminished, and there is likely to be impairment of expiratory flow rates.

CYANOSIS

Central cyanosis may be due to alveolar hypoventilation, uneven distribution of ventilation and perfusion, venous-to-arterial shunt, or to a combination of these factors. The cause is usually evident from the clinical and radiological findings, and can be confirmed by the appropriate tests of pulmonary function. A simple test of *venous-to-arterial shunt* is to measure arterial oxygen saturation after pure oxygen is breathed: failure to obtain 100 per cent saturation is an indication of abnormal shunt. A more precise test is to calculate the total shunt as a percentage of cardiac output from a measurement of the alveolar-arterial oxygen tension difference after the patient has breathed oxygen for at least 25 minutes: under these circumstances even the worst ventilated alveoli become filled with oxygen, and the remaining alveolar-arterial oxygen tension difference is only attributable to shunted blood.

Hypoventilation may be a cause of cyanosis in patients with otherwise normal lung function. Measurement of the blood gases shows a reduction in arterial oxygen saturation (or tension) and an increase in carbon dioxide tension; these changes can be partially or completely restored to normal by encouraging the patient to hyperventilate for 30 seconds.

The possibility of methaemoglobinaemia or sulphaemoglobinaemia should be borne in mind.

THE CAUSE OF DYSPNOEA

In assessing a patient with dyspnoea for which no satisfactory explanation has been reached by clinical or radiological examination it is necessary to perform a large series of pulmonary function tests to enable the *pattern* of disability to be recognised. In this way an abnormality in one test of pulmonary function gains added significance when it is found in association with another functional abnormality. As an example, two common patterns of functional abnormality characteristic of obstructive lung disease (e.g. bronchial asthma or chronic bronchitis) and restrictive lung disease (e.g. fibrosing alveolitis) are shown in Table 7.1.

Table 7.1

Test	*Obstructive*	*Restrictive*
1. Lung volumes	TLC and VC normal or increased; RV and FRC often increased due to hyperinflation	Reduced
2. Maximal flow rates	FEV1, FEV1/FVC ratio, PEFR and MVV reduced	FEV1 reduced FEV1/FVC ratio normal MVV normal or reduced
3. Airway resistance	Reduced	Normal
4. Compliance	Normal or increased	Reduced
5. Distribution of ventilation	Impaired	Impaired
6. Arterial oxygen	Sa,O_2, Pa,O_2 reduced	Sa,O_2, Pa,O_2 normal or slightly reduced, greatly reduced on exercise
7. Arterial carbon dioxide	Pa,CO_2 normal or increased	Pa,CO_2 normal or reduced
8. Arterial pH	Decreased during exacerbations	Normal
9. Diffusion	T_L,CO normal or reduced	$T_L CO$ often reduced

EXERCISE TESTING

It is not always easy to assess the severity of breathlessness from the history and clinical examination alone although valuable information can often be gained by making first-hand observations on the patient's degree of breathlessness and on the pulse and respiratory rate after walking him up several flights of stairs. More objective tests of cardiopulmonary function have been devised for the laboratory, using a bicycle ergometer or a treadmill to impose measurable work loads

on the patient. The main value of such tests is to prove cardiorespiratory normality in patients suspected of having lung or heart disease.

A simple screening test consists of measuring ventilation with a gas meter and heart rate by continuous recording of the electrocardiogram while the patient performs three or more levels of exercise at progressively increasing work loads. Normal standards are available which allow the observed performance to be compared with predicted values based on age, weight and physical fitness. A more sophisticated analysis of exercise performance may be obtained by adding expired gas and arterial blood collections, rapid gas analysis at the mouth and blood lactate estimations.

8

The Circulation and Lymphatic Drainage of the Lungs

Structure and Function

ANATOMY OF THE PULMONARY VASCULAR BED

The main pulmonary arteries arise at the bifurcation of the pulmonary trunk and divide into a variable number of branches that supply each lobe. These vessels are classified as 'elastic arteries', having a media that consists mainly of elastic fibrils with some smooth muscle fibres and collagen. The lobar branches follow the course of the main bronchi and their subdivisions, dividing irregularly into progressively smaller vessels down to the level of the smaller bronchioles where they gradually merge into muscular pulmonary arteries, characterised histologically by a media consisting of circular smooth muscle bounded by internal and external elastic laminae. The muscular arteries range in size from 1,000 to 100 microns, lying close to the bronchioles, respiratory bronchioles, and alveolar ducts. They are end-arteries from which the pulmonary arterioles arise as terminal or side branches. The normal arteriole, a vessel of diameter less than 100 microns, has smooth muscle only at its origin, derived from the medial coat of the parent artery; the arteriolar wall consists of an endothelial lining with a single elastic lamina.

At alveolar level the capillaries arise as side branches or terminations of the arterioles, lying in the alveolar septa and separated from the alveolar space by only a small amount of interstitial tissue and the alveolar lining cells. The alveolar capillaries are so numerous and diffuse that the capillary bed may usefully be thought of as a thin sheet of blood flowing along an enormous number of parallel channels between two layers of endothelium. The alveolar capillaries drain into pulmonary vessels which are histologically identical to the arterioles, and then into pulmonary veins which tend to be situated away from the bronchial tree, the larger veins lying in the alveolar septa.

The small muscular pulmonary arteries and arterioles are thought

to be the main site of resistance to pulmonary blood flow, at least in conditions of alveolar hypoxia. In hypoxic conditions of the lung (e.g. in dwellers at high altitude, or patients with alveolar hypoventilation) the muscular media of the arteries becomes hypertrophied and smooth muscle extends even into the walls of the arterioles, a development thought to account for the pulmonary hypertension encountered in such individuals.

PULMONARY BLOOD FLOW

The pulmonary circulation is a low-resistance circuit, for it receives the same blood flow as the systemic circulation but at one sixth the blood pressure: a representative value for pulmonary arterial pressure in a normal subject at rest is 20/9 mm Hg with a mean of 15 mm Hg. Exercise may double or even quadruple pulmonary blood flow but mean pulmonary arterial pressure increases at most by a few mm Hg, showing that the normal pulmonary vascular bed is able to accommodate a considerable increase in flow without a significant rise in pressure, partly by recruitment of blood vessels which are closed during the resting state and also by dilation of already opened vessels.

Pulmonary Vascular Resistance. There is at present some un-certainty as to where in the pulmonary vascular bed lies the main site of resistance to blood flow. Evidence based on measurements of blood vessel size made on casts of the pulmonary vascular tree indicates that more than half the total pressure drop across the pulmonary vascular bed occurs proximal to the capillaries. On the other hand, it is generally accepted that blood flow through the lungs is regulated at capillary level according to the relationship between arterial, venous, and alveolar pressures, which is responsible for differences in resting blood flow in different parts of the upright lung (page 63). A rise in intra-alveolar pressure would be expected to increase pulmonary vascular resistance at the level of the alveolar capillaries, and it has been suggested that the pulmonary hypertension occurring in acute exacerbations of chronic bronchitis may be partially attributable to this mechanism.

On histological grounds it has long been supposed that the main site of resistance to blood flow lies in the small (100–1,000 microns diameter) muscular arteries since these vessels would be expected to be capable of constriction or dilatation by virtue of their muscular walls. Although they receive both sympathetic and parasympathetic nerve fibrils the calibre of these vessels does not seem to be controlled by the autonomic nervous system in man, but they are capable of dilation and constriction under the influence of certain chemical

stimuli, the most important being the vasoconstrictive effect of hypoxia.

Vascular resistance is usually calculated according to the equation:

$$\text{resistance} = \frac{\text{driving pressure}}{\text{blood flow}}$$

where the driving pressure is the pressure difference across the resistance, in this case, pulmonary arterial pressure—left atrial pressure.

Changes in Pulmonary Arterial Pressure. Pulmonary hypertension may be caused either by an obstruction to the flow of blood through the pulmonary vascular bed, or by a large, sustained increase in the volume of blood flowing through the pulmonary circulation. The pathogenesis of pulmonary hypertension and cor pulmonale is further considered in Chapter 9 (page 109).

Distribution of Pulmonary Blood Flow is affected chiefly by three factors: gravity, hypoxia, and occlusive or destructive disease of the pulmonary vascular bed. The effect of gravity in producing a slight relative preponderance of flow to the bottom of the lung in the upright position has been described previously (page 63). During exercise when pulmonary blood flow is increased, or in conditions characterised by congestion of the lungs such as mitral stenosis or atrial septal defect the distribution of blood flow becomes more uniform. Hypoxia appears to be an important determinant of flow distribution in diffuse pulmonary disease because arterial vasoconstriction occurs in areas of lung that are hypoxic due to alveolar hypoventilation; as a result, flow is diminished to areas where ventilation is diminished, an effect that reduces unevenness of ventilation : perfusion distribution and therefore improves gas exchange.

THE BRONCHIAL CIRCULATION

The bronchial arteries arise from intrathoracic systemic vessels, usually the aorta, and act as nutrient arteries to the walls of the tracheobronchial tree and to the supporting framework of the lungs. Bronchial venous blood drains mainly into the azygos veins but some also enters the pulmonary veins. It is extremely difficult to find evidence of broncho-pulmonary anastomoses in the normal lung but in disease the bronchial circulation may enlarge and proliferate, and precapillary anastomoses between the two circulations may become evident. This is particularly liable to happen in areas of chronic inflammation such as empyema and lung abscess, in bronchiectasis and sometimes in association with pulmonary carcinoma. The drainage of bronchial veins into the pulmonary venous system makes a small contribution to the true venous-to-arterial shunt in normal

individuals, but this contribution may be substantially increased in disease; for example, in right heart failure when pressure in the right atrium exceeds that in the left, thus diverting bronchial venous blood into the pulmonary veins.

LYMPHATIC DRAINAGE OF THE LUNGS

There are three main groups of pulmonary lymphatics in man. The first group begins in the visceral pleura or in the interlobular septa, draining the periphery of the lung lobules by channels that follow the course of the pulmonary veins to the hilum of the lung. The second group of lymphatics begins as blind-ended tubes in the acini around the alveolar ducts, draining to the hilum via the peribronchial lymphatics. The third group forms anastomotic channels between the perivenous and peribronchial lymphatics. Normally the lymphatics of the upper part of the left lung drain into the thoracic duct while those from the remainder of the left lung and from the whole of the right lung drain into the right lymphatic duct.

The pulmonary lymphatics play an important role in removing protein molecules that have accumulated to excess in the pleural fluid as a result of increased capillary permeability due to inflammatory conditions of the pleura. Lymphatic absorption probably occurs almost entirely into the lymphatics of the lower mediastinal folds.

Pleural Fluid. The passage of fluid into or out of any capillary depends on a balance of forces between the plasma colloid pressure which tends to draw water and electrolytes into the capillary, and the hydrostatic pressure in the capillaries which tends to drive them out. In the systemic circulation these forces are approximately equal, with plasma colloid pressure predominating slightly; in the pulmonary circulation capillary hydrostatic pressure is only about one third that in the systemic capillaries, so that it is generally exceeded by plasma colloid pressure. At the pleural surface, which forms an interface between the pulmonary and systemic circulations, the net effect is a pressure gradient from the interstitial tissue on the parietal side of the pleura to the interstitial tissue of the lung on the visceral side, producing a net absorptive force of about $1 \cdot 7$ kPa (13 mm Hg) into the visceral pleura.

This pressure gradient is responsible for the sucking force that normally keeps the two pleural surfaces in apposition. It is also the cause of pleural effusions that occur as complications of ascites, for example in Meig's syndrome (pleural effusion with ascites associated with ovarian fibroma) or in cirrhosis of the liver, presumably following a small rupture of the diaphragm.

An excess of fluid in the pleural space can therefore be attributed to an upset of the mechanisms that maintain a normal balance of water,

electrolytes, and protein: excessive capillary pressure in cardiac failure, increased capillary permeability in inflammatory conditions, or impaired clearance of protein when the pulmonary lymphatics are obstructed.

Investigation of the Pulmonary Circulation

MEASUREMENT OF PRESSURES AND FLOW

Measurement of the pressures in the right side of the heart and the pulmonary arteries is achieved by inserting a catheter into an antecubital vein and manipulating it through the cavities of the right side of the heart and into the lumen of the pulmonary vessels. At any site the pressure at the tip of the fluid-filled catheter may be recorded by attaching the proximal end to a sensitive manometer. Pressure in the pulmonary capillaries is obtained when the tip of the catheter is 'wedged' in a peripheral pulmonary arteriole. Mixed venous blood can be obtained by sampling through the catheter, and its oxygen content measured in order to calculate blood flow by the *Fick method,* according to the equation:

$$\text{blood flow (1/min)} = \frac{\text{oxygen uptake (ml/min)}}{\text{arteriovenous oxygen difference (ml/1)}}$$

Alternatively, blood flow may be measured by a *dye dilution method.*

Cardiac catheterisation is not without serious side effects, the most important being the occasional precipitation of cardiac arrhythmias which include ventricular fibrillation. A procedure that appears to carry less risk is the use of a 'floating catheter', a relatively soft nylon tube of small diameter which can be positioned with the minimum of manipulation and enables pressure and flow measurements to be made even in seriously ill patients. It has the added advantage that the procedure can be carried out in the ward. Cardiac catheterisation does not play an important part in the clinical investigation of pulmonary disease although a precise estimate of pulmonary arterial pressure is occasionally of prognostic value in chronic diffuse pulmonary disease.

RADIOLOGY OF THE PULMONARY VESSELS

In the *plain radiograph* of the chest pulmonary hypertension is suggested by:

1. Increase in heart size due to right ventricular enlargement.
2. Increased prominence of the hilar vascular shadows. In chronic airways obstruction a transverse distance of more than 10 cm between the bifurcations of the right and left main pulmonary arteries

(the 'transpulmonary' or 'transhilar' distance) is highly suggestive of pulmonary hypertension.

3. Generalised prominence of the pulmonary vascular shadows associated with abnormal pulsation of the hilar vessels on fluoroscopy ('hilar dance') indicating greatly increased pulmonary blood flow (e.g. left-to-right intracardiac shunts).

In contrast, increased translucence of the lung fields with thinning and attenuation of the vascular shadows, which peter out before reaching the periphery of the lungs, is one of the main diagnostic signs of emphysema.

Pulmonary angiography is valuable in outlining defects of the pulmonary circulation, usually in the investigation of suspected pulmonary embolism. Radio-opaque contrast medium is injected into a peripheral vein, or for better delineation through a catheter into the right atrium, the passage of the material through the pulmonary circulation being followed with rapid serial radiographs. Pulmonary angiography is not without risk of causing fatal cardiac arrhythmias when it is carried out in the investigation of pulmonary hypertension e.g.; due to chronic pulmonary thrombo-embolism.

RADIOSCANNING

A newer technique, known as *pulmonary scanning,* is to inject macro-aggregates of ^{131}I-labelled human serum albumin into a peripheral vein; the material is carried to the lungs where it impacts in the small pulmonary vessels, being distributed according to the blood flow in the pulmonary arteries at the time of the injection. The thorax is scanned with a scintillation counter which produces a 'picture' of the distribution of radioactivity within the lungs, areas of obstructed or diminished flow appearing as blank spaces against a background of radioactivity. After a few hours the macro-aggregates break up and the radioactive iodine is excreted, the total radiation received by the lungs being comparable to that received during a routine chest radiograph. Since the subject has to lie still for 15 minutes the test is unsuitable for those who are seriously ill. A scintillation camera is a better alternative for such patients.

The technique is most useful in the diagnosis of pulmonary embolism, and in determining the extent of pulmonary involvement. It must be used in conjunction with the clinical and radiographic findings since similar appearances may result from other diseases such as lung cysts, carcinoma, pneumonia, and pleural effusions. It is less hazardous a technique than pulmonary angiography although sudden death has been described in patients with severe pulmonary hypertension, and is more effective in demonstrating abnormalities at the periphery of the lung fields. It may be useful in the investigation of

pulmonary carcinoma, in determining the extent of the lesion and, therefore, the resectability of the tumour.

ELECTROCARDIOGRAPHY

In obstructive disease of the pulmonary circulation, whatever its cause, the work of the right ventricle is increased, resulting in hypertrophy and sometimes dilatation of the right ventricle, and commonly overloading of the right atrium. Particularly when there is emphysema, but also because of right ventricular hypertrophy, the heart rotates in a clockwise direction about its antero-posterior and longitudinal axes, producing the signs of *right axis deviation*: the major QRS deflection being downward in leads I and aVL, and upwards in leads III and aVF. The *electrocardiographic diagnosis of cor pulmonale* is possible in only about one third of cases, the distinguishing features being:

1. P pulmonale: tall, spiky P waves in leads II, III and aVF.
2. Signs of right ventricular hypertrophy:
   R tall and S small in V1,
   R small and S deep in V5–6,
   T biphasic or negative and S–T depressed in V1–3.
3. Signs of incomplete right bundle branch block:
   RSR′ in leads III, a VF and V1–2,
   Wide S in leads I, aVL and V5–6.

An acute and sudden rise in pulmonary arterial pressure occurs most commonly as the result of *pulmonary embolism*. It causes acute dilatation of the right ventricle, clockwise rotation of the heart and right atrial overloading. The electrocardiographic changes are:

1. 'S1 Q3 T3' pattern:
   S in lead I, deep Q in lead III,
   S–T segment depression in leads I, II, aVL, elevation in III, aVR, aVF,
   T inversion in lead III.
2. Signs of incomplete right bundle branch block.
3. Chest leads:
   Predominant S waves in all leads to V5 or V6,
   S–T elevation and T inversion in leads V1–3.
4. Rarely, P pulmonale.
5. Arrhythmias, including sinus tachycardia, extrasystoles and atrial fibrillation.

These changes may be of short duration, so that the typical electrocardiographic appearance is often incomplete. It may be confused with that of *inferior myocardial infarction,* which is marked by the identical behaviour of leads II and III, and a deep Q in aVF.

9

Disordered Function
in Lung Disease

A knowledge of the physiological basis of lung function and an understanding of pulmonary function tests are relevant to the assessment and management of lung disease. In treatment particularly, it is important to recognise the processes that lead to disturbance of function so that appropriate steps may be taken to prevent or correct the functional abnormality. In this chapter certain common patterns of disturbed function are considered in relation to the clinical syndromes that cause them.

Ventilation Perfusion Abnormalities

AIRWAYS OBSTRUCTION

The essential feature of this disease pattern is irregular narrowing or obstruction of the airways so that ventilation becomes non-uniform. This in itself causes uneven distribution of ventilation and perfusion which leads to the type of impairment of gas exchange described in Chapter 6 (page 58), but in most clinical causes of airways obstruction the physiological disturbance is aggravated by destructive or obliterative changes in the pulmonary vascular bed.

1. *Bronchial Asthma.* The clinical condition is characterised by episodes of acute dyspnoea and wheezing resulting from narrowing of the airways. This is due to a combination of bronchoconstriction, thickening of the bronchial mucous membrane and increased bronchial secretions. The functional effect of these changes is to cause a large increase in airway resistance and in the work of breathing, associated with air-trapping and hyperinflation of the lungs. Distribution of inspired gas is non-uniform but pulmonary blood flow is relatively undisturbed. The effect of these abnormalities on gas exchange is to lower arterial oxygen tension because of uneven distribution of ventilation/perfusion ratios, but arterial carbon dioxide tension is maintained at normal or subnormal levels by hyperventilation. If airways narrowing persists the patient may become exhausted

by the effort of breathing, alveolar ventilation diminishes, and cyanosis and carbon dioxide retention develop.

The correction of these functional abnormalities is directed towards the relief of airways obstruction. Bronchodilator drugs, physiotherapy to promote the expectoration of secretions, corticosteroids to reduce the hyperactive response of the bronchial mucosa, and rehydration to reduce the viscosity of bronchial secretions are the basic forms of therapy. When respiratory failure threatens it is necessary to maintain ventilation artificially in order to relieve the patient of the work of breathing until the bronchial reaction has had time to subside.

2. *Chronic Bronchitis and Emphysema.* In this condition the symptoms of progressive exertional dyspnoea and chronic productive cough are due to narrowing of the airways resulting from inflammatory swelling of the bronchial mucosa, and from expiratory collapse of the bronchi due to loss of the normal elastic supporting tissues of the lungs. Active bronchoconstriction plays a relatively minor role. Acute exacerbations of the chronic disorder frequently follow upper respiratory tract infections which lead to bacterial invasion of the bronchi.

The functional effect of these changes is similar to that seen in bronchial asthma except that the inflammatory and destructive changes in the airways and lung parenchyma progressively limit ventilation, so that little ventilatory response is possible when gas exchange becomes acutely impaired by an infective exacerbation of the disease. Uneven distribution of ventilation/perfusion ratios is here due to non-uniformity of perfusion as well as ventilation, largely because chronic hypoxia leads to narrowing of the small pulmonary arteries and arterioles. Damage to the alveolar walls probably also contributes to the unevenness of blood flow. Carbon dioxide retention and cyanosis eventually occur as a result of the ventilation/perfusion imbalance, usually during an episode of acute bronchitis, and are often accompanied by congestive cardiac failure. This is due to the increase in pulmonary vascular resistance which results from hypoxic pulmonary vasoconstriction.

The measures required in treatment are: (1) improvement of ventilation/perfusion imbalance by relieving airways obstruction, using antibiotics to control infection, physiotherapy to remove secretions, and bronchodilators; and (2), the partial relief of hypoxia by giving gas mixtures containing sufficient oxygen (24 to 28%) to improve arterial oxygen saturation significantly without at the same time depressing the hypoxic respiratory drive.

3. *Bronchiectasis and Other Residual Inflammatory Conditions.* Destructive changes in the bronchiolar walls and lung parenchyma occur as a complication of pulmonary infection, particularly

tuberculosis and pneumonia caused by *Klebsiella pneumoniae, Streptococcus pyogenes* and the staphyloccus. Similar changes may result from lung abscess or from bronchial obstruction; for example, in cystic fibrosis and postoperative pulmonary collapse. These sequelae lead to uneven distribution of ventilation and perfusion with physiological consequences similar to those of chronic bronchitis and emphysema. It is important that the incidence of residual pulmonary disability should be minimised by prompt, effective treatment of such infections, particularly when they occur as a consequence of surgery.

RESTRICTIVE LUNG DISEASE

In this pattern of pulmonary disease the cause of non-uniformity of ventilation/perfusion ratios lies in variation in the degree of distensibility (and therefore of ventilation) of alveolar units in different parts of the lung. The pathological basis for this variation may be obvious, for example severe thoracic cage deformity causing gross mechanical unevenness of ventilation between different areas, or it may be apparent only microscopically, as when diffuse interstitial pulmonary fibrosis causes differences in distensibility of individual lung units; the overall effect is to produce impairment of gas exchange characterised mainly by hypoxia since excretion of carbon dioxide is maintained by an increased share of ventilation in the more distensible parts of the lung.

1. *Diffuse Pulmonary Fibrosis.* This disorder occurs in a number of diseases of varied aetiology, including sarcoidosis, occupational diseases due to the inhalation of organic and inorganic dusts and fumes, certain collagen diseases and cryptogenic fibrosing alveolitis. It is characterised by progressive exertional dyspnoea often accompanied by cyanosis, and the chest radiograph commonly shows diffuse mottled shadowing of the lung fields, especially in the lower zones. Pulmonary hypertension and cor pulmonale occur as late complications. The characteristic pathological change is widespread thickening of the alveolar septa by fibrous tissue and cellular infiltration, the airways being unaffected.

The functional effect of these changes is reduction in the lung volumes without alteration in airway resistance. Marked diminution of lung compliance occurs and is probably responsible for the sensation of dyspnoea and for the adoption of a rapid, shallow pattern of breathing. The transfer factor for carbon monoxide is reduced. Unevenness of the interstitial fibrosis throughout the lung leads to variation in compliance of different alveolar units so that their ventilation also varies. In addition, the pathological changes in the alveolar walls lead to non-uniform obliteration of the pulmonary capillary bed so that uneven distribution of both ventilation and

perfusion contributes to impairment of gas exchange. Excretion of carbon dioxide is maintained by the well-ventilated units, but arterial oxygen desaturation develops, particularly on exercise. Alveolar hypoxia and capillary obliteration both ultimately contribute to an increase in pulmonary vascular resistance which leads to pulmonary hypertension and cor pulmonale.

It seems unlikely that diffusion of oxygen into the pulmonary capillary blood is limited by thickening of the alveolar-capillary membrane—'alveolar-capillary block'—since the rate of oxygen diffusion through tissues is so very rapid. Nevertheless, there is some experimental evidence which shows that arterial hypoxaemia in some patients with diffuse pulmonary fibrosis can be attributed to uneven distribution of diffusion in relation to perfusion.

Oxygen is valuable in the therapy of such patients, e.g. in the treatment of intercurrent infections. In the absence of coincidental chronic bronchitis it is appropriate to use a relatively high concentration of oxygen in the inspired gas since there is no risk of carbon dioxide retention.

2. *Thoracic Cage Deformity.* When the thoracic cage is severely deformed by kyphoscoliosis the rigidity of the chest wall leads to an increase in the work of breathing and, therefore, to dyspnoea. Chronic bronchitis and recurrent pulmonary infections are common complications, and cor pulmonale occurs late in the disease. The functional effect of the rigid chest wall is to diminish lung volumes although airway resistance remains normal in the absence of complicating bronchitis. Uneven distribution of ventilation and perfusion is mainly due to variations in ventilation that result from compression of parts of the lungs within the distorted thoracic cage. Alveolar hypoventilation plays a part in the impairment of gas exchange, which is aggravated by airways obstruction due to co-existent chronic bronchitis. Hypoxaemia is the characteristic blood gas abnormality, but carbon dioxide retention is likely to develop in the event of complicating airways obstruction. Cor pulmonale is due to pulmonary vasoconstriction resulting from chronic hypoxia.

To prevent functional deterioration due to infection it is important to give prompt antibiotic therapy, accompanied by intensive physiotherapy. Oxygen should be given in low concentration when hypercapnia is suspected.

3. *Disease of the Pleura.* Pleural fibrosis and pleural effusion both limit function by restricting expansion of the underlying lung, the degree of functional impairment depending on the extent of the pleural fibrosis or the size of the effusion. Some reduction in vital capacity may occur but airway resistance is unaffected. Because of contraction or compression there may be regional variation in the distensibility of

the lung, leading to uneven distribution of inspired gas and consequent non-uniformity of ventilation/perfusion ratios. Some hypoxaemia may develop but hypercapnia is prevented by increased ventilation of the remaining alveoli unless, as may well be the case, the condition is complicated by coexistent obstructive disease of the airways.

PULMONARY VASCULAR OBSTRUCTION

Widespread obstruction of the pulmonary vascular bed occasionally results from repeated scattered emboli originating from venous thrombosis in the legs or pelvis. The clinical effect of these changes is to produce progressive dyspnoea on exertion and, ultimately, pulmonary hypertension and cor pulmonale due to increased pulmonary vascular resistance. Total ventilation tends to increase considerably, but pulmonary compliance usually remains normal. Perfusion, however, becomes uneven, causing imbalance of ventilation and perfusion which leads to hypoxaemia, carbon dioxide tension being maintained at normal level by hyperventilation. The transfer factor for carbon monoxide may be decreased if the alveolar-capillary interface is significantly diminished in area by obliteration of the pulmonary capillary bed. Pulmonary hypertension occurs only when about two-thirds of total pulmonary vascular bed is occluded.

In the natural course of this disease small pulmonary emboli are rapidly absorbed and the vascular lumen becomes re-canalised. Anticoagulant therapy is given to prevent further thrombus formation so that the pulmonary circulation may not be further jeopardised by repeated embolisation. During the acute stage of the condition oxygen may be given in high concentration since carbon dioxide retention does not occur.

VENOUS-TO-ARTERIAL SHUNT

Any venous blood that bypasses ventilated alveoli and mixes with 'arterialised' blood coming from the lungs is termed a shunt. The effect of this admixture on arterial blood is to lower its oxygen content and increase its carbon dioxide content, but a shunt must be at least 20 per cent of the cardiac output to cause a significant increase in arterial carbon dioxide tension since hyperventilation usually maintains it at normal level. The characteristic physiological abnormalities of a large shunt are therefore increased ventilation and hypoxaemia.

Large extrapulmonary shunts occur clinically in congenital disorders of the heart or great vessels, but a small admixture of venous blood occurs in normal individuals due to the drainage of part of the coronary circulation through the Thebesian veins into the chambers of the left side of the heart. A rare cause of intrapulmonary

shunt is pulmonary arteriovenous fistula, but in clinical practice venous-to-arterial shunting is seen much more commonly when perfusion is maintained in areas of lung that have been deprived of ventilation by disease. This occurs in pneumonic consolidation, lobar collapse due to bronchial obstruction, and in spontaneous pneumothorax.

Hypoxaemia due to shunt can be reduced by inhaling oxygen in high concentration, but it cannot be fully corrected. When pure oxygen is breathed the arterial oxygen tension does not reach the maximal value (more than 80 kPa (600 mm Hg) attained in normal subjects or in patients with other forms of pulmonary disease, and this test is used to distinguish venous-to-arterial shunt from other causes of hypoxaemia such as alveolar hypoventilation or uneven distribution of ventilation and perfusion.

Alveolar Hypoventilation

In its widest sense the term 'alveolar hypoventilation' implies that the volume of inspired gas reaching the alveoli, and hence taking part in pulmonary gas exchange, is inadequate to maintain normal levels of arterial blood oxygen and carbon dioxide tension. Although it contributes to the failure of gas exchange that occurs in severe chronic bronchitis and emphysema or restrictive lung disease, alveolar hypoventilation as a *clinical* concept usually refers to those patients who show evidence of impaired gas exchange without underlying disease of the lungs. Alveolar hypoventilation should therefore be suspected in a patient who shows signs of carbon dioxide retention and cyanosis, sometimes accompanied in the chronic case by secondary polycythaemia, without evidence of lung disease but often with external signs relating to ventilatory inadequacy such as muscular weakness or deep coma.

CAUSES

Alveolar hypoventilation may be due to a mechanical defect in the function of the thoracic cage, to an abnormality affecting the respiratory centre, or it may be 'primary', i.e. occurring in patients who can ventilate normally by conscious effort but who habitually hypoventilate.

Mechanical defects

1. Neurological disorders. These include poliomyelitis, spinal cord lesions at or above the level of the phrenic nerve outlet (C3,4,5), polyneuritis, botulism, and neuromuscular block produced by curare or by ganglion-blocking agents.

2. Muscular disorders, such as myasthenia gravis, dermato-myositis, and muscular dystrophy.

3. Crush injuries of the chest. Multiple fractures of the ribs or costochondral junctions produce a 'flail chest' in which the affected part of the thoracic cage moves paradoxically inwards on inspiration. thus reducing effective ventilation of the alveoli. An associated phenomenon is 'pendeluft' ('swinging air') due to paradoxical movement of the affected lung, causing dead space gas to shunt from the abnormal to the normal side on inspiration and back on expiration, so that the patient, in effect, inspires with each breath a portion of his expired gas, leading to further hypoxia and hypercapnia. In severe cases the mediastinum itself may swing to and fro with respiration and interfere with venous return to the heart.

Respiratory Centre Depression

1. Narcotic overdose. Alveolar hypoventilation leading to cyanosis and carbon dioxide retention is a common complication of poisoning with narcotics such as the barbiturates or morphine. It may also be an additional cause of respiratory failure in patients with chronic obstructive lung disease who are incautiously sedated.

2. Oxygen overdose. The injudicious administration of oxygen in high concentration to patients with hypercapnic respiratory failure aggravates hypoventilation by removing the hypoxic drive to the respiratory centre, and leads to further carbon dioxide retention.

'Primary' Alveolar Hypoventilation

Patients with this condition show evidence of hypoxaemia and hypercapnia although all objective tests of pulmonary function are normal. When encouraged to hyperventilate these individuals are able to restore the blood gas tensions to normal levels although they quickly relapse into their accustomed hypoventilatory state when the stimulus ceases. Somnolence is a common accompaniment of the condition.

1. Excessive obesity (Pickwickian syndrome). Some individuals who are excessively obese are especially liable to episodic somnolence and develop cyanosis with secondary polycythaemia, hypercapnia and often, pulmonary hypertension leading to cor pulmonale. A number of factors have been suggested to account for the impairment of gas exchange in these patients, including mechanical impairment of respiration or of the distribution of ventilation due to fatty infiltration of the respiratory muscles, decreased compliance of the thoracic cage, and excessive elevation of the diaphragm in the supine posture. Concomitant chronic bronchitis sometimes appears to be a

contributory factor. Massive weight reduction may be effective in restoring blood gas tensions to normal levels.

2. Hypoventilation in the non-obese. Very rarely, patients of normal stature have been described as having alveolar hypoventilation in the absence of lung disease. Most of these patients appear to have had widespread disease of the central nervous system and it seems possible that respiratory centre depression may have been the cause of the ventilatory abnormality.

RECOGNITION OF ALVEOLAR HYPOVENTILATION

Acute. In patients whose ventilation is jeopardised by neurological or muscular disease or by trauma to the thoracic cage, the signs of respiratory embarrassment should be looked for assiduously at regular intervals. An increase in respiratory and cardiac rate, anxiety and restlessness on the part of the patient, and a progressive increase in the measured arterial carbon dioxide tension should lead to the prompt introduction of mechanical ventilation.

Chronic. Primary alveolar hypoventilation should be suspected in a patient with polycythaemia who appears cyanosed, particularly when drowsy or sleeping, and who becomes pinker when he awakes or when he is encouraged to hyperventilate. Examination of the blood shows raised carbon dioxide tension and plasma bicarbonate, and use of the ear oximeter shows that hyperventilation on air produces prompt elevation in arterial saturation. A pulmonary cause for the blood gas abnormalities should be excluded by demonstrating a normal ventilatory capacity and normal distribution of inspired gas, and the size of the venous-to-arterial shunt should be measured to exclude this cause of arterial desaturation.

PRINCIPLES OF TREATMENT

If the underlying lesion is reversible, alveolar hypoventilation may be relieved by the appropriate corrective treatment; e.g. surgical fixation of the thoracic cage may be necessary in crush injuries of the chest, and intensive weight reduction is obligatory in patients with hypoventilation of obesity. Any contributory respiratory cause of ventilatory impairment such as pneumonia or bronchitis should be appropriately treated.

Patients with alveolar hypoventilation of limited duration, such as narcotic overdose, poliomyelitis, polyneuritis, flail chest, and spinal cord injuries, must be supported by mechanical ventilation until the acute phase of the underlying disorder has passed and sufficient ventilatory capacity has returned to allow normal blood gas levels to be maintained.

Respiratory Failure

In the foregoing sections it has been shown that disturbances of pulmonary function characterised by uneven distribution of ventilation and perfusion, alveolar hypoventilation, venous-to-arterial shunt, or a combination of two or more of these abnormalities can lead to changes in the levels of arterial blood oxygen and carbon dioxide tension. In the initial stages of the underlying disease these blood gas disturbances are corrected by an increase in ventilation and, possibly, by some redistribution of pulmonary ventilation and perfusion, but if the disease progresses or if it is complicated by superadded pulmonary infection these compensatory mechanisms become inadequate and hypoxaemia (Pa,O_2 less than $8\,kPa$ or $60\,mm\,Hg$), with or without accompanying hypercapnia (Pa,CO_2 more than $6\cdot6\,kPa$ or $50\,mm\,Hg$), occurs. A patient in this state is in respiratory failure.

Respiratory failure may be characterised by:

1. Hypoxaemia without hypercapnia. This occurs in diffuse interstitial pulmonary fibrosis and in extensive pulmonary consolidation or collapse, carbon dioxide excretion being maintained in these conditions by hyperventilation.

2. Hypoxaemia with hypercapnia. This is the condition most commonly understood by the term respiratory failure, and it occurs as a result of maldistribution of ventilation and perfusion or in alveolar hypoventilation, usually as a complication of severe airways obstruction.

The importance of distinguishing these two types of respiratory failure lies mainly in the use of oxygen as a therapeutic agent. In the absence of hypercapnia high concentrations of oxygen can be given in the inspired gas for a limited period with impunity, but in the presence of significant carbon dioxide retention oxygen inhalation reduces the hypoxic respiratory drive and therefore aggravates underventilation and carbon dioxide retention.

PRINCIPLES OF THERAPY IN RESPIRATORY FAILURE

To treat respiratory failure effectively it is necessary to recognise the underlying physiological disturbances. This is likely to become apparent from the clinical history and examination, by far the commonest cause being chronic bronchitis and emphysema exacerbated by an acute infection. Treatment should be guided by the following considerations:

Recognition of Precipitating Factors. Certain subsidiary factors may precipitate respiratory failure. They include:

1. Alveolar hypoventilation due to respiratory centre depression,

when injudicious oxygen therapy has been given or when the patient has been carelessly sedated.

2. Alveolar hypoventilation due to mechanical limitation of respiratory movement; for example, following thoracic or abdominal surgery, or in the presence of gross ascites.

3. Aggravation of ventilation/perfusion abnormalities by bronchopneumonia, spontaneous pneumothorax or a large pleural effusion.

Relief of Ventilatory Obstruction. This is usually due to a combination of bronchial mucosal thickening caused by inflammation, increased bronchial secretions, and bronchoconstriction. In bronchial asthma particularly, scattered areas of the lung may become completely unventilated due to plugging of the bronchi. The measures available to correct these obstructive changes are:

1. Physiotherapy, to promote expectoration and drainage of secretions.
2. Rehydration, to reduce sputum stickiness.
3. Bronchoscopy and bronchial lavage, to remove bronchial plugs.
4. Bronchodilator drugs.
5. Antibiotic therapy, to control secondary bronchial infection.

Relief of Hypoxia. This is achieved by giving inspiratory gas mixtures containing oxygen in increased concentration. The choice of oxygen mixture and the mode of administration is discussed below. It is important that a patient with hypercapnia should not be given oxygen in high concentration for fear of exacerbating his carbon dioxide retention, and oxygen masks that increase the patient's respiratory dead space should be avoided for the same reason.

Maintenance of Ventilation. When the patient's ability to ventilate his lungs effectively fails, due to muscular weakness, to exhaustion, or to the depressant central effects of carbon dioxide or narcotic drugs, it may be necessary to maintain ventilation artificially until there has been time for the other therapeutic measures to take effect. The clinical signs of impending respiratory and peripheral circulatory collapse are increasing respiratory rate, tachycardia, hypotension, anxiety and restlessness progressing to drowsiness and mental confusion, cyanosis, and evidence from the blood gas estimations of rising arterial carbon dioxide tension and falling oxygen tension. Ventilation by mechanical means should not be undertaken unless there is a reasonable expectation that the underlying cause of respiratory failure will subside, or be controlled by simpler therapeutic measures within a few days, or at most, two or three weeks.

Artificial ventilation may be maintained for up to 3 or 4 days through an endotracheal tube, but for longer periods it is necessary to

perform tracheotomy because subglottic oedema, granuloma of the cords or tracheal stenosis may result from prolonged endotracheal intubation. The advantages that may be derived from mechanical ventilation are:

1. Adequate, controlled ventilation.
2. Relief of hypoxia, without danger of aggravating hypercapnia.
3. Relief of the patient's work load of breathing.
4. Access to the airways, to enable removal of secretions and instillation of saline or other agents to liquefy the sputum.

It is important that the aspiration of secretions should be carried out using a sterile technique, that the inspired gas should be humidified, and that the patient's nutrition and fluid balance should be carefully maintained throughout the period of ventilatory dependence. The management of such patients requires special skills and a high level of training, and is usually carried out in an intensive care unit.

OXYGEN THERAPY

The administration of oxygen makes an important contribution to the therapy of patients with respiratory disease complicated by hypoxia; in particular, it is required to prevent myocardial hypoxia, which promotes the cardiac arrhythmias and myocardial failure liable to occur in severe pulmonary infections or respiratory failure.

The following principles should be observed in the administration of oxygen—

1. In hypoxaemia due to shunt (e.g. pneumonia uncomplicated by airways obstruction) or to restrictive lung disease, a high concentration of oxygen up to 60 per cent of the inspired gas may be given without fear of causing carbon dioxide retention.

2. In hypoxaemia associated with hypercapnia (e.g. in airways obstruction or alveolar hypoventilation) the concentration of oxygen in the inspired gas should not be more than 30 per cent, and serial estimates of arterial carbon dioxide tension should be carried out before and during oxygen therapy to ensure that ventilation is not sufficiently depressed to cause significant carbon dioxide retention.

3. The mode of administration of oxygen to patients with carbon dioxide retention should be chosen to avoid an increase in the respiratory dead space, since this leads to further hypercapnia.

4. Oxygen in high concentration (e.g. more than 60 per cent oxygen given to a patient maintained by artificial ventilation) should not be administered continuously for more than a few hours because of the danger of causing toxic damage to the alveolar epithelium.

Method of Administration. The need for a high concentration of

oxygen in the inspired gas arises only when there is no danger of causing respiratory depression due to carbon dioxide retention; for example, when hypoxaemia occurs in the acute phase of pneumonia or following major pulmonary collapse. Concentrations of 50 to 60 per cent oxygen in the inspired gas can be achieved by using a close-fitting oro-nasal mask (e.g. BOC Polymask) or by means of an oxygen tent. The oro-nasal mask has the disadvantage that it increases the respiratory dead space so that the patient tends to rebreathe part of the expired gas, and it also impedes the ingestion of fluids and may be intolerably uncomfortable to the ill, restless patient. The oxygen tent is unwieldy and makes nursing procedures difficult, being used in adult practice only for the treatment of those patients who cannot tolerate a mask or nasal catheter.

In hypercapnic respiratory failure oxygen can be safely administered only in low concentration. In the severely hypoxaemic patient, however, even small increments of oxygen in the inspired gas will raise the arterial blood oxygen content significantly, because of the steep slope of the oxyhaemoglobin dissociation curve at these oxygen tensions, and it is usual to administer oxygen in concentrations of 24 or 28 per cent, using a mask that incorporates the Venturi principle: a stream of oxygen entrains a large quantity of air to produce a gas mixture of fixed oxygen concentration which flows over the patient's face.

The use of a nasal catheter to administer oxygen in low concentration is much less reliable than the Venturi-type mask since the concentration of oxygen inspired by the patient is less predictable; the method has the advantage that it is better tolerated by the patient, but it can only be safely used during recovery when the inspired oxygen concentration is less critical. Once oxygen therapy is started it must be continuous, since hypoventilation aggravates hypoxaemia during the periods when no oxygen is given. Regular estimates of the arterial carbon dioxide tension must be made before and during the period of oxygen administration to ensure that it is not causing excessive carbon dioxide retention.

Oxygen Toxicity. Continuous ventilation with a gas mixture containing more than 60 per cent oxygen has two important detrimental effects upon the lung:

1. When the nitrogen normally present in the lung is largely replaced by oxygen, collapse of poorly-ventilated alveoli or lung segments occurs because the rate of uptake of oxygen by the blood perfusing such areas exceeds the rate at which it can be replaced by oxygen diffusing from the airways.

2. Oxygen in high concentration has a direct toxic effect on the

cells of the alveoli, causing destruction of the cell membrane leading to capillary congestion, alveolar haemorrhage, oedema, fibroblastic proliferation, and the shedding of lining cells into the alveolar lumen. These changes cause gross disturbance of alveolar gas exchange and decreased pulmonary compliance.

Such complications can be avoided by administering oxygen in concentrations high enough only to provide adequate oxygenation of the arterial blood, and to discontinue oxygen administration in high concentration as soon as possible. Concentrations of oxygen in excess of 60 per cent should not be given for longer than a few hours.

Pulmonary Hypertension and Cor Pulmonale

PATHOGENESIS

Either obstruction to blood flow through the pulmonary vascular bed or a large, sustained increase in the volume of pulmonary blood flow may lead to pulmonary hypertension. Any obstruction 'downstream' from the right ventricle initially prevents complete emptying during systole and causes a slight increase in its diastolic size; the ventricular muscle responds by increasing the force of its contraction (Starling's Law of the heart), thus raising pulmonary arterial pressure progressively until it reaches a point at which normal flow can be maintained in spite of the obstruction. A sustained increase in the work of the right ventricle leads to hypertrophy of the ventricular muscle, and, ultimately, to ventricular dilation and congestive heart failure if the obstruction is so severe as to prevent the right ventricle maintaining its output.

Many factors, singly or in combination, may lead to a rise in pulmonary artery pressure. They include:

1. Pulmonary arterial vasoconstriction and medial muscular hypertrophy due to alveolar hypoxia; e.g. chronic bronchitis and emphysema, the hypoventilation syndrome of obesity, residence at high altitude.

2. Pulmonary vascular occlusion or destruction; e.g. thromboembolism, diffuse pulmonary fibrosis, chronic inflammatory disease such as bronchiectasis.

3. Loss of lung tissue; e.g. pneumonectomy associated with chronic airways obstruction in the remaining lung.

4. Increased blood viscosity; e.g. in polycythaemia secondary to chronic hypoxic lung disease.

5. Pulmonary venous hypertension; e.g. in mitral stenosis or left ventricular failure.

6. A large, sustained increase in pulmonary blood flow; e.g. in

congenital left-to-right intracardiac shunts (VSD, ASD), patent ductus arteriosus and aorto-pulmonary septal defect.

Pulmonary hypertension should be suspected as a complication of any of the above conditions when the signs of right ventricular hypertrophy and congestive heart failure are found in association with the characteristic signs of raised pulmonary arterial pressure described on page 38. The diagnosis is confirmed by the radiographic and electrocardiographic changes described on pages 94−96, and by direct measurement of pulmonary arterial pressure by right heart catheterisation.

RELIEF OF PULMONARY HYPERTENSION

The correction of the abnormality depends upon the underlying cause and on its duration. In some forms of pulmonary hypertension, notably mitral stenosis and those congenital cardiovascular lesions associated with greatly increased pulmonary blood flow, the sustained increase in pulmonary arterial pressure causes morphological changes to the walls of the pulmonary vessels which are initially reversible if the underlying disease is corrected surgically, but ultimately are destructive and irreversible leading to permanent pulmonary hypertension. In hypoxic pulmonary disease, on the other hand, the arterial constriction and medial muscular hypertrophy of the arterial walls which leads to pulmonary hypertension can be reversed if the hypoxia can be relieved.

Relief of hypoxia in hypoxic lung disease (e.g. in chronic bronchitis and emphysema) is therefore important not only to improve tissue oxygenation but also to reverse the pulmonary vascular narrowing that contributes so largely to the development of cor pulmonale. It seems that hypoxia plays a dual role in the pathogenesis of pulmonary hypertension; in the short term by causing pulmonary vasoconstriction and in the long term by reducing the capacity of the pulmonary vascular bed due to muscular hypertrophy and narrowing or closure of the small pulmonary arteries and arterioles. The logical treatment of an acute rise in pulmonary arterial pressure due to an acute exacerbation of chronic bronchitis would therefore be the inhalation of a gas mixture containing oxygen in increased concentration. In the long term, however, treatment must be directed towards the relief of the underlying hypoxic state; for example, the improvement of alveolar ventilation with physiotherapy and antibiotics, or effective weight reduction in a patient suffering from hypoventilation associated with obesity.

It remains a possibility that other factors may contribute to pulmonary hypertension in chronic lung disease. An increase in blood carbon dioxide tension may, by increasing blood acidity, potentiate

the pulmonary hypertension produced by hypoxia. There are theoretical reasons for supposing that the combination of increased blood acidity, hypoxia, and increased haematocrit may cause a considerable increase in blood viscosity which would be expected to aggravate pulmonary hypertension, although large changes in haematocrit alone appear to have only a small effect on pulmonary arterial pressure. Another factor that may play a part in the pulmonary hypertension of chronic airways obstruction is an increase in total blood volume, and it has also been suggested that a rise in alveolar pressure caused by broncho-constriction may increase alveolar capillary pressure and so influence pulmonary arterial pressure.

Pleural Effusion

A pleural effusion signifies a disorder of function caused by a number of diseases. Although a large effusion may accumulate quite silently, the *symptoms* that may indicate its presence are a history of pleuritic pain or dyspnoea; the *signs* may be summarised as a reduction in chest expansion on the side of the effusion, shift of the mediastinum to the opposite side, dull percussion note over the effusion, reduced breath sounds and voice sounds, and sometimes bronchial breathing with increased voice sounds in a limited area at the upper border of the effusion. Very large effusions sometimes cause bulging of the intercostal spaces in thin persons and, if left-sided, may obscure the apex beat and heart sounds.

FUNCTIONAL DISORDER

As described on page 93, the small volume of fluid normally present in the pleural space is maintained by an absorptive force that causes fluid to flow from the interstitial tissue on the parietal side of the pleura to the interstitial tissue of the lung on the visceral side. Pleural effusion can therefore be explained in terms of an imbalance in the forces that maintain the normal flow of water, electrolytes and protein into and out of the pleural space:

1. *Increased capillary pressure:*
   Heart failure, hypervolaemia.
2. *Increased capillary permeability:*
   Pleural inflammation (pneumonia, pulmonary tuberculosis, collagen diseases);
   Pleural malignancy (lung carcinoma, mesothelioma, reticulosis);
   Pulmonary infarction;
   Subdiaphragmatic disease (subphrenic abscess, amoebic abscess of liver, acute pancreatitis).
3. *Impaired lymphatic clearance of protein:*

Lymphangitis carcinomatosa;
Developmental lymphatic abnormalities.

In addition, an excess of pleural fluid may be due to flooding of the pleural space by bleeding due to trauma or to an aneurysm of the aorta, or by leakage of chyle due to traumatic damage or malignant disease involving the thoracic duct.

DIAGNOSIS AND MANAGEMENT

Investigation should be directed towards determining the extent and nature of the effusion with a view to diagnosing the underlying disease. Chest radiography makes it possible to detect effusions of about 100 ml, which appear as a shadow filling the costophrenic angle. Larger effusions appear in the postero-anterior radiograph as triangular shadows lying against the lateral chest wall, or against the posterior chest wall in a lateral view. Sometimes an effusion, particularly if exudative, is loculated to a limited part of the pleural space and may be confined to an interlobar fissure where it appears on the lateral radiograph as an elliptical thickening of the normal hairline shadow of the fissure. The lung fields should be carefully inspected both before and after aspiration for signs of an intrapulmonary lesion which may be responsible for the effusion.

The aspirate may have the milky opalescence of chyle or it may be pure blood, but it is usually a yellow serous fluid that may be bloodstained. Bloodstaining is suggestive but not diagnostic of underlying malignancy. If it clots easily it is likely to have a high protein content. This should be estimated to distinguish a transudate from an exudate, the latter containing more than 3 g protein per 100 ml. Pus may be apparent macroscopically, but a specimen should always be examined microscopically for its red blood cell and leucocyte content, and for the presence of bacteria, including tubercle bacilli. Cultures should be set up, and a specimen examined for malignant cells.

Pleural Biopsy. This procedure may give histological information about the cause of undiagnosed pleural effusion. It is a safe and easy technique which enables a small piece of parietal pleura to be sampled using a special needle. It is of greatest value in diagnosing malignant disease of the pleura and tuberculous pleurisy.

Treatment is mainly a question of diagnosing and treating the underlying disease, but it may occasionally be necessary to relieve disabling dyspnoea by aspiration. Removal of a large effusion too quickly occasionally leads to pulmonary oedema or shock, and aspiration should be discontinued if the patient begins to cough or complains of tightness in the chest. Persistent effusions, i.e. those that respond poorly to treatment, are usually due either to chronic heart disease or to malignant invasion of the pleural cavity.

PART III

Varieties of Lung Disease

10

Bronchial Asthma

Incidence

Bronchial asthma is a common disease characterised by spasmodic attacks of wheezing and shortness of breath. About one-third of cases present in the first decade and the majority before the age of forty, but there is a recognisable group of cases in whom asthma-like symptoms first present in middle age; this group is often difficult to distinguish clinically from chronic bronchitis and emphysema. The overall incidence is equally divided between the sexes although childhood asthma is somewhat commoner among boys than girls, whereas asthma of later onset is more frequent in women. It occurs in all races, in all parts of the world.

Pathogenesis

Patients with asthma fall into two broad groups; those who show evidence of hypersensitivity to external antigens ('extrinsic' asthma) and those who do not ('intrinsic' asthma).

ATOPY

The term 'atopic' is commonly applied to people who give a history of allergic illnesses that often develop in the first few years of life, and are manifested in various ways such as infantile eczema, skin sensitivities, food allergies, hay fever, allergic rhinitis, asthma or sensitivity reactions to drugs. There is commonly a similar history in other members of the patient's family. The patient may himself be aware of factors that precipitate symptoms such as seasonal incidence relating to the increased presence of pollen or fungal spores in the atmosphere, physical proximity to a specific animal or plant, or engagement in an occupation that results in the inhalation of organic dust.

Atopic subjects customarily show a positive Type I, immediate skin reaction to a wide variety of allergens, elicited by pricking the skin through a drop of antigenic extract. Such reactions indicate the presence of IgE antibody, which is usually present in higher concentration in the serum of atopic subjects, especially those with multiple sensitivities, than in non-atopic individuals.

Although the terms atopic and non-atopic have been widely used synonymously with extrinsic and intrinsic asthma respectively, it is now recognised that extrinsic asthma may occur in non-atopic subjects as a result of Type III, immune-complex reactions in the bronchi. It therefore seems best at present to use the term atopic to describe individuals with the typical constitutional characteristics, and to group asthmatics into those in whom causal allergens are demonstrable (extrinsic) and those in whom they are not (intrinsic).

EXTRINSIC ASTHMA

Most, but not all, patients with extrinsic asthma are atopic, showing hypersensitivity to one or more of a wide range of antigenic materials. Among the substances that commonly provoke an asthmatic attack are feathers, animal fur, house dust and the house-dust mite, *Dermatophagoides pteronyssinus,* pollen grains and fungal spores, various foods such as milk, eggs, fish and chocolate, alcoholic drinks (due to the congeners of the alcohol rather than the alcohol itself) and many drugs of which aspirin is an important example.

Hypersensitivity Mechanisms. Two types of allergic reaction are of special importance in respiratory disease; these are the Type I reaction, relating particularly to asthma, allergic rhinitis and hay fever, and the Type III reaction associated mainly with extrinsic allergic alveolitis (*see* page 227) but also occasionally with asthma. The *Type I, immediate reaction* is due to interaction between the antigen and tissue cells previously sensitised passively by antibody, leading to the release of pharmacologically active substances. The antibody, originally known as reagin, is the immunoglobulin IgE, which is present in normal serum. In atopic subjects, production is stimulated by exposure to common allergens, resulting in allergen-specific IgE and, often, abnormally high levels of the immunoglobulin. It becomes fixed to mast cells, leading to the release by enzymatic reactions of bronchoconstrictor substances such as histamine, slow-reacting substance—Anaphylaxis (SRS–A), bradykinin and perhaps serotonin, whenever a subsequent exposure to the allergen occurs.

The *Type III, immune-complex reaction* may produce asthma in atopic or non-atopic subjects. The initial exposure to antigen leads to the production of circulating precipitin antibody which reacts with the antigen on subsequent exposure to produce fever, polymorphonuclear leucocytosis and rather prolonged and refractory asthma after four or five hours. The reaction appears to take place in the vascular walls and surrounding tissue, causing damage to cells and blood vessels. There is evidence to suggest that the Type III asthmatic reaction develops only after an introductory Type I, immediate reaction has occurred, mediated by IgE in the case of atopic individuals and

possibly by a special IgG antibody in non-atopic subjects. This 'dual response' can be demonstrated by exposing susceptible individuals to the relevant antigen, either by prick tests or inhalation tests. Type III asthmatic reactions, with or without a dual response, occur in allergic bronchopulmonary aspergillosis, allergy to avian proteins and house-dust mite sensitivity.

Eosinophilia in the blood and sputum is a characteristic accompaniment of extrinsic asthma, but may also occur in asthmatics who show no other evidence of an allergic aetiology.

INTRINSIC ASTHMA

Spasmodic asthma occurring in the absence of demonstrable skin sensitivity and usually without an allergic history is said to be intrinsic. It is commonly of later onset than extrinsic asthma and the attacks tend to become persistent and continuous, responding poorly to bronchodilator drugs. The level of IgE is not increased in the serum but it is possible that a local increase in the concentration of IgE may play a part in intrinsic asthma. The fact that eosinophilia may occur in both sputum and blood, and that such patients often show a good response to corticosteroid drugs, suggests that some unrecognised allergic mechanism may be present.

PRECIPITATING FACTORS

Apart from the allergic phenomena mentioned above, a number of other stimuli may provoke asthma in susceptible individuals. They include:

1. Upper respiratory infections.
2. Exercise.
3. Air pollutants, including 'smog' and tobacco smoke.
4. Emotional factors. Asthmatic attacks are sometimes precipitated by a psychological upset, and occasionally the onset of asthma appears to date from a particular emotional incident.
5. Drugs. Certain pharmacological agents may provoke broncho-constriction in asthmatic individuals. They include histamine, and β-adrenergic blocking agents such as propranolol and practolol.

Pathology

During an attack of asthma the airways become narrowed by broncho-constriction, oedema of the bronchial mucous membrane, and secretion of viscid mucus which contains numerous eosinophils and spiral casts of the smaller bronchi. The lungs of patients dying in status asthmaticus are grossly hyperinflated, the small and medium-sized airways being blocked with mucus plugs. Small areas of pneumonic consolidation may be present in the periphery of the lung.

The mucous membrane of the bronchi shows a great increase in the number of mucus-secreting cells which largely replace the normal ciliated epithelium, and areas of squamous metaplasia occur. Hypertrophy of the bronchial musculature is another characteristic feature.

Clinical Presentation

An attack of bronchial asthma may be brought on by any of the precipitating factors mentioned above, or it may occur without any obvious cause. An infection of the upper respiratory tract is one of the commonest introductory features. The onset may be gradual or extremely sudden, occasionally frighteningly abrupt. One of the dominant features of asthma, at least in the early stages of the disease, is its spasmodic nature, the patient being relatively normal between attacks and often showing a normal tolerance to exercise. In severe and persistent disease, however, the airways and lung parenchyma become gradually affected by mucus obstruction and recurrent infection which lead to impaired gas exchange because of uneven distribution of ventilation and perfusion. Even at their best these patients suffer from exertional dyspnoea, with intermittent attacks of reversible bronchospasm superimposed on the underlying respiratory disorder. This pattern of disease is very characteristic of the middle-aged asthmatic and is often indistinguishable from chronic bronchitis and emphysema.

SYMPTOMS OF EXACERBATION

The patient complains of *severe dyspnoea* and in extrinsic asthma can sometimes attribute the onset to a specific cause. He is aware of *wheezing* and is troubled by coughing, often paroxysmal, which aggravates the breathlessness and is usually effective only in producing a little viscid, whitish sputum. Many patients notice that the sputum becomes 'looser' and more easily expectorated as the attack begins to subside. Chest pain is not a feature of asthma itself, but may be an indication of spontaneous pneumothorax which occurs as a complication of the disease. *Exercise tolerance* is grossly impaired during an attack, and may be diminished to a greater or lesser extent when the disease is quiescent. The duration of attacks is extremely variable, ranging from less than an hour to several days or longer, severe and prolonged episodes being known as *status asthmaticus*.

CLINICAL SIGNS

The most obvious sign is *respiratory distress*. The patient sits upright or leans forward, using the accessory muscles particularly to assist

expiration, which is unduly prolonged and laboured. The *respiratory rate* is somewhat increased but is limited by the need for a prolonged expiratory phase of respiration; only when respiratory failure is imminent does the rate of breathing rise excessively. Speech is often difficult, and the smallest extra exertion such as removal of a garment may be exhausting. *Wheezing* may be heard at the bedside, most marked in expiration, and the chest appears hyperinflated. The percussion note is hyperresonant and the auscultatory signs consist of widespread rhonchi of varying pitch, loudest during expiration. In the severest cases air entry is so reduced that wheezing may diminish or even disappear. In unrelieved *status asthmaticus* the patient ultimately becomes exhausted and dehydrated, central cyanosis occurs, and signs of peripheral circulatory failure may be apparent.

Course and Complications

Onset in Childhood. Wheeziness is a common symptom in infancy, usually related to minor respiratory tract infections or sometimes to more severe infections such as acute bronchiolitis due to the respiratory syncytial virus. The distinction between this type of wheeziness and true asthma is difficult in the small child although the recurrent nature of attacks, which are often unrelated to infection, is an indication that they are in fact asthmatic. Non-asthmatic wheeziness usually settles as the child grows but the outlook in true asthma is less good, especially in those with other allergic manifestations or with a familial predisposition to allergic disease. Only about one quarter of those children with severe asthma, and half of those with mild asthma, are symptom-free by the age of fifteen. Severe asthma appears to carry a mortality of about 1 per cent in childhood, but the morbid effects of the disease may be considerable, resulting in progressive pulmonary damage which may lead to respiratory failure and cor pulmonale in later life, and retardation of growth and considerable disruption of the child's upbringing and education.

Onset in Adult Life. Asthma coming on in adult life or persisting from childhood varies greatly in severity and in frequency of attacks, but is often a troublesome and disabling disease. Such patients are prone to *recurrent bronchitis* and *pneumonia* which inevitably cause impairment of pulmonary function over a period of years, frequently leading to disablement in later life. *Respiratory failure,* due to uneven distribution of pulmonary ventilation and perfusion, and *cor pulmonale* are sometimes seen as the sequels to severe, chronic asthma and appear to be particularly common when the disease first makes its appearance in middle age. There is an increased risk of spontaneous pneumothorax which may precipitate respiratory failure

in patients whose respiratory reserve is already affected by chronic asthma.

Status asthmaticus is a serious hazard, consisting of a persistent, severe, refractory asthma that is resistant to treatment with agents such as adrenaline or aminophylline. If it persists it leads to respiratory and circulatory failure, and it has a high mortality. *Sudden death* due to asthma increased significantly in the United Kingdom in the 1960s and was attributed to the misuse of isoprenaline-containing aerosol inhalants (page 123).

Investigation

DIAGNOSTIC TESTS

The diagnosis of bronchial asthma is based essentially on the clinical findings. Confirmatory investigations include the *chest radiograph* which may show evidence of hyperinflation during an attack (elevation of the rib cage, depression of the diaphragm and increased translucency of the lung fields) although it may appear entirely normal. Radiographic signs of segmental or lobar collapse, or patchy shadows due to pneumonic consolidation may be evident, resulting from bronchial obstruction and infection. Rarely, mucoid impaction of a bronchus occurs in chronic asthmatics, causing collapse and peripheral bronchiectatic changes which are usually in the upper or middle lobes. The radiographic appearance of a dense opacity is readily confused with bronchial carcinoma or tuberculosis. The *sputum* is normally mucoid or mucopurulent and contains bronchial casts (Curschmann's spirals) and large numbers of eosinophils; in asthma resulting from infection it may contain bacteria and pus cells, and it should be cultured to discover the sensitivities of the infecting organisms. *Eosinophilia* is also apparent in the peripheral blood films.

Asthma is a common symptom in some of the conditions that are associated with pulmonary infiltrations, fever and eosinophilia. In the British Isles *allergic bronchopulmonary aspergillosis* is the cause in 80 per cent of such cases, the diagnosis being confirmed by culturing *A. fumigatus* from the sputum and by demonstrating precipitins in the serum. A similar syndrome may occur as a result of hypersensitivity to intestinal *parasitic infestations* such as filariasis, schistosomiasis and ascariasis; the diagnosis may be made by finding ova or parasites in the stools and by complement fixation tests. Asthma or sinusitis may be presenting features of *polyarteritis nodosa* which is also sometimes associated with pulmonary infiltrations and eosinophilia and should be suspected if the erythrocyte sedimentation rate is persistently raised with hypergammaglobulinaemia (page 256).

Asthma due to the carcinoid syndrome, resulting from carcinoid tumour of the ileum with hepatic metastases or, occasionally, from bronchial carcinoid (page 245), may be suspected on clinical grounds and the diagnosis confirmed by finding 5-hydroxyindoleacetic acid in the urine.

TESTS FOR HYPERSENSITIVITY

Evidence of an allergic basis for asthma is usually best obtained by taking a careful history, but this can sometimes be supported by *skin testing,* using a series of specially prepared solutions containing antigenic material from a wide variety of sources, which are pricked or scratched into the skin of the forearm. A Type I response (wheal and erythematous flare) to the appropriate antigen occurs in hypersensitive individuals within a few minutes. Intradermal injection of the antigen is liable to cause more severe reactions. *Inhalation tests* may be carried out by giving the antigen in aerosol form but can provoke a dangerous asthmatic attack.

FUNCTIONAL INVESTIGATIONS

Since airways obstruction is the dominant feature of bronchial asthma the most characteristic disorder found on functional testing is increased *airway resistance.* The FEV1, FEV1/FVC ratio and PEFR are the most useful simple tests, and airway resistance may be measured directly if a body plethysmograph is available. During an asthmatic attack values for all these parameters are reduced, and serial measurements of FEV1 or PEFR are useful in determining the natural reversibility of the bronchospasm when the attack subsides. The effect of *bronchodilator drugs* should be assessed by making measurements before and after the inhalation of a bronchodilator aerosol such as 2 per cent isoprenaline, as a guide to the likely value of subsequent therapy. The *lung volumes* may be abnormal because of the pulmonary hyperinflation and air trapping that occur during an attack of asthma; the total lung capacity (TLC) is normal or increased, often associated with an increase in residual volume (RV) and functional residual capacity (FRC) but a diminution in vital capacity. These changes revert to normal after the attack although some increase in RV may persist.

In severe asthma *pulmonary gas exchange* is affected by the uneven distribution of ventilation resulting from generalised bronchospasm. Single or multiple breath tests of gas distribution are abnormal, and physiological dead space is increased. In the initial stages, increased ventilatory effort maintains a normal or increased total ventilation, the major physiological abnormality being gross unevenness of ventilation/perfusion distribution; this leads to a moderate fall in

arterial oxygen tension, but arterial carbon dioxide tension is initially maintained at a normal or low value due to the increased wash-qut of carbon dioxide from alveoli with high $\dot{V}A/\dot{Q}$ ratios. If bronchoconstriction increases or the patient becomes exhausted and dehydrated, the distribution of ventilation becomes more uneven and total alveolar ventilation falls, leading to cyanosis and carbon dioxide retention. The latter change is a very significant sign of deterioration in severe asthma, and even a small rise in carbon dioxide tension to 6·7–7·3 kPa (50 or 55 mm Hg) should be taken as a sign of impending respiratory and circulatory failure.

In the *long-term management* of bronchial asthma serial recordings of FEV1 or PEFR are a useful means of judging progress and assessing the effect of various therapeutic agents, especially in judging the genuineness of a response to corticosteroid therapy.

Treatment

PREVENTIVE MEASURES

Although an allergic basis for asthmatic attacks may be identified in a small proportion of cases, treatment by hyposensitisation with the appropriate antigen or with a mixture of antigens is disappointing. This form of therapy is most effective in seasonal asthma due to gross pollen sensitivity, the antigen being given as a preseasonal course of injections which vary in number according to the type of preparation used. Aqueous extract of pollen antigen is administered in twenty injections, but occasionally causes adverse reactions which include anaphylactic shock. Depot preparations are also available. Hyposensitisation with other antigens such as house dust, animal danders, moulds and insect antigen is even less effective, but is worth trying in the individual who shows an obvious sensitivity to an antigen which cannot be avoided. The use of bacterial vaccines for patients whose asthma appears to result from bacterial infection is of no value.

Having identified a likely source of hypersensitivity, a more effective step may be to remove as far as possible all sources of the antigen from the patient's environment. This may include the removal of household pets, the substitution of foam rubber for feathers in pillows and the replacement of regular bed clothes with those woven entirely from man-made fibres. Patients whose asthma is commonly preceded by upper respiratory tract infection may obtain some protection from polyvalent influenza vaccine given regularly in the autumn.

The use of disodium cromoglycate (Intal) and corticosteroids in preventing or reducing the frequency of severe asthma is discussed in a subsequent section.

BRONCHODILATOR DRUGS

Bronchodilation can be produced both by stimulating beta adrenergic receptors and by blocking cholinergic receptors or alpha adrenergic receptors. Beta receptors are of two forms, beta 1 and beta 2; beta 1 stimulation enhances myocardial contraction and increases heart rate, whereas beta 2 stimulation causes bronchodilation, vasodilation and tremor of skeletal muscle.

In asthma and bronchitis the drugs most commonly used are the adrenergic (sympathomimetic) drugs and the theophylline group of drugs. Both groups have their effect by increasing the level of intracellular 3′,5′-AMP, leading to bronchodilation, vasodilation and inhibition of histamine release. The main unwanted effects of the sympathomimetic drugs arise from coincidental alpha stimulation (causing constriction of blood vessels and of the sphincters of the bladder and gastro-intestinal tract), and the effects of beta 1 stimulation on the heart.

Adrenaline has alpha and beta effects which result in effective bronchodilation, but also troublesome side-effects such as tachycardia, hypertension, anxiety and cardiac arrhythmias which are particularly dangerous in hypoxia. It is given subcutaneously in a dose of 0·1 ml per minute of a 1 : 1,000 solution up to a total of 1 ml.

Ephedrine has alpha and beta actions which may cause sleeplessness due to central nervous stimulation, and urinary retention in elderly men. It is a mild oral bronchodilator drug, given in a dose of 30 to 60 mg three times daily.

Isoprenaline has both beta 1 and beta 2 sympathomimetic effects but no alpha effects. It is usually given as a pressurised aerosol, producing prompt but rather short-lived bronchodilation. Excessive use of isoprenaline-containing aerosols has led to sudden death in some patients due to cardiac depression associated with severe hypoxia, and it is therefore important to give strict instructions limiting the dose to 2 'puffs' only, repeated after 4 hours if necessary. Loss of efficacy of the aerosol in the event of an unusually severe attack of bronchospasm should be an indication to seek medical advice, *not* to take further isoprenaline aerosol indiscriminately.

Selective beta 2 adrenergic drugs include *orciprenaline, salbutamol, isoetharine* and *terbutaline*. These are similar in action to isoprenaline but their effect is slower in onset and of longer duration. Both tablet and aerosol preparations are available, but cautionary advice should be given to prevent overdose with the aerosol because of the risk of cardiac depression similar to that from isoprenaline. Muscle tremor and tremulousness are common side-effects from oral therapy, especially in elderly patients, but are quickly relieved by reducing the dose.

Aminophylline by intravenous injection is often very effective in the acute asthmatic attack, given at a rate not exceeding 2 ml per minute up to a total of 500 mg in 20 ml. It may also be given as a suppository, sometimes providing useful relief from nocturnal wheezing.

Choline theophyllinate is a useful oral bronchodilator although absorption is rather variable; the usual dose is 200 mg three times daily.

THE ACUTE ATTACK

In the early stages of an asthmatic attack, when simple oral or aerosol preparations have failed to alleviate bronchospasm, either aminophylline or adrenaline may be given, although the latter is now seldom used except in children because of its troublesome side-effects. Aminophylline is effective as a respiratory and cardiac stimulant as well as producing bronchodilation. Its effectiveness may be short-lived, in which case repeated intravenous injections every four hours or a continuous slow intravenous infusion may maintain adequate bronchodilation.

Persistence or worsening of severe bronchospasm for several hours or days in spite of the above measures constitutes *status asthmaticus.* The excessive work of breathing increases oxygen consumption and carbon dioxide output, airway narrowing causes ventilation/perfusion inequality which is aggravated by retention of dry, inspissated bronchial secretions, and dehydration and physical exhaustion contribute to the patient's inability to cough or maintain the excessive ventilatory effort. In these circumstances the arterial oxygen tension begins to fall, carbon dioxide is retained, and signs of peripheral circulatory failure develop.

Rehydration should be instituted by giving intravenous fluids. Oxygen may safely be given in low concentration (24 to 30%) by means of a Venturi-type face mask, and in high concentration provided there is no risk of carbon dioxide retention. Hydrocortisone acetate should be given in massive dosage, e.g. 1 g in 24 hours by intravenous infusion, with 100 mg prednisolone by mouth in divided doses over the same period. Adrenocorticotrophic hormone (ACTH) is effective but less reliable since the adrenal cortical response is variable and unpredictable; it should not be used for patients who are already taking long-term corticosteroid therapy. Provided a response is obtained the dose of steroids may be reduced gradually in the convalescent period following the attack.

Assisted Ventilation. Corticosteroids are not effective for 6 to 8 hours, and during that period the patient may deteriorate into respiratory or peripheral circulatory failure. These complications are

indicated by increasing exhaustion and unresponsiveness, rising respiratory and heart rate, fall in blood pressure, cyanosis, and respiratory acidosis. In these circumstances the patient must be relieved of the work of breathing by mechanical means. Endotracheal intubation is performed under general anaesthesia, and mechanical ventilation established. Bronchial lavage with 1 per cent sodium bicarbonate solution may be carried out via the endotracheal tube, allowing the removal of tenacious bronchial plugs and consequent improvement in ventilation. Once ventilation is controlled by mechanical means oxygen-enriched gas mixtures can be given to combat hypoxia without fear of carbon dioxide retention, respiration being maintained artificially until bronchospasm subsides. It is important that the decision to institute mechanical ventilation is taken early, before the patient's general condition has become desperate. If started in good time this form of treatment is often quickly effective and intubation need only be maintained for 24 to 48 hours. It requires great skill and should preferably be undertaken by an expert team in a special unit where all the necessary facilities are available.

LONG TERM MANAGEMENT

Most patients with asthma of mild to moderate severity can be successfully treated with bronchodilators of the sympathomimetic or theophylline groups which are used intermittently to suppress attacks as they occur. For this purpose ephedrine or one of the selective beta 2 adrenergic drugs, given either by mouth or by pressurised aerosol, have proved most useful. Recognition and *avoidance of precipitating factors* may be an important aspect of management, especially in extrinsic asthma when the antigenic stimulus is recognisable. In asthma precipitated by respiratory tract infection prompt treatment with a wide-spectrum antibiotic may shorten the illness. Physiotherapy has a place, especially in childhood, in teaching the asthmatic to control his breathing pattern in order to improve ventilation. The value of *psychotherapy* in the control of asthma remains equivocal although some patients appear to obtain relief by hypnosis.

In more severe asthma in which the bronchospasm is persistent and incapacitating, some reduction in the frequency and severity of the attacks may be obtained by regular inhalation of *disodium cromoglycate*. This material is said to suppress the release of the humoral factors that mediate the allergic response and therefore to have a preventive role in asthma. It appears to be most effective in extrinsic asthma, nevertheless some patients with the intrinsic type also seem to improve. As disodium cromoglycate is poorly absorbed from the gastro-intestinal tract it has to be given as an inhaled

powder, the standard dose being four capsules a day (20 mg disodium cromoglycate in each capsule). The positive effect of this drug is variable and should be reviewed critically; a reduction in the frequency of asthmatic attacks or in the requirement of bronchodilator drugs or corticosteroids observed during a trial period would be an indication for long-term therapy.

In the severe asthmatic, *corticosteroid drugs* may be the only means of maintaining a reasonable mode of life, by reducing bronchospasm and exertional dyspnoea, and diminishing the frequency of acute asthmatic attacks. The indications for regular steroid treatment are:

1. Chronic asthma causing severe respiratory disability.
2. A history of one or more near-fatal episodes of status asthmaticus.
3. Chronic asthma associated with pulmonary eosinophilia and transient pulmonary infiltrates.

Either an oral preparation (e.g. prednisolone) or intramuscular adrenocorticotrophic hormone (ACTH) may be given, the disadvantage of the former being that it suppresses the adrenal cortex so that sudden withdrawal leads to adrenal failure, while ACTH seems more likely to cause hypertension, water retention, and potassium loss.

The *side-effects* of long-term corticosteroid therapy include:

1. Cushingoid symptoms (moon face, obesity, hypertension, osteoporosis leading to fracture of vertebral bodies, bruising and skin damage, diabetes mellitus, salt retention).
2. Increased liability to infections, including opportunist infection.
3. Hazard of adrenal failure following accident, infection or surgery, when the need for additional corticosteroid therapy is unrecognised by the medical attendant.
4. Mental symptoms, including depression which may be suicidal.
5. Increased liability to peptic ulceration and gastric bleeding.
6. In children, stunting of growth.

In order to avoid these side-effects it should be the aim to maintain the patient on 10 mg prednisolone daily or less, increasing the dose only when an exacerbation of asthma or an unrelated acute illness make it necessary.

The recent introduction of topical preparations has increased the potential of corticosteroid therapy in resistant asthma. Betamethosone, either as the valerate or dipropionate, is administered as an aerosol in metered doses of 50 µg per 'puff', the usual maintenance dose being 200 to 400 µg per day. In larger dosage

there is a considerable likelihood of troublesome laryngitis and pharyngitis due to *Candida* infection. Corticosteroid therapy for asthma in this form appears to be effective, without producing the systemic side-effects, and is therefore particularly useful in the treatment of severe childhood asthma and for patients who would otherwise need large doses of oral prednisolone. It should be borne in mind that an exacerbation of asthma requires prompt recourse to oral or parenteral corticosteroids to control the bronchospasm.

11

Chronic Obstructive Lung Disease

The non-specific term 'chronic obstructive lung disease' is here used to group together certain common conditions characterised by a chronic, slowly progressive course, obstruction to bronchial airflow which is poorly reversible, and destruction of the pulmonary parenchyma. At the present time the cause of these changes is imperfectly understood but it is apparent that multiple factors are responsible for the development of these diseases. These factors include familial predisposition, genetically-determined enzyme defects, inhaled particles, and infection.

CHRONIC BRONCHITIS AND EMPHYSEMA

The syndrome of chronic bronchitis and emphysema has two pathological elements, a destructive one affecting the lung parenchyma, and an inflammatory one that affects the airways. These processes have led to two separate definitions of the disease: that of chronic bronchitis, which is defined *clinically* as 'the condition of subjects with chronic or recurrent excessive mucus secretion in the bronchial tree'; and that of emphysema, which is defined *pathologically* as 'a condition of the lung characterised by increase beyond normal in the size of the air spaces distal to the terminal bronchiole with destructive changes in their walls'. Although 'pure' chronic bronchitis or 'pure' emphysema can occur separately it is more usual for both processes to exist together in the same patient, and for this reason it seems better to use the comprehensive term 'chronic bronchitis and emphysema' to describe the condition.

The functional result of this dual process is impaired distribution of inspired gas and pulmonary blood flow so that gas exchange becomes progressively less efficient, leading to increased ventilatory effort, hypoxaemia, and carbon dioxide retention. The clinical effects are

bronchial hypersecretion with cough and purulent sputum, shortness of breath on exertion and, ultimately, respiratory failure. Within the wide spectrum of the disease there is considerable variation in the clinical manifestations and functional disability of individual patients so that distinct 'types' of the disease can be recognised, e.g. a 'bronchitic type' or an 'emphysematous type'. In the majority of cases, however, such clear-cut distinctions are impossible and it must be assumed that both emphysema and chronic bronchitis co-exist.

Aetiology
The cause of chronic bronchitis and emphysema is not clearly understood, but certain relevant factors have been demonstrated by epidemiological surveys. The disease commonly manifests itself in middle age and its incidence increases with advancing age; it is more likely to occur in smokers, particularly of cigarettes, and among those exposed to urban and industrial air pollution or engaged in dusty occupations. It seems likely that the pathological changes in the lungs occur slowly, becoming clinically apparent only when a considerable amount of damage has been done over a period of perhaps twenty or thirty years; the cause of the damage may be inhaled foreign particles of dust, smoke, or industrial fumes.

The role of infection in producing these chronic changes is uncertain although there is no doubt that such patients are more liable to recurrent bronchial infection and that infections produce gross temporary derangement of pulmonary function, which may be lethal. There is, however, no evidence that a patient who has recovered from some such acute infective exacerbation shows any abrupt deterioration in function inconsistent with the gradual progression of the underlying disease.

Notwithstanding the relevance of age, smoking, and air pollution in the pathogenesis of chronic bronchitis and emphysema, there remains a group of cases in which none of these factors is applicable and yet all the features of the condition occur. It seems likely that some may have an inherent predisposition to the disease, and there is good evidence in a few patients that severe emphysema coming on at an unusually early age is genetically linked to deficiency of alpha 1-antitrypsin in the serum.

Alpha 1-antitrypsin is a protein with the property of inactivating proteolytic enzymes such as leucocyte collagenase and elastase. It is produced by liver cells and is an acute phase reactant, the normal serum concentration of approximately 240 mg per 100 ml being increased two- or three-fold in inflammatory and infective states. The normal serum level of alpha 1-antitrypsin is governed by a series of specific alternative genes, known as the Pi (protease-inhibitor) system,

which behave as fully-penetrant co-dominant alleles. About 30 phenotypes have so far been distinguished by serum electrophoresis and labelled alphabetically according to their electrophoretic mobility, 90 per cent of the population having the MM phenotype and most of the remainder MS or MZ with somewhat diminished alpha 1-antitrypsin levels. About one person in 2,500 is of phenotype ZZ, which leads to gross deficiency of alpha 1-antitrypsin, and these people have a greatly increased liability to pulmonary emphysema of early onset, apparently affecting predominantly the lower lobes of the lungs. It does not seem that people with partial deficiency of alpha 1-antitrypsin, e.g. those of phenotype MS or MZ, are more liable to lung disease than those of phenotype MM with normal levels. The proportion of individuals with chronic bronchitis and emphysema whose disease can be attributed to alpha 1-antitrypsin deficiency is therefore small, but the concept that the destruction of tissue in emphysema may be due to an imbalance between naturally-occurring proteolytic enzymes and their antagonists is currently the subject of wide-ranging research.

The factors concerned in the production of chronic bronchitis and emphysema may therefore be summarised as:

1. Age.
2. Cigarette smoking.
3. Air pollution due to industrial fumes and dust.
4. Inherent predisposition, including genetically-determined alpha 1-antitrypsin deficiency.

The role of infection in initiating the pathological changes remains uncertain, although it clearly plays an important part in clinical exacerbations of the disease.

Pathology

MORPHOLOGICAL CHANGES

The pathological hall-mark of *chronic bronchitis* is hypertrophy of the mucous glands throughout the trachea and bronchi associated with a great increase in the number of goblet cells, particularly in the bronchioles. The increased secretion of the mucous glands and goblet cells is responsible for the excessive production of sputum which is so characteristic of chronic bronchitis. The thickened mucous membrane and excessive mucus production cause airway narrowing and obstruction, aggravated by bronchospasm due to an excessive reaction of the bronchial tree to infection or to inhaled irritant particles. The clearance of infected material from the bronchi is impaired, causing chronic or recurrent inflammation of the bronchial

tree which presents clinically with an increased production of purulent sputum and wheezy dyspnoea. Infection often becomes persistent in the airways, and pneumonia due to involvement of the lung parenchyma is not unusual. Such infections are slow to resolve and often leave residual fibrosis because of the defective bronchial drainage.

Two types of *emphysema* are recognised in relation to the condition; centrilobular, in which the lesion consists of dilatation and destructive changes in the small airways at the level of the respiratory bronchioles, leaving the alveoli themselves relatively unaffected; and panlobular (or panacinar) emphysema in which the alveoli themselves are dilated and their walls disrupted. Both types frequently co-exist in the same individual.

In severe longstanding disease associated with chronic hypoxia muscular hypertrophy develops in the media of the small pulmonary arteries and extends even into the arterioles which normally have no muscular coat. These changes are thought to be a consequence of persistent hypoxic vasoconstriction, and they lead to increased pulmonary vascular resistance and raised pulmonary arterial pressure, resulting in right ventricular hypertrophy and dilation.

FUNCTIONAL PATHOLOGY

Emphysema and chronic bronchitis most commonly occur together, although the relative extent of each pathological process varies greatly in different individuals. The effect of narrowing and obstruction of the bronchial tree is to impair the distribution of inspired gas, while disruption of the peripheral gas-exchanging zone by bronchiolitis and emphysema causes gross maldistribution of ventilation and perfusion. The rise in airway resistance causes a great increase in the work of breathing and in the oxygen requirement of the respiratory muscles, so that the amount of oxygen available for other activities may be limited. Impairment of gas exchange causes hypoxaemia and carbon dioxide retention which may eventually lead to respiratory failure and cor pulmonale.

There is some evidence to suggest that the functional disability varies according to the dominant pathological change in the lung. Patients with predominant emphysema (Type A, or 'Pink Puffers') are characterised by severe shortness of breath with little cough or sputum, only slight derangement of the blood gases except in the terminal stages, radiological evidence of generalised emphysema, increased thoracic gas volume, reduction in carbon monoxide uptake (T_L,CO) and a tendency to develop arterial oxygen desaturation on exercise. Those with predominant bronchitis (Type B or 'Blue Bloaters') have pronounced productive cough but are less troubled by

shortness of breath, are subject to frequent chest infections, and show radiographic evidence of chronic parenchymatous inflammation rather than emphysema, show marked changes in blood gas tension, and tend to develop cor pulmonale and respiratory failure more readily. Nevertheless the majority of patients appear to be somewhere between these two extremes, showing the characteristics of both to a greater or lesser extent.

Clinical Presentation

SYMPTOMS

Patients with chronic bronchitis and emphysema present with a *productive cough* associated with *wheezy dyspnoea*. These symptoms often follow an upper respiratory tract infection such as a cold or an attack of influenza which fails to settle within a few days. The *sputum* is usually purulent and fairly copious but only rarely does it show blood streaking. On questioning, the patient admits to having a slight cough even when he is well, and to bringing up a little sputum each day, usually in the morning after smoking his first cigarette. It is very uncommon not to obtain a *history of cigarette smoking* over many years in chronic bronchitis. By definition, chronic bronchitis is diagnosed from a history of cough with sputum on most days for at least three months of the year, for at least two years.

Dyspnoea on exertion is a symptom that varies considerably in severity, some patients being hardly aware that their exercise tolerance is diminished until asked closely about their ability to climb stairs, to hurry or to undertake unaccustomed exertion. In others, dyspnoea is the major symptom, often developing fairly rapidly in middle age over a period of two or three years and converting the unfortunate individual from being an active wage-earner to a respiratory cripple. Such an abrupt turn of fortune often causes severe *depression,* especially when the patient realises how little can be done for him. Severely incapacitated patients often describe increased breathlessness when lying flat (*orthopnoea*), due to limitation of diaphragmatic movement in that position. *Swelling of the legs or feet* due to oedema may be a major complaint of those suffering from cor pulmonale, and a slight degree of ankle swelling in the evenings, often noticed as tightness of the shoes, may be an early indication of incipient right heart failure.

A history of recurrent attacks of acute bronchitis is often obtained, tending to increase in frequency as the years go by. Childhood chest illnesses, bronchial asthma and rheumatic fever should be enquired for. Pneumonia or pleurisy may have occurred previously as complications of the chronic bronchial infection. The patient's

occupational history may be relevant to his bronchitis, specifically with regard to work in the linen or cotton industry which may have led to byssinosis as the cause of his chronic airways obstruction, and to cadmium poisoning (an occupational hazard in scrap-metal cutters) which may cause severe emphysema.

CLINICAL SIGNS

External Appearance. 'Emphysematous' (Type A) patients commonly have a thin, asthenic appearance, while 'bronchitic' people (Type B) are usually short and stocky. Loss of weight and a cachectic appearance are not uncommon in patients with advanced chronic airways obstruction, especially when dyspnoea is the dominant symptom. Cyanosis, rarely associated with digital clubbing, is seen mainly in patients with bronchitic symptoms.

Airways Obstruction. This is indicated externally by: (1) alteration of the breathing rhythm due to prolonged expiration; (2) pursing of the lips during expiration; (3) contraction of the accessory muscles of respiration; (4) fixation of the scapulae by clamping the arms to the bedside, thus allowing the latissimus dorsi to act in assisting expiration; and (5) indrawing of the supraclavicular fossae and intercostal tissues during inspiration, and jugular venous distension during expiration, due to excessive swings of intrathoracic pressure.

The Chest. The chest sometimes appears barrel-shaped because of a relative increase in the antero-posterior diameter, and the percussion note is hyperresonant, with loss of cardiac and hepatic dullness and depression of the diaphragm. The characteristic breathing sound is widespread wheezing (rhonchi) of variable pitch, usually most marked in expiration. In patients with excessive bronchial secretions crepitations are heard, especially at the lung bases. Both wheezing and crepitations may be altered in character by coughing. In patients with severe airways obstruction, due to expiratory collapse of large bronchi, occasional crepitations may be heard *early* in inspiration, attributable to sudden opening of the collapsed airways.

The Heart. The apex beat is often impalpable and the heart sounds diminished or inaudible because of the interposition of hyperinflated lung tissue between the heart and the chest wall, and because of the deafening background noise of wheezing. If appreciable, a left parasternal heave with an exaggerated pulmonary second sound suggests right ventricular enlargement and pulmonary hypertension, which may be associated with hepatic and jugular venous distension and dependent oedema.

Course and Complications

The typical course of the disease is a long one, beginning in the

twenties or thirties with 'smoker's cough', i.e. a small amount of mucoid sputum expectorated in the mornings, aggravated in winter time or following a cold. Minor upper respiratory infections tend to persist rather longer than usual, and frequently extend to cause attacks of acute bronchitis. Although there is some impairment of the patient's exercise tolerance this is often hardly noticed because the patient naturally becomes less energetic with the passage of time. He first notices that he is ill when he gets a severe attack of bronchitis that prevents him from working, characterised by purulent sputum and dyspnoea. Thereafter such attacks return at irregular intervals, usually in winter time, and the patient's working capacity deteriorates so that some time in his fifties or early sixties he finally has to give up his work, especially if it is an outdoor, physically-demanding occupation. It seems possible that abandonment of the smoking habit or reduction of environmental air pollution may slow down progression of the disease, but evidence on these points is still inadequate.

During the course of the illness the patient is more than usually liable to acute bronchitic attacks. Pneumonia and pleurisy are common in the later stages of the disease and spontaneous pneumothorax is an occasional complication. During one of the recurrent exacerbations of bronchitis occurring in the advanced stages of the disease the first signs of respiratory failure or congestive heart failure may be observed. These complications tend to become gradually more persistent and the patient eventually succumbs during a severe bronchitic exacerbation, often accompanied by pneumonia, which causes a degree of respiratory insufficiency and cardiac failure too severe to be overcome.

In patients of the predominantly emphysematous type the course of the disease often appears rather less protracted, the symptoms of severe dyspnoea often coming on in middle age without a significant previous history of productive cough. Such patients often become quite incapacitated by breathlessness on exertion within two or three years although the signs of respiratory failure and cor pulmonale are slow to appear.

Investigations

Evidence of emphysema on the *chest radiograph* is indicated by hypertranslucency of the lung fields, elevation of the ribs, depression of the diaphragm, a thin, elongated heart shadow and, most characteristically, attentuation and disappearance of the vascular shadows at the periphery of the lung fields. Rounded areas of hypertranslucency with thin, hair-line shadows forming the margin suggest emphysematous bullae. These are seen most commonly at the lung apices, but in emphysema associated with alpha 1-antitrypsin

deficiency the bullae characteristically occur in the lower zones. When bronchitic changes predominate, evidence of hyperinflation of the lungs is not so marked, and the lung fields may even appear normal. Patchy shadows of irregular distribution often occur in bronchitis at the lung bases, due to areas of broncho-pneumonia and fibrosis. If pulmonary hypertension has developed, the vascular shadows at the hilum are enlarged and the transverse diameter of the heart may be increased due to right ventricular enlargement.

The *sputum* is white and mucoid when bronchitis is quiescent but becomes purulent during exacerbations. In some patients whose disease has an asthmatic component eosinophils may be found. The commonest infecting organisms are *Streptococcus pneumoniae* and *Haemophilus influenzae*.

The *blood count* often shows a polymorphonuclear leucocytosis during acute infective exacerbations, and secondary polycythaemia occurs in patients with chronic hypoxaemia.

Tests of *pulmonary function* demonstrate increased airway resistance with reduction in FEV1, FEV1/FVC ratio, and PEFR, which may be relieved to some extent by the inhalation of 1 per cent isoprenaline aerosol. The FRC, RV, and RV/TLC ratio are generally increased. Tests of distribution of inspired gas show marked unevenness of ventilation, and blood gas measurements in severe chronic bronchitis usually show a fall in arterial oxygen tension and an increase in arterial carbon dioxide tension, changes that are most marked in exacerbations of the disease when respiratory failure threatens. In the emphysematous type of disease these changes in blood gas tension occur in the late stages only, although arterial desaturation characteristically occurs on exercise.

Prevention

Some success is being achieved in reducing the level of air pollution in the larger cities of industrial countries but it is too early to assess the effect of these changes on the prevalence of chronic bronchitis. Little progress is being made in the reduction of cigarette smoking, but doctors can play an important part in actively discouraging the habit in patients with respiratory symptoms, and especially in the young. The prevention of chronic bronchitis and emphysema due to byssinosis can be achieved by measures to reduce dust in mills and factories, and by annual clinical examination and recording of the forced expiratory spirogram in all exposed workers.

The methods currently available for assessing physiological function such as FEV1, closing volume and flow-volume measurements, do not seem to be sufficiently sensitive to distinguish the early changes of chronic bronchitis and emphysema, and

widespread epidemiological surveys designed to identify potential bronchitics by these methods are likely to be unproductive.

Treatment

LONG-TERM MANAGEMENT

General Measures. Surprisingly, patients with chronic bronchitis and emphysema often seem unaware that smoking contributes to their disability. They should be advised against it in the strongest terms. Weight reduction may be a valuable way of improving exercise tolerance in the obese patient, and breathing exercises sometimes afford marginal relief to the severely disabled.

Infection. Respiratory tract infections are the commonest cause of acute deterioration of the patient's condition, and require early treatment with antibiotics. It may be possible to reduce the frequency of such infections by giving polyvalent influenza vaccine at the beginning of each winter, since secondary bacterial bronchitis often complicates viral infections of the upper respiratory tract. The patient should be warned to treat seriously minor infections such as colds or sore throat, and to approach his doctor for a course of antibiotic therapy as soon as he observes an increase in the quantity or purulence of the sputum, accompanied by wheezing and dyspnoea. Since the infecting organism is commonly either *Haemophilus influenzae* or *Streptococcus pneumoniae* the initial antibiotic regimen should be one of the following:

1. Ampicillin 1 g 6-hourly by a parenteral route if the infection is a serious one.
2. Co-trimoxazole 2 tablets, twice daily by mouth.
3. Amoxycillin 250 to 500 mg 6-hourly, by mouth.
4. Oxytetracycline 250 to 500 mg 6-hourly, by mouth.

It is usually necessary to continue treatment for about a week only, but long-term antibiotic therapy is occasionally indicated in the rare patient who becomes unwell with purulent sputum whenever antibiotics are discontinued. Failure of therapy with one of the above regimens should not be followed by changing indiscriminately to an alternative antibiotic; sputum culture should enable a diagnosis of the infecting organism and its sensitivities to be made so that the appropriate antibiotic can be chosen.

Dyspnoea. Wheezy dyspnoea is improved by effective antibiotic treatment which reduces the inflammation and hypersecretion of the bronchial mucous membrane. Bronchoconstriction plays a variable part in the production of airways obstruction, and the probable value of bronchodilator agents can be usefully assessed by measuring the FEV1 before and after the inhalation of an isoprenaline aerosol. Any

of the bronchodilator drugs described for the treatment of bronchial asthma (page 123) may be tried in chronic bronchitis and emphysema although the effect is usually much less impressive. Pressurised aerosol bronchodilators such as isoprenaline or salbutamol are found useful to relieve troublesome spasms of wheezing, and an aminophylline suppository often gives nocturnal relief. Combined preparations containing a bronchodilator and a sedative such as barbiturate should be avoided because of the risk of carbon dioxide retention due to respiratory centre depression, and because patients become dependent and addicted to ineffective medication by using this type of preparation.

Corticosteroid drugs are not usually very effective in chronic bronchitis and emphysema unless there is a definite asthmatic element, and have the disadvantage of aggravating fluid retention in cor pulmonale. In patients with dominant wheezing associated with eosinophils in the sputum a trial of prednisolone may be given in a dose of 20 mg twice daily for a week, measuring the FEV1 before and during the period of treatment. Only if there is objective evidence of improvement should corticosteroid treatment be continued on a maintenance dose, and in most cases it seems advisable to discontinue such therapy once the patient has recovered from an acute exacerbation.

Cough is often a troublesome symptom, especially at night. So that the patient may obtain adequate rest it is often necessary to suppress nocturnal coughing with a cough linctus such as Codeine Linctus, BNF 5 ml.

MANAGEMENT OF ACUTE RESPIRATORY FAILURE

An acute exacerbation of chronic bronchitis is usually heralded by an increase in the quantity, purulence, and stickiness of the sputum due to respiratory infection and aggravated by dehydration. Exhausted by persistent coughing the patient becomes unable to clear his airways, with resulting exacerbation of ventilatory insufficiency. The essential physiological outcome is a fall in arterial oxygen tension, a rise in arterial carbon dioxide tension and a fall in pH. Hypoxia leads to further pulmonary hypertension and congestive cardiac failure while hypercapnia results in drowsiness and a disinclination or inability to cough up secretions. The basic aim of treatment must be to reduce hypoxia and to improve alveolar ventilation.

Initial Assessment. It is important to discover from the patient or a close relative the degree of disability that existed before the onset of the present illness. This information may be needed later to assess the patient's suitability for mechanical ventilation should more conservative treatment prove ineffective. It is also necessary to

consider the reason for the patient's present deterioration; in the majority of cases the cause will be an acute respiratory infection, but occasionally some other cause, for example injudicious oxygen therapy or sedation, may be found. Pneumothorax occasionally occurs, and the diagnosis should be excluded by chest radiography. Treatment should be preceded by certain base-line observations; a note must be made of the patient's state of consciousness, his ability to cough, the presence or absence of cyanosis and of congestive heart failure, and the level of blood carbon dioxide tension. A purulent specimen of sputum should be taken for culture.

Relief of Bronchial Obstruction. Of all forms of treatment vigorous and frequent attempts to clear the patient's airways is the most necessary. In the seriously ill patient coughing should be encouraged every fifteen minutes, assistance being given by the medical or nursing staff if the patient is unable to bring up sputum unaided. Postural drainage may be helpful. It is undoubtedly true that many patients may be revived from near unconsciousness by a few hours' attentive, persistent work by the ward staff. It is important to keep frequent periodical records of whether the patient is able to cough and bring up sputum with or without assistance, since the investigation of the patient's response is itself therapeutic.

Expectoration may be improved if the bronchial secretions can be made less tenacious. If the patient is dehydrated, rehydration by intravenous infusion is essential. Bronchodilators are only of marginal value in improving ventilation, which is limited by obstructive sputum rather than by bronchospasm. Aminophylline may be given intravenously, either by intermittent injection of 0·25 g every 4 to 6 hours, or by continuous infusion of 1 to 1·5 g in 24 hours. The intermittent use of a Wright nebuliser for a few minutes in every hour is a satisfactory way of administering 1 per cent isoprenaline.

Antibiotic therapy is important in controlling infection and hence in reducing bronchial secretions. The choice of antibiotic depends partly on knowledge of the patient's previous medication but also upon guessing the organism most likely to be responsible for the exacerbation. Undoubtedly the organisms most commonly responsible are *Haemophilus influenzae* and *Streptococcus pneumoniae,* and the antibiotic regimen of choice is either co-trimoxazole, amoxycillin, oxytetracycline, or ampicillin (page 136). In the seriously ill patient parenteral therapy is preferable in order to avoid the uncertainty of impaired gastro-intestinal absorption. If sputum culture subsequently shows that the causative organism is insensitive to the chosen antibiotic and provided the patient is not improving, a change may be made to the appropriate antibiotic indicated by the culture sensitivities.

Hypoxia. Correction of hypoxia is very important and requires careful supervision to ensure that administration of the oxygen-enriched gas mixture does not increase carbon dioxide tension enough to cause further depression of consciousness. For this reason the concentration of the inhaled gas mixture should not be greater than 24 or 28 per cent oxygen. Once oxygen therapy is initiated it must be continued, since intermittent oxygen aggravates the hypoxaemia and is consequently more harmful than no oxygen at all. For the patient whose initial arterial carbon dioxide tension is less than 8·0 kPa (60 mm Hg) it is probably safe to give a 28 per cent oxygen mixture, either by a mask of the Venturi type which is the most accurate and reliable method, or by nasal catheter at an oxygen flow rate of 2 litre/min. The nasal catheter is much better tolerated by the patient and gives a sufficiently accurate oxygen concentration at this flow rate but is unreliable at lower flow rates. For the patient with an initial arterial carbon dioxide tension higher than 8·0 kPa (60 mm Hg) a 24 per cent oxygen mixture should be given by Venturi mask. By whatever method and in whatever concentration the oxygen is administered, the patient's arterial carbon dioxide tension must be estimated after two hours of therapy. Some rise in carbon dioxide tension is to be expected but provided it does not exceed 13·4 kPa (100 mm Hg) and provided that the patient remains rousable and able to cough when encouraged it is probable that he can be maintained for long enough to allow the infection to be suppressed and the airways obstruction to be relieved.

Cor pulmonale. The relief of airways obstruction and the administration of oxygen both contribute to the treatment of the accompanying congestive heart failure which is in part due to pulmonary hypertension resulting from hypoxic pulmonary vasoconstriction. Diuretic therapy has been shown to be valuable, and frusemide, 40 mg, should be given intravenously at the beginning of treatment and repeated daily if necessary. At the same time oral diuretic therapy may be started, using a thiazide diuretic such as bendrofluazide 2·5 to 10 mg daily, or chlorothiazide 0·5 g twice daily. If fluid retention persists, a diuretic response may sometimes be achieved with spironolactone 25 mg four times daily by mouth. Digitalis is frequently given although its value seems doubtful and there is some evidence that patients with severe hypoxia are particularly likely to develop cardiac arrhythmias on digitalis therapy.

Deterioration. If the measures described are inadequate and the patient becomes more deeply unconscious with a rising blood carbon dioxide tension, respiratory stimulants should be tried. Excessive dosage causes vomiting or convulsions, particularly when given by continuous intravenous infusion, and this method of administration should be avoided. It is better to give nikethamide intravenously at

half-hourly intervals in a dose sufficient to arouse the comatose patient for long enough to encourage him to cough and expectorate. An initial dose of 3 to 5 ml of a 25 per cent solution may be given, increasing the dose until satisfactory arousal is achieved.

In the last resort assisted ventilation may be required. This method demands expert attention, usually in an intensive care unit, and enables a high concentration of oxygen to be administered along with adequate alveolar ventilation, using intermittent positive pressure, preferably with a constant volume machine. The airways can be cleared efficiently by suction, and bronchial secretions diluted by the instillation of saline. Patients should not be chosen for assisted ventilation, however, unless their history indicates a reasonably high degree of activity, for example, ability to be at work, until shortly before their current illness.

Such patients may benefit from a short period of assisted ventilation which gives temporary relief from the work of breathing and affords an opportunity for bronchial suction to remove tenacious secretions. In the more severely disabled patients, however, treatment by assisted ventilation has a high mortality.

SURGICAL TREATMENT OF EMPHYSEMATOUS BULLAE

Large apical cysts or bullae, which are not uncommon in patients with chronic bronchitis and emphysema, occasionally enlarge sufficiently to cause compression of the airways leading to relatively healthy lung and, therefore, diminish overall lung function disproportionately. In such cases surgical excision of the bullae may improve exercise tolerance provided that the remaining lung is not too severely affected by generalised disease. Operative mortality can be as high as 12 per cent and postoperative improvement is often disappointingly transient, so that careful preoperative assessment and selection is necessary.

BRONCHIECTASIS

Drainage of the bronchial tree is normally achieved by ciliary action and by expiratory contraction of the bronchial muscles which propels secretions towards the trachea. Bronchiectasis is a condition characterised by chronic dilation of one or more bronchi which impairs the drainage of bronchial secretions and leads to persistent infection in the affected segment or lobe. Chronic infection causes further destructive injury to the bronchial walls and a vicious cycle is set up, often leading to spread of infection along the airways and into the lung parenchyma.

Pathogenesis

The aetiology of bronchiectasis is not always clear, and there is

evidence that it may sometimes be *congenital,* for example, when it is associated with dextrocardia and sinusitis (Kartagener's syndrome). In most instances, however, it is probably *acquired* due to the association of bronchial obstruction and infection:

1. Pulmonary tuberculosis, due to the involvement and destruction of bronchial walls by the tuberculous inflammatory process. This is particularly liable to cause bronchiectasis of the upper lobes, which is often asymptomatic because bronchial drainage is achieved by gravity.

2. Cystic fibrosis, due to obstruction of the bronchi by plugs of viscid mucus, followed by secondary bacterial infection.

3. Infectious diseases of childhood, including bronchiolitis, measles and whooping cough, which are frequently complicated by secondary bacterial infection of the lower respiratory tract and by obstructive collapse of a lobe or segment.

4. Bronchial obstruction by a tumour or an aspirated foreign body, followed by secondary infection of the distal bronchial tree.

5. Hypogammaglobulinaemia, due to the tendency for persistent or recurrent respiratory infections.

Functional Abnormality

The degree of functional disturbance depends upon the extent of involvement of pulmonary tissue, localised bronchiectasis of one or two segments or of a single lobe causing little impairment of pulmonary function. Some degree of hypoxaemia due to ventilation/perfusion abnormality is likely to occur in diffuse disease especially if there is significant chronic bronchitis, but carbon dioxide elimination is usually maintained by hyperventilation of uninvolved portions of the lung. Because of the development of large precapillary bronchopulmonary anastomoses in bronchiectasis, mixed venous blood obtained by sampling from the pulmonary artery is often more oxygenated than normal, and this may account for the relatively normal values for arterial oxygen saturation which are found in such patients, despite the apparent severity of their disease.

In assessing the suitability of a patient for surgery it is particularly important to determine the severity of airways obstruction; if it is present to a significant degree it is likely that the results of surgery will be disappointing.

Clinical Presentation

The *symptoms* often date back to childhood, commonly beginning with a respiratory illness. *Cough* is usually present all the year round but becomes particularly troublesome following a cold or other respiratory tract infection. The *sputum* is usually purulent and

copious, even amounting to 200 ml daily in severe cases. *Haemoptysis* is common, usually consisting of blood streaks in the purulent sputum although occasionally it is severe, particularly in bronchiectasis of the middle lobe. It may be the only symptom of bronchiectasis in the upper lobes since free bronchial drainage prevents the usual symptoms of cough and sputum. *Dyspnoea* and *wheezing* may be encountered because of associated chronic bronchitis, particularly when it is aggravated by an intercurrent respiratory infection. The symptoms of *chronic sinusitis* are a common accompaniment of bronchiectasis, and *stunting of growth* is sometimes seen in children severely affected by the disease. Deafness due to keratosis obturans is occasionally associated with bronchiectasis.

The most characteristic of the *physical signs* is the presence of coarse crepitations heard over the affected area of the lung. Localised *rhonchi* are often audible, most marked on expiration and usually altered or cleared by coughing. Signs of pulmonary *consolidation* or *collapse* may be observed as complications of the underlying bronchiectasis. *Digital clubbing* is commonly seen, and *cyanosis* sometimes occurs in severe cases when gas exchange is gravely disturbed.

Complications

The commonest complications are due to spread of infection from the bronchiectatic focus: they include *chronic bronchitis,* recurrent *pneumonia* and *pleurisy,* and sometimes *empyema* and *lung abscess.* *Haemoptysis* is occasionally severe and may be a special indication for surgical treatment. *Brain abscess* and *secondary amyloidosis* are classical complications which are occasionally encountered.

Investigations

The diagnosis of bronchiectasis is often indicated by changes in the plain *radiograph of the chest*: crowding and haziness of the vascular shadows in the affected area, cyst-like shadows which sometimes contain fluid levels, and increased translucency of normal areas of lung due to hyperinflation. Confirmation may be obtained by the technique of *bronchography,* whereby the lumen of the bronchial tree is outlined by radio-opaque contrast medium instilled into the trachea, usually by dripping or injecting it over the back of the tongue having previously anaesthetised the pharynx and larynx with lignocaine. The various bronchi can then be outlined by positioning the patient appropriately. This technique is indicated:

1. In the investigation of haemoptysis which is unexplained on clinical grounds or by other investigations, including bronchoscopy.

2. As a preliminary to the surgical treatment of bronchiectasis, to define precisely the extent of the disease.

Sputum examination should be carried out to exclude a diagnosis of underlying pulmonary tuberculosis, and specimens should be cultured to identify and obtain the sensitivities of the infecting organism as a guide in chemotherapy. *Bronchoscopy* may be indicated to exclude bronchial tumour or an aspirated foreign body as underlying causes of the bronchiectasis.

Management

MEDICAL TREATMENT

Medical treatment is successful in controlling infection and reducing symptoms in most cases of bronchiectasis, based on the principles of adequate postural drainage and effective chemotherapy.

Postural drainage is achieved by locating the site of infection by clinical or radiological examination, and positioning the patient so that the affected segment or lobe is drained by gravity. The patient is taught to adopt the appropriate position and to expectorate as much sputum as possible by deep breathing or coughing, assisted by percussion or pressure over the affected area. To maintain good health it is important that this procedure should become a routine part of the patient's daily life.

Chemotherapy should be given to control acute exacerbations of infection which are most commonly due to *Haemophilus influenzae,* the pneumococcus and *Staphylococcus pyogenes.* The choice of antibiotic is based on the same principles as those followed in treating chronic bronchitis (page 136), using sputum cultures and sensitivities as a guide. In the more severe cases continuous chemotherapy may be necessary during the winter months or even throughout the year. Oxytetracycline in a dose of 0·5 g twice daily is an effective and practicable form of suppressive therapy, although ampicillin or co-trimoxazole may be used as alternatives.

SURGICAL TREATMENT

Surgery should be considered when:

1. Medical treatment has failed to control the symptoms effectively.
2. The bronchiectatic changes are confined to a single segment or lobe.
3. The patient is less than 40 years of age.
4. Respiratory function is good.

It is also usually indicated when the disease presents with severe haemoptysis, especially if it is recurrent. Bronchography should

always be carried out as a preliminary to surgery, to ensure that the full extent of the disease has been defined.

In more diffuse disease surgery offers little advantage over careful medical treatment, and in any case it is probably wise to withhold surgery for at least a year while the effects of carefully controlled medical treatment are assessed. Surgery is most commonly contra-indicated by the presence of generalised airways disease.

CYSTIC FIBROSIS

Cystic fibrosis is an inherited disorder that affects exocrine glands, causing excessive activity and hyperplasia of mucus-secreting glands and an abnormally high concentration of sodium chloride in sweat. The condition is carried by an autosomal recessive gene, the homozygous state which causes clinical disease occurring about once in every 2,500 live births, while the incidence of the heterozygous or 'carrier' state is about one in 25 live births.

Pathology

The mucus blanket that lines the epithelium of the respiratory tract has a number of important functions which include the prevention of fluid loss in the expired air, the entrapment of foreign particles, and an anti-infective action against inhaled micro-organisms. It is normally carried by ciliary action to the trachea and larynx whence it is coughed up and swallowed, but in cystic fibrosis the movement of mucus along the airways is impaired, and as a result the small bronchi and bronchioles, although normal at birth, become blocked by mucus which becomes secondarily infected by inhaled bacteria, causing destructive changes to the bronchial walls and subsequent bronchiectasis. These changes lead to alveolar hypoventilation and uneven distribution of ventilation and perfusion, and finally to respiratory failure and cor pulmonale. Emphysema appears to be a relatively infrequent finding in this disease, although the observation of alveolar dilatation especially in the more longstanding cases may be an indication that panacinar emphysema is likely to develop in those who survive into adult life. Nasal polyposis and obstruction of the paranasal sinuses also occur, and chronic sinusitis is a common complication.

Elsewhere in the body abnormal secretions cause obstruction in the bowel, the pancreatic ducts, the bile ducts, and the tubules of the testis. Bowel obstruction occurs in infancy as *meconium ileus,* i.e. obstruction of the terminal ileum arising from the abnormally viscid nature of the meconium. Fibrotic damage with cyst formation and failure of pancreatic secretion occur as a result of obstruction to the pancreatic ducts, contributing to the development of meconium ileus

in infancy and leading to intestinal malabsorption later. Obstruction of the vas deferens due to fibrosis apparently causes almost universal infertility in homozygous males.

Clinical Features

RESPIRATORY MANIFESTATIONS

Chronic or recurrent infections of the respiratory tract are a characteristic feature of the disease, usually beginning in infancy, although very occasionally the respiratory and pancreatic defects are mild or delayed so that the disease only becomes apparent later in childhood or in adolescence. Cough with purulent sputum occurs, the quantity of sputum increasing with age as the airways become bronchiectatic. Wheezing and dyspnoea on exertion are common, and in severe cases the child becomes increasingly crippled as recurrent episodes of bronchitis, pneumonia and pulmonary collapse lead to a steady deterioration in lung function. Cyanosis often occurs and clubbing of the digits is associated with bronchiectasis or lung abscess. The patient's state of nutrition suffers both from the chronic respiratory illness and from intestinal malabsorption, so that stunting of growth is a common manifestation. Respiratory failure and cor pulmonale occur in advanced disease.

NON-RESPIRATORY MANIFESTATIONS

In infancy intestinal obstruction due to meconium ileus occurs in about 10 per cent of cases, while intussusception, faecal impaction, and rectal prolapse sometimes affect older children. Malabsorption due to deficiency of pancreatic secretion leads to steatorrhoea associated with slow growth, poor stature, and a markedly protuberant abdomen. Cirrhosis of the liver has been observed as a complication of the disease, occasionally associated with jaundice and hypersplenism. Circulatory failure due to heat stroke may result from excessive sodium chloride loss in the sweat, especially among infants and small children.

Diagnosis

The diagnosis of cystic fibrosis should be considered whenever the child suffers from persistent or recurrent respiratory infections, especially if there is a family history of similar illness. A history of gastro-intestinal symptoms and steatorrhoea, particularly an increase of total free fatty acids in the stool, gives supporting evidence of pancreatic involvement. The most reliable screening test is the estimation of sodium and chloride in the sweat, using the pilocarpine iontophoresis method for stimulating local sweat production.

Concentrations of sodium and chloride in excess of 70 mmol/litre are diagnostic in children, but the upper level of these electrolytes in sweat is less uniform in adults or adolescents. In doubtful cases spironolactone should be given for several days in a dose of 0·1 mg/kg; in normals this treatment causes a fall in sweat sodium level, but in cystic fibrosis patients the high sodium level is maintained.

The sweat test is not precise enough for identifying the heterozygote and at the present time no reliable test is available for this purpose.

Management

Until recently, children with cystic fibrosis died from respiratory complications before reaching their teens, but early recognition of the disease, intensive physiotherapy and antibiotics have prolonged their life expectancy although the number surviving into adult life is still small. Pulmonary dysfunction is the overriding factor in determining survival, and the successful management of this aspect of their disease is therefore critical.

Removal of bronchial secretions is a crucial aspect of treatment. Postural drainage should be carried out twice daily in each of the several positions necessary to achieve gravity drainage of the various lung lobes. Drainage is assisted by clapping with the cupped hand and vibration over the appropriate area. It is valuable to precede postural drainage with a ten-minute period of aerosol therapy given by oronasal mask using an effective compressor which can produce droplets small enough, i.e. 1 to 10 microns in diameter, to reach the small airways in order to liquify tenacious mucus. The aerosol can also be used to transport bronchodilators such as 1 per cent isoprenaline, or local antibiotics such as neomycin, bacitracin, or polymyxin. The use of mist tent therapy during sleep has many advocates but it poses considerable social problems for the child and its efficacy is a matter for controversy. It is more widely favoured in the U.S.A. than in Britain.

Treatment of Infection. Chronic low-grade infection of the bronchial tree and intermittent exacerbations of acute bronchitis or bronchopneumonia form the respiratory background to this disease. Cystic fibrosis patients are particularly susceptible to infection by *Staphylococcus pyogenes* but Gram-negative organisms may also be encountered. Acute exacerbations of pulmonary symptoms should be treated according to the bacteriology and sensitivities of the pathogens cultured from the sputum, but in the absence of definite bacteriological information antistaphylococcal antibiotics such as erythromycin, clindamycin or cloxacillin should be given, the treatment being continued for one to two months after the infection

has cleared. In patients with more advanced pulmonary involvement *Pseudomonas aeruginosa* is frequently cultured and should be treated with sulphadiazine or co-trimoxazole. Gentamycin and carbenicillin may be given in severe infections.

Preventive treatment. Antistaphylococcal antibiotics should be given to all cystic fibrosis infants throughout the first year of life, and to patients with minimal pulmonary involvement who develop an upper respiratory infection. Prophylactic polyvalent influenza vaccine should be given at the beginning of each winter, and children should be vaccinated early against whooping cough and measles. Chronic sinusitis may be the source of recurrent infections of the lower bronchial tree, and should be treated actively with irrigation, antibiotics, and surgery where necessary.

Pancreatic Insufficiency. The treatment of pancreatic insufficiency should consist of a low fat, high protein diet, supplementary fat soluble vitamins and pancreatic enzyme replacement. The amount of fat restriction and the quantity of pancreatic enzyme required must be suited to the fat tolerance of each individual.

12

Spontaneous Pneumothorax

Pneumothorax is the presence of air in a pleural cavity, causing the lung on that side to collapse to a greater or lesser extent depending on the volume of air admitted. The introduction of air may be accidental, as the result of a penetrating injury of the chest wall or by mischance during the aspiration of intrapleural fluid, or it may occur spontaneously due to the escape of air from the air passages of the lung into the pleural space through a hole in the visceral pleura.

The definition of *primary spontaneous pneumothorax* is that the pneumothorax occurs in the absence of any clinical evidence of underlying pulmonary disease; *secondary spontaneous pneumothorax* occurs as a consequence of a manifest disease process; for example, chronic airways obstruction or pulmonary tuberculosis. The reported incidence of primary spontaneous pneumothorax has varied from 2·4 to 17·8 per 100,000 population per year, 85 per cent of cases occurring in young adult males between the ages of twenty and forty years. Secondary spontaneous pneumothorax is much less common and occurs in an older age group, the underlying disorder most frequently encountered being chronic airways obstruction.

Pathogenesis

DYNAMICS

During normal breathing the pressure within the pleural space—the intrathoracic pressure—is always negative relative to the pressure in the airways—the intrapulmonary pressure—although the difference between these two pressures varies at different times in the respiratory cycle, from $-0·44$ to $-1·3$ kPa (-3 to -9 mm Hg). During shouting or coughing the intrapulmonary pressure may increase to $9·4$ kPa (70 mm Hg) or more, and extreme fluctuations are liable to occur during strenuous physical exercise.

The underlying factors that appear to contribute to the development of a pneumothorax are:

1. Rapid and large fluctuations in intrapulmonary pressure, causing transient increases in the pressure gradient across the pleural surface of the lung.

2. Increase in pressure in the subpleural air spaces, due to localised air trapping as a result of airways obstruction.

3. The presence of large alveoli, lung cysts, blebs and bullae which, because of their large diameter, sustain more tension in their walls than do normal alveoli when distended by a given intrapulmonary pressure (Laplace's law states that the tension sustained by the curved surface of a space is proportional to the diameter of curvature and to the pressure gradient across the surface).

Once rupture has occurred, air continues to escape into the pleural space from the lungs until the pressure gradient reaches zero, or until the aperture is sealed by collapsing lung tissue. Occasionally, a valvelike mechanism occurs, whereby air enters the pleural space during inspiration but cannot escape during expiration, so that pressure within the pneumothorax steadily increases—a *tension pneumothorax*—leading to mediastinal shift and compression of the opposite lung.

AETIOLOGY

In the majority of cases of *primary spontaneous pneumothorax,* rupture of the lung surface probably occurs at the site of a pulmonary bleb, a small air-filled cystic structure closely underlying the visceral pleura. The abnormality appears to be localised to a small area at the lung apex, consisting of focal fibrosis, patchy chronic inflammation and one or more fibrous-walled cysts. It is not known whether these cysts are congenital in origin, or result from stress, injury or degenerative change in the lung. Rarely, the condition is familial. The association of spontaneous pneumothorax with Marfan's syndrome and the Ehlers-Danlos syndrome is due to the rupture of pulmonary cysts which are presumably formed as a result of the inherited disorder of connective tissue. In a few cases of primary spontaneous pneumothorax treated by open thoracotomy no bleb has been found at the point of rupture, but tears of the visceral pleura at the site of an adhesion have been incriminated.

Secondary spontaneous pneumothorax most commonly occurs in *chronic bronchitis and emphysema* due to rupture of subpleural emphysema or an emphysematous bulla. Focal emphysema secondary to *pulmonary fibrosis* is similarly responsible for the occasional occurrence of spontaneous pneumothorax in sarcoidosis, in the pneumoconioses, and in other forms of diffuse pulmonary fibrosis. Acute *pulmonary tuberculosis* is responsible for a significant

number of cases of secondary spontaneous pneumothorax, and other causes include *asthma, pneumonia, lung abscess* and *bronchial carcinoma.*

Functional Abnormality

The immediate effect of partial or complete collapse of one lung is to cause a gross disturbance of ventilation/perfusion distribution on the affected side. For a time perfusion continues through unventilated tissue, resulting in a large venous-to-arterial shunt which produces arterial hypoxaemia. Within a few hours pulmonary blood flow through the collapsed lung diminishes, probably as a result of active pulmonary vasoconstriction which causes right ventricular output to be largely transferred to the ventilated side. Some unevenness of ventilation/perfusion ratios however persists, the mixed venous-to-arterial shunt remaining higher than normal until some time after the pneumothorax has been reabsorbed. A reduction in lung volumes and in carbon monoxide transfer factor occurs, to a degree that would be expected from the loss of functioning tissue in one lung.

The functional consequences of unilateral pneumothorax depend upon the degree of pulmonary collapse and upon the presence of underlying lung disease. In a healthy adult complete collapse of one lung produces mild arterial hypoxaemia and moderate impairment of exercise tolerance, but a serious threat to life occurs only in the presence of a tension pneumothorax which causes progressive compression of the opposite lung and also obstructs venous return to the heart by distortion of the mediastinum. A simple pneumothorax has much more serious consequences for patients with chronic lung disease such as chronic airways obstruction or pulmonary fibrosis because the sudden aggravation of an underlying ventilation/perfusion defect is liable to lead to acute respiratory failure.

Clinical Features

SYMPTOMS AND SIGNS

Spontaneous pneumothorax should be suspected in patients with chronic airways obstruction who present with evidence of acute respiratory failure, and in any young adult presenting with chest pain and dyspnoea. The onset of symptoms is abrupt in two-thirds of cases, but gradual in the remainder, being related to strenuous activity in about 20 per cent.

Chest pain is the commonest symptom. It is usually constant but may be of a pleuritic nature, and is commonly described as a sharp, tight or pulling type of pain. *Dyspnoea* occurs almost as commonly as pain, but *cough* is only an occasional symptom, usually unproductive

but rarely associated with slight *haemoptysis*. In patients with chronic airways obstruction the symptoms of spontaneous pneumothorax may appear to be no more than an acute infective exacerbation of the underlying disease.

The classical *clinical signs* of air in the pleural cavity consist of reduction in chest expansion on the affected side, shift of the mediastinum to the opposite side, hyperresonance over the pneumothorax with loss of cardiac dullness or downward displacement of hepatic dullness, and distant or absent breath sounds. It will be appreciated that these signs are extremely difficult to distinguish in a patient with chronic airways obstruction who has diffuse pulmonary emphysema, and diagnosis in such cases depends upon the radiological appearances. Even in the previously healthy patient a small pneumothorax may cause little in the way of abnormal clinical signs.

Accompanying signs may include the presence of subcutaneous emphysema in the neck or over the chest, and a succussion splash when there is an associated pleural effusion. Tension pneumothorax is suggested by signs of peripheral circulatory failure or cyanosis, asymmetrical enlargement of the chest due to over-distension of the affected hemithorax, and a hyperresonant percussion note.

THE CHEST RADIOGRAPH

The diagnosis of spontaneous pneumothorax is confirmed by a postero-anterior chest radiograph, which shows the lung partially collapsed towards the hilum with a peripheral area of increased translucency due to air in the pleural space. The mediastinum is shifted towards the opposite side and the hemidiaphragm on the affected side may be depressed. Small pneumothoraces at the lung apex may be difficult to detect even radiologically because the lung margin is concealed by skeletal shadows. A triangular shadow in the costophrenic angle is a common finding, due to an associated small pleural effusion.

In patients with emphysema the distinction between a localised pneumothorax and a large emphysematous cyst is sometimes difficult to make.

COURSE AND COMPLICATIONS

Air in the pleural cavity is gradually reabsorbed, a 50 per cent pneumothorax taking about six weeks to re-expand fully. Many patients are treated simply by rest, but *recurrent pneumothorax* is a common and annoying complication. After re-expansion, adhesions often form between the visceral and parietal pleura, and these are liable to bleed if torn by a subsequent recurrence, resulting in a

haemopneumothorax. Such bleeding is occasionally severe, requiring prompt and adequate blood replacement. Pneumothorax quite commonly occurs on the side opposite to previous episodes, and *bilateral pneumothoraces* occasionally arise simultaneously.

Tension pneumothorax is an important complication that may rapidly lead to death from peripheral circulatory failure and respiratory failure. The danger of *respiratory failure* is particularly acute in patients suffering from underlying chronic pulmonary disease who develop either a simple or a tension pneumothorax, since their reserves of pulmonary function are already in jeopardy.

Pneumomediastinum and *subcutaneous emphysema* occasionally occur, due to leakage of air via the interstitial tissues of the lung into the mediastinum and neck. *Bronchopleural fistula* and *empyema* are rare complications.

Treatment

The aim of treatment should be to re-expand the lung, to prevent recurrence of the pneumothorax, and to restore the patient to normal activities as soon as possible. With these objects in view, two courses are open to consideration in the uncomplicated case:

1. A small pneumothorax, which is not progressing and is not associated with respiratory insufficiency, may be allowed to re-expand without surgical interference. Bed rest is unnecessary but physical activity of more than moderate degree should be avoided, and serial chest radiography is needed to ensure that re-expansion of the lung is complete.

2. A large pneumothorax should be treated by inserting an intercostal tube, to achieve re-expansion quickly and to avoid the slight risk of contralateral pneumothorax.

INSERTION OF INTERCOSTAL TUBE

A large catheter is introduced through the chest wall under local anaesthesia, using an introducer which is passed through a cannula in the 4th or 5th intercostal space just posterior to the anterior axillary line, or anteriorly through the 2nd intercostal space. Alternatively, an Argyll thoracic catheter which has numerous side holes near its end may be introduced in the axilla and inserted upwards towards the lung apex. The distal end of the catheter is merely attached to an underwater seal, for it is seldom necessary to apply suction in order to achieve satisfactory expansion. Incautious suction may re-expand the lung too rapidly, causing unilateral pulmonary oedema.

The intercostal tube is left in place for 24 hours longer than the time required to obtain full expansion of the lung, usually a period of

several days. Analgesics should be given to relieve any pain. The tube must be removed and replaced if it becomes obstructed by pleural exudate.

PREVENTION OF RECURRENT PNEUMOTHORAX

The use of an intercostal tube in itself assists in the prevention of subsequent pneumothoraces because the inflammatory reaction set up by the catheter helps to stick the pleural surfaces together. Nevertheless, recurrence can become a nuisance to some patients and a serious hazard to those with underlying lung disease. The methods available for treatment are:

1. Chemical pleurodesis, whereby adhesion between the parietal and visceral layers of the pleura is achieved by the instillation of pleural irritants (commonly iodised talc) through a cannula into the pleural space, but at the risk of causing progressive impairment of ventilation due to pleural fibrosis. For this reason the method is now out of favour except in patients with extensive underlying lung disease who are unsuitable for thoracotomy.

2. Parietal pleurectomy, performed through a small thoracotomy which allows any bullae or blebs to be ligated or resected. The parietal pleura is then stripped off the chest wall leaving the diaphragmatic and mediastinal pleura intact.

3. Wedge resection of the lung apex has recently been advocated as an effective means of preventing recurrence of pneumothorax. This procedure is based on the observation that, in a series of patients with recurrent primary spontaneous pneumothorax, the only pulmonary abnormality was confined to a small area at the lung apex. Further experience is needed to determine whether apical wedge resection is the treatment of choice for primary spontaneous pneumothorax which persists or recurs after initial management by intercostal tube drainage.

TREATMENT OF COMPLICATIONS

Tension pneumothorax is treated in an emergency by inserting a needle through an intercostal space, the subsequent treatment being the introduction of an intercostal tube. *Massive haemopneumothorax* may require open thoracotomy to obtain haemostasis and to remove blood clot so that the lung can subsequently re-expand completely. *Infection* of the pleural space, due either to tuberculosis or to pyogenic organisms, requires the appropriate antibiotic regimen.

13

Acute Infections of the Respiratory Tract

Acute Virus Infections

The majority of acute upper respiratory infections and some infections of the lower respiratory tract are due to viruses. The identification of individual types of virus with specific clinical syndromes has proved a complicated task, partly because of the wide variation in antigenic character shown by many viruses but also because of the tendency for viruses to affect more than one anatomical area of the respiratory tract so that the clinical syndromes resulting from infection are difficult to define. These problems have been simplified by developments in the techniques of culturing viruses, in recognising their morphological characteristics, and in diagnosing viral infection by serological methods so that a broad outline of the clinical syndromes most characteristic of the various different viral infections can be recognised. It should be appreciated, nonetheless, that infection with a specific virus, for example one of the influenza A viruses, although usually causing the well-known acute epidemic infection called influenza may occasionally cause clinical syndromes as trivial as a mild 'common cold' or as catastrophically severe as acute influenzal pneumonia.

Identification of a virus infection on clinical grounds is therefore liable to error. Recognition of the virus particle itself can usually be achieved by culturing the organism obtained from throat swabs or nasal washings in the appropriate tissue, either by egg or tissue culture inoculation or by isolation in organ cultures. The virus may be identified by various methods which include its morphological appearance on electron microscopy and certain serological characteristics. From the clinical point of view, however, serological diagnosis of viral infections is usually retrospective since it depends on demonstration of a fourfold or greater rise in the patient's antibody titre in paired sera collected in the acute and late stages of the illness. Table 13.1 shows the pattern of disease most commonly caused by individual virus groups.

154

Table 13.1

Respiratory Viruses

Virus Group	Diameter (mµ)	Antigenic Types	Main Disease Pattern
Myxoviruses Influenza A	80–120	Constantly varying	Major influenza epidemics; croup in infants during epidemics; high mortality in the elderly from cardio-respiratory complications
B		Constantly varying	Recurrent influenza outbreaks
C		One only	Sporadic mild upper respiratory illnesses
Parainfluenza	150–220	4 types	Croup and pneumonia in children
Respiratory syncytial virus	120–130	Little variation	Bronchiolitis and pneumonia in infants and children
Coronavirus	80–120	Several types	Colds in children and adults
Adenovirus	70–90	Many types	Feverish cold, sore throat and occasional pneumonia in children and young adults
Picornaviruses Rhinovirus	22–27	Many types	Common cold; acute exacerbations of chronic bronchitis
Enteroviruses		Many types	Febrile colds and pharyngitis

PATHOLOGY

Respiratory viral infections cause necrosis and degeneration of the ciliated columnar epithelium of the respiratory tract, associated with excessive mucus production by the goblet cells. The cellular damage induces a submucosal inflammatory reaction with polymorphonuclear exudation but, later, mononuclear cells predominate. During recovery the underlying inflammatory changes resolve and the denuded areas of epithelium are resurfaced, first by stratified squamous and then by normal columnar epithelium.

PATHOGENESIS

The replication of virus particles in respiratory epithelial cells upsets

the normal metabolic cellular processes, leading to degeneration and death of the cells. Although this process is probably the major cause of the pathological changes described above there is reason to believe that an allergic inflammatory response is an important factor in some viral infections, notably the acute bronchiolitis of infants due to respiratory syncytial virus. It is now considered that this condition is due to an immunological reaction occurring on the epithelium between the infecting virus and IgG antibodies passively acquired from the mother.

VIRAL SYNDROMES

The Common Cold. Usually caused by rhinoviruses which form part of the picornavirus group, a similar syndrome to the common cold is occasionally due to infection by any of the other virus groups listed. It is characterised by sneezing, nasal discharge, 'scratchiness' rather than soreness of the throat, chilliness and headache. Nasal obstruction and slight cough develop over the next day or two, the whole illness subsiding within six or seven days. Fever is usually absent. Colds are commoner among smokers than non-smokers but their incidence is not increased by exposure to cold, damp, draughts or other minor environmental changes. Neither antibiotics nor vitamin preparations are shown to be of any value in their prevention or treatment.

Sore Throat. The main viral cause of febrile sore throats (pharyngitis and tonsilitis) is the adenovirus group although the influenza and picornavirus groups are responsible for a considerable proportion of infections. No clinical distinction can be made, however, between viral infections and those caused by haemolytic streptococci. The most prominent symptom is severe sore throat accompanied by redness of the pharynx and redness and swelling of the tonsils. In severe cases a purulent exudate appears on the surface of the tonsils and cervical lymph node enlargement is present. General symptoms such as fever, malaise, muscular aching, and headache are quite common, and a rise in temperature may be observed. Cough often occurs.

Influenza. Epidemic influenza is caused by influenza viruses A and B but influenza-like illnesses are also caused by the adenoviruses and by the echo and coxsackie groups of the picornaviruses. The illness begins acutely with malaise, backache, nasal symptoms, shivering, headache and fever, although in some instances the attack may be ushered in by a cough, cold or sore throat for a few days beforehand. The pyrexia is variable in form, continuing irregularly for three to five days, and is accompanied by constitutional symptoms such as muscular aching, prostration, anorexia and dry cough which often

becomes productive later. The eyes look injected and watery, the throat is reddened, and sometimes occasional crepitations and scattered rhonchi may be heard in the chest. Although the illness is usually over in about ten days some degree of lassitude and mental inertia is often felt for a week or two. In debilitated patients or in those suffering from underlying chronic chest or heart disease an attack of influenza often precipitates acute bronchitis or pneumonia complicated by secondary bacterial infection.

Complications of Influenza. The development of wheezing, dyspnoea and productive cough in patients with influenza suggests the diagnosis of *acute influenzal bronchitis* which tends to be most common in those with a previous history of chronic bronchitis and emphysema or organic heart disease. The illness takes rather longer to subside than simple influenza and may be complicated by secondary bacterial infection. In a few cases, apparent recovery from an attack of simple influenza is set back in the early convalescent period by the development of secondary pneumonia which is nearly always pneumococcal in origin. The most severe and fulminant type of *acute influenzal pneumonia* is associated with a synchronous staphylococcal infection although occasionally only viral lesions have been shown at necropsy. It is encountered most commonly in the early stages of influenzal pandemics and is most likely to occur among patients with underlying chronic cardiorespiratory disease. The abrupt onset is similar to that of uncomplicated influenza, but is quickly followed by a productive cough, often haemoptysis, and rapid breathing with cyanosis. Fever is irregular and swinging, and delirium may accompany the hypoxia. The chest signs indicate a diffuse process with patchy dullness, reduced breath sounds and scattered crepitations, the signs of consolidation being usually absent. Recovery is slow, and complications such as lung abscess, empyema and bronchiectasis are typical of those seen in staphylococcal infection of the lung. Cardiac arrhythmias, myocarditis, polyneuritis, and encephalitis are among the rare complications of influenza that are occasionally encountered.

Croup (acute laryngotracheobronchitis). This usually occurs in children under the age of three years, and is due to infection by parainfluenza virus, commonly Type 1. It begins with slight cough, fever, and nasal discharge, followed after about one day by increasing cough and dyspnoea due to inspiratory obstruction which causes stridor and indrawing of the chest wall on inspiration, particularly in the suprasternal and subcostal areas. In mild cases the inflammation and oedema of the airways settle down after a few days, but when respiratory obstruction due to congestion of the larynx is severe, cyanosis and carbon dioxide retention are liable to occur, aggravated

by bronchitis. In such cases tracheotomy is urgently indicated to prevent asphyxiation.

A number of other viruses including measles, adenoviruses, and enteroviruses can cause croup, and obstructive laryngotracheitis in older children may be due to influenza virus infection. Secondary bacterial infection sometimes occurs.

Acute bronchitis is due to an extension of upper respiratory viral infections to the bronchi, causing a productive cough which is often associated with retrosternal pain or discomfort due to mucosal inflammation. No particular virus is responsible.

Acute bronchiolitis typically affects infants under the age of two years, usually in winter epidemics. It begins with cough and nasal discharge for two or three days, followed suddenly by exacerbation of the cough, dyspnoea, inspiratory stridor, and wheezing. Rhonchi and crepitations are heard at the bases or sometimes over the whole lung, and the chest becomes overinflated. After three or four days the illness subsides gradually, usually with no more than a transient rise in temperature. The mortality is low but it is important to distinguish the development of bronchopneumonia, which is indicated by the appearance of homogeneous or mottled opacities of lobar or segmental distribution on the chest radiograph. The major cause of acute bronchiolitis is the respiratory syncytial virus although the influenza and parainfluenza groups may also occasionally be responsible. Secondary bacterial infection may occur and affects the outlook unfavourably, especially when it is due to the staphylococcus.

MANAGEMENT OF VIRAL INFECTIONS OF THE UPPER RESPIRATORY TRACT

Prevention. The virus infections of the respiratory tract are spread by droplet transmission resulting from close contact between individuals. It appears impossible to prevent spread of infection except by isolation of individuals one from another, an impractical proposition in view of the ubiquity of the respiratory viruses. Individual resistance to infection may, however, be promoted by vaccination with inactivated or with living but attenuated virus vaccine, provided that the vaccine contains the antigens likely to be encountered in the expected epidemic. It is also important that the timing of vaccination should be judged accurately in relation to the arrival of the epidemic since the antibody response tends to fall quite rapidly after a few months.

Application of these methods in the prevention of influenza has led to only partial success, the order of protection being at best only 70 per cent and the duration of protection being short. In addition, the antigenic structure of the influenza viruses changes periodically.

Attempts to protect whole populations by influenza vaccination are therefore not justified, but there is an accepted place for polyvalent vaccination of groups specially subject to infection or to unusually severe consequences of infection. These include:

1. Patients with chronic disease of the lungs, heart or kidneys.

2. Patients with diabetes, and some other endocrine disorders such as Addison's disease.

3. Patients with impaired immunological response, such as recipients of organ transplants and others on immunosuppressive therapy or on steroids.

4. Hospital and health workers during widespread epidemics.

Inactivated vaccines have been prepared from some of the adenovirus group, and have been shown to give some protection against epidemic infection, but it is probably true to say that vaccination as a preventive measure against respiratory virus infection is likely to be displaced by the development of effective chemotherapeutic agents. At the present time only amantadine has been extensively investigated in the treatment of respiratory viral infection, and trials of its effectiveness have not shown consistent results.

Treatment in adults is directed towards the relief of symptoms and the prevention, recognition, and treatment of secondary bacterial infection. Bed rest is unnecessary for minor colds or sore throats but should be insisted upon in febrile illnesses for the patient's comfort, at least until the fever has subsided. Headache, muscular pains, and sore throat are relieved by paracetamol, or by acetylsalicylic acid, although the latter tends to cause uncomfortable sweating and carries some hazard because of gastric irritation and occasional gastro-intestinal bleeding. Cough may be suppressed with Linctus Codeine provided that the amount of sputum is small and that there is no indication for ensuring adequate bronchial drainage. Insomnia may be managed with hypnotics such as dichloralphenazone or Nitrazepam 5 mg. Antibiotics should not be used in the treatment of un-complicated viral infections but if there is any indication that the infection is due to haemolytic streptococci (i.e., severe sore throat with tonsillar exudate and enlarged, tender cervical lymph nodes) treatment with oral penicillin (phenoxymethylpenicillin) should be instituted. Prophylactic chemotherapy is justified in patients with a history of previous chronic chest or cardiac disease, a five-day course of a wide-spectrum antibiotic such as oxytetracycline being given. Ampicillin should not be used in the treatment of severe sore throat without carefully considering whether the symptoms are due to glandular fever; in this condition a troublesome allergic skin reaction to the drug is likely to occur.

Treatment in children should follow the same principles as those outlined for the management of adult upper respiratory viral infections. The narrowness of the airways in infants calls for special care in observing signs of deterioration such as increasing stridor, pallor, restlessness, respiratory difficulty, and cyanosis, especially as these changes can develop quite rapidly. In infants with croup the possible need for tracheotomy should be borne in mind, and if performed it should be followed by repeated aspiration of retained secretions in the trachea and main bronchi.

Extension of infection down the airways of small children may result in bronchopneumonia or in lobar or segmental consolidation. Such complications are suggested by general deterioration, rapid pulse and respiratory rate, coughing with grunting respirations and diffuse or localised crepitations. These changes may be due to viral pneumonia, particularly in infants, but, as in adults, pneumococci, staphylococci, haemolytic streptococci, *Klebsiella pneumoniae,* and *Haemophilus influenzae* are the chief causes of pneumonia in children. The use of oxytetracycline should be avoided in children because of the danger of permanent damage to developing teeth, but treatment with penicillin should be initiated, together with methicillin or cloxacillin if the organism is suspected of being or shown to be a penicillin-resistant staphylococcus. Ampicillin may be used in the treatment of Gram-negative infections.

PNEUMONIA

Pneumonia is an acute inflammatory reaction in the lung parenchyma with an outpouring of inflammatory exudate into the alveoli, commonly resulting in respiratory and systemic symptoms. It is usually of *infective* origin but may also be caused by inhaled *chemical* irritants such as gases and vapours (e.g. ammonia, nitrogen dioxide or cadmium, page 217), fatty or oily material causing lipoid pneumonia, and vomit in the unconscious patient or refluxed gastric secretions in patients with hiatus hernia. Pneumonia may also occur in pulmonary hypersensitivity states such as Loeffler's syndrome (page 272), and in pulmonary polyarteritis nodosa (page 256).

This section deals with the commoner types of pneumonia of infective origin: tuberculous and fungal pneumonias are mentioned in the appropriate chapters.

CAUSAL AGENTS

The micro-organisms most commonly encountered as pathogens in pneumonia are as follows:

1. Bacterial   *Streptococcus pneumoniae*
                      Staphylococcus pyogenes
                      Klebsiella pneumoniae

2. Mycoplasmal   *Mycoplasma pneumoniae*

3. Rickettsial   *Rickettsia burneti*

4. Viral   *Adenovirus*
                      Chlamydia (Psittacosis-ornithosis group)

Pneumonia due to *Haemophilus influenzae* occurs as a complication of chronic lung disease since this organism and *Streptococcus pneumoniae* are the commonest pathogens in chronic bronchitis and bronchiectasis. Other Gram-negative organisms such as *Pseudomonas aeruginosa, Escherichia coli* and *Proteus* are uncommon but likeliest to occur in a hospital setting in patients debilitated by chronic disease and with impaired immunity. Prolonged antibiotic therapy is liable to suppress the sensitive commensal organisms and favour resistant species such as Pseudomonas.

PATHOLOGY

The inhalation of virulent bacteria sets up an inflammatory reaction that is usually centred in the larger bronchi at the hilum of the lung. The inflammation may spread rapidly through a lobe towards the periphery, producing characteristic 'lobar' pneumonia. However, commonly the spread is more limited around the bronchi but extends down the airways, producing patches of inflammation of bronchial distribution. In severe bronchopneumonic infections adjacent patches of pneumonia may become confluent, so that the greater part of a lobe becomes involved, a picture very similar to that of true lobar pneumonia.

The inflammatory reaction consists of a phase of local vasodilation followed by an outpouring of exudate, comprising red cells, leucocytes and macrophages, fibrin and oedema fluid into and around the alveoli and small airways. The affected part of the lung becomes airless and solid—'consolidated'—and extension of the inflammation to the pleural surface causes an exudate and often a pleural effusion that occasionally becomes purulent. Virulent organisms may invade the bloodstream in sufficient numbers to cause a septicaemia with the possibility of metastatic abscess formation in distant organs such as the brain or kidneys. Local spread from the hilum may result in acute pericarditis and even involvement of the myocardium. Resolution of the pneumonia begins with ingestion and removal of bacteria and the exudative debris by leucocytes and macrophages, which finally clear the air spaces and in uncomplicated cases leave the lung tissue in its

previously normal condition. Nevertheless, local complications such as lung abscess, bronchiectasis and local fibrosis may result when resolution is incomplete, particularly when the infection is due to *Staphylococcus pyogenes* or *Klebsiella pneumoniae.*

In adenovirus pneumonia the pathological changes consist of marked alveolar exudation with hyaline membranes in the alveoli and respiratory bronchioles, oedematous thickening of the alveolar interstitium with lymphocyte infiltration and epithelial necrosis of the trachea and bronchi. Similar changes have been described in patients dying from rickettsial infections.

PREDISPOSING FACTORS

A variety of factors predispose to bacterial infection of the lung parenchyma. They may be grouped as follows:

1. Factors that lower the resistance of the individual to infection.
2. Viral infections of the upper respiratory tract.
3. Diameter of the airways.
4. Chronic infection of the airways.
5. Impairment of bronchial drainage.
6. Aspiration of infected material.

Lowered resistance appears to be an important predisposing factor to pneumonia in old age, partly because frailty and weakness reduce the effectiveness of the cough and presumably also because of a general impairment of the body's defence mechanisms. Chronic debilitating diseases such as uncontrolled diabetes mellitus and glomerulonephritis may have a similar effect, while conditions such as hypogammaglobulinaemia and multiple myelomatosis specifically interfere with the normal production of antibody. Corticosteroid therapy is also likely to suppress the normal immune mechanisms.

Viral infections commonly precede secondary bacterial pneumonia, including not only the respiratory viruses such as influenza and the respiratory syncytial virus but also the viruses of smallpox, chicken pox and measles.

Diameter of the Airways. The small size of the airways in infancy predisposes to bronchopneumonia in that age group.

Chronic airways obstruction, due to chronic bronchitis, bronchiectasis and cystic fibrosis, often predisposes to spread of bacterial infection into the lung parenchyma.

Impairment of bronchial drainage may be a factor in the development of pneumonia complicating chronic bronchitis or bronchiectasis, but it is also an important cause of pneumonia distal to a local obstruction such as bronchial carcinoma or adenoma, or an inhaled foreign body. Obstruction also frequently plays a part in the

production of postoperative pneumonia, due to a failure to expectorate infected bronchial secretions.

Aspiration pneumonia occurs in patients affected by chronic infection of the upper airways such as chronic sinusitis. It may also be due to the inhalation of ingested food material in patients with oesophageal obstruction, particularly achalasia of the cardia.

CLINICAL PRESENTATION

Acute bacterial pneumonia occurs in all age-groups, but the incidence tends to increase from middle age onwards, due partly to the presence of pre-existing illnesses such as chronic airways obstruction and chronic heart disease, and partly to the increasing frailty of the elderly. The incidence of acute pneumonia in healthy, well-nourished adolescents and adults is low in economically developed countries, possibly because of the widespread use of antibiotics in the treatment of minor respiratory infections. Viral and mycoplasmal pneumonias, on the other hand, are by no means uncommon in healthy young adults, and minor epidemics tend to occur among closely-knit communities such as military encampments and schools. Some modern forms of treatment have increased the liability of patients to acute infections such as pneumonia, including corticosteroid therapy and immunosuppressive agents. A brief enquiry into the patient's current medication may therefore be a relevant aspect of the history.

The *onset* of pneumonia is often sudden although it sometimes follows a minor upper respiratory infection of a few days duration. The major *symptoms* are:

1. General symptoms of infections, such as malaise, fever, rigors, vomiting, shivering and chilliness, and in the elderly, often confusion and disorientation.

2. Pulmonary symptoms of dyspnoea, cough, and sputum which is often bloodstained, viscid and difficult to expectorate.

3. Pleural symptoms of severe pain, aggravated by cough, deep breaths and movement, usually localised to the site of the inflammation but sometimes referred to the tip of the shoulder (from diaphragmatic inflammation) or to the abdomen when a lower lobe is involved.

It is difficult to differentiate between bacterial and non-bacterial pneumonias on clinical grounds. Viral, mycoplasmal and rickettsial infections tend to be dominated by non-pulmonary symptoms such as rhinitis, fever, myalgia and headache, but these features are by no means diagnostic.

On *general examination* the patient appears to be ill with sinus tachycardia, rapid respiratory rate and a high fever, flushed dry skin

and often herpes labialis. The pulmonary signs depend on the extent of the lesion; chest expansion is generally reduced on the side of the lesion but the mediastinum is central except in the presence of a large pleural effusion or pulmonary collapse. Where consolidation extends all the way from the large bronchi to the pleural surface the classical signs will be found: impaired percussion note, bronchial breath sounds, increased voice sounds with aegophony and whispering pectoriloquy. In less extensive inflammation, however, the percussion note may be barely altered, the breath sounds being either vesicular or having a muffled bronchial quality. Crepitations are heard over the affected area, and a pleural rub may be present.

In examining the cardiovascular system care should be taken to exclude underlying chronic heart disease, and evidence of possible complications should be looked for: atrial fibrillation or other arrhythmia suggesting the possibility of cardiac or pericardial infection; congestive cardiac failure or peripheral circulatory failure as indications of general deterioration. In examining the abdomen care must be taken to exclude a possible abdominal cause for the pulmonary inflammation, bearing in mind the occasional presentation of subphrenic infection by upward extension into the thorax. In acute infections such as pneumonia, urinary examination often reveals a small quantity of albumin, but the presence of excessive amounts of protein or of glucose may be an indication of chronic underlying disease such as glomerulonephritis or diabetes.

COURSE AND COMPLICATIONS

The course of acute bacterial pneumonia depends upon the infecting organism, its virulence, and the resistance of the affected individual. In minor infection of healthy people the response to antibiotic therapy is usually dramatic within twenty-four hours, all toxic signs having disappeared, the fever subsided, and the pulmonary signs begun to resolve. Virulent infections may cause septicaemia which increases the toxaemia and prostration although only rarely do distant septic foci develop into metastatic abscesses. If the lung infection is widespread the patient is liable to become cyanosed due to uneven distribution of pulmonary ventilation and perfusion, and the combination of hypoxia and toxaemia may lead to myocardial failure with peripheral circulatory failure, complications that indicate a very poor prognosis.

Pneumonia of viral, mycoplasmal or rickettsial origin usually follows a benign course which lasts for 10 or 14 days, although the radiological shadows may persist for some time after the symptoms have subsided. *Chlamydia* and Q fever infections are occasionally severe and prolonged with a significant mortality, and a few cases of fatal adenovirus pneumonia have been described in young adults.

Recovery from the primary lung infection does not necessarily imply complete resolution, since lung abscess, bronchiectasis, and pleural thickening due to empyema may leave a residue of distorted and damaged lung which is likely to be the cradle of chronic lung infection and respiratory disability in the future. For this reason infections with *Klebsiella pneumoniae* and *Staphylococcus pyogenes* are more likely to cause subsequent chronic lung disease, compared with pneumococcal and viral infections which commonly leave the affected areas of lung undamaged. In healthy middle-aged men pneumonia is not infrequently the presenting feature of bronchial carcinoma, and this possibility should be excluded before a confident prognosis is given.

SPECIFIC CLINICAL FEATURES

Streptococcus pneumoniae Infection. The particular features to be remembered about pneumococcal pneumonia, considered against the general background described above, are:

1. It is the commonest form of pneumonia (80% of cases) and tends particularly to affect infants and the aged, in whom it often takes the *broncho*pneumonic form.

2. Lobar pneumonia due to the pneumococcus, although the 'classical' form of pneumonia in adults is now relatively uncommon, and if seen should arouse the suspicion of bronchial obstruction as an underlying cause.

3. Resolution of pneumococcal pneumonia is good, and there are usually no sequelae. The organism is almost always sensitive to penicillin, although tetracycline-resistant infections have become increasingly recognised in some areas.

4. Septicaemia is an important complication and is usually associated with Type III pneumococcus. Before the introduction of antibiotics or sulphonamides in the treatment of pneumonia the most effective method was the use of type-specific antisera, and for this reason the typing of the infecting strain of pneumococcus became standard practice. Type III has always been known as a particularly lethal strain, and as recently as 1968 figures from the USA showed that it is still likely to cause a high mortality in spite of the use of antibiotics and modern supportive measures.

5. The pneumococcus is one of the two most common infective agents in chronic bronchitis (the other is *Haemophilus influenzae*), and it is therefore frequently responsible for secondary pneumonia superimposed on chronic airways obstruction.

Staphylococcol Pneumonia. Although this can occur as a primary infection it is more commonly seen as a secondary invader. The

following characteristics should be noted:

1. It is a common cause of secondary pneumonia in patients debilitated by chronic lung disease, such as cystic fibrosis, in which antibiotics have been used for long periods.

2. In influenza epidemics it may be responsible for acute, short-lived and lethal pneumonia.

3. Response to antibiotics is unpredictable—often the organism may have developed resistance, particularly to penicillin.

4. The spread of infection is usually bronchial rather than lobar in distribution, with damage to bronchial and bronchiolar walls which may lead to subsequent bronchiectasis.

5. Severe sequelae are common, lung abscess and empyema being frequent complications, and tissue destruction is characteristic of the infection.

Klebsiella pneumoniae (Friedlander's bacillus) Infection. This is an infrequent cause of pneumonia (1% of all causes), but important because the infection is destructive, mortality is high and sequelae are common.

1. The onset is particularly acute and prostration is severe; the sputum is usually blood-stained and often gelatinous, having a 'red-currant jelly' appearance.

2. The organism is *not* sensitive to penicillin, so that early bacteriological diagnosis is essential in order to start effective treatment with streptomycin plus oxytetracycline.

3. In spite of antibiotics the mortality is 40 per cent, and is particularly high in elderly or weakly people.

4. Bronchiectasis, abscess formation, cavitation and empyema are common destructive sequelae which lead to subsequent chronic respiratory difficulty.

5. The infection may become chronic with severe progressive destruction of lung tissue and a protracted illness that may ultimately convert the patient into a respiratory cripple.

Mycoplasma Pneumoniae Infection (primary atypical pneumonia). Mycoplasmata are small organisms, of the same order of size as the influenza viruses (80 to 120 mμ), but can be cultivated on artificial media. *Mycoplasma pneumoniae* commonly causes a minor infectious illness of the upper and lower respiratory tract, pneumonia being its most serious manifestation. It is most likely to affect children and young adults, particularly those living in closed communities. It has the following clinical characteristics:

1. Constitutional symptoms such as headache, malaise and fever often precede the respiratory symptoms for a few days, crepitations

and radiological abnormalities of the chest appearing some days after the onset of the illness.

2. The most common radiological signs are patchy areas of consolidation and evidence of pleural reaction. Hilar lymphadenopathy occasionally occurs in young people.

3. The illness usually settles within ten days, but protracted illness and lethargy with recurrent abnormal signs in the chest are not uncommon. A few patients relapse after making an initial improvement.

4. The organism is sensitive *in vitro* to a number of antibiotics including tetracycline, streptomycin, and erythromycin, but not to penicillin. The clinical response to antibiotic therapy is often disappointing in spite of apparent *in vitro* sensitivity, and new symptoms or radiological signs may continue to appear in spite of such treatment.

5. Infection may be recognised serologically by means of a specific complement fixation test. Significant titres of cold agglutinins to human Group O red cells develop in about 50 per cent of cases, but a similar reaction is not unknown in patients with other forms of pneumonia.

6. A number of non-respiratory complications of the infection are seen occasionally, including haemolytic anaemia associated with a high titre of cold agglutinins, rashes such as erythema multiforme and Stevens-Johnson syndrome, and occasional neurological complications such as meningo-encephalitis, aseptic meningitis, and acute peripheral neuritis. More rarely, acute pericarditis and acute febrile arthralgia or arthropathy occur.

7. The prognosis is almost uniformly good.

Q Fever. The causative organism, *Rickettsia burneti,* primarily infects cattle, sheep and goats, and many infections in man originate from contact with these animals, probably by the inhalation of dust containing the rickettsiae, or from drinking raw milk. Nevertheless, there are many records of infection among persons who had had no known contact with any animal.

1. The disease most commonly appears as atypical pneumonia but with headache and myalgia as prominent symptoms.

2. There is a prolonged incubation period of up to 28 days.

3. The infection may be confirmed by finding complement-fixing antibody against *R. burneti,* a rise in titre between the acute and convalescent stages of the illness being suggestive of infection.

4. The course of the illness is usually short (up to 8 days) and benign, but chronic and recurrent infection can occur. Rickettsial

endocarditis is a rare complication in patients suffering from underlying valvular disease, and is frequently fatal.

5. The infection responds to treatment with the tetracyclines but prolonged therapy may be necessary to avoid relapse.

Adenovirus Pneumonia. Although adenoviruses may cause an acute and sometimes fatal pneumonia in infants, in adults and older children the infection is nearly always benign and does not seem to lead to secondary bacterial infection. The clinical presentation and behaviour of adenovirus infection does not differ in any significant respect from that due to *Mycoplasma pneumoniae,* the main differentiating features being the absence of the cold agglutinin reaction and the identification of the virus by serological methods. Adenovirus pneumonia occurs typically in minor epidemics among service personnel and in residential schools.

Chlamydia Infection. The psittacosis-ornithosis group of viruses were originally recognised as causing severe and often fatal pneumonia among patients who had been in direct contact with sick birds, particularly those of the parrot family. It has since been recognised that about 10 per cent of cases of benign 'viral' pneumonia show serological evidence of infection with one or other of the *Chlamydia* group, and serological signs of infection may occur in the absence of any respiratory illness. Infection in man is acquired by inhalation of the excreta of birds, but may be passed on by direct droplet spread.

1. The infection should be suspected among patients showing the symptoms and signs of pneumonia who have a history of contact with birds, especially parrots and, occasionally, pigeons.

2. The infection may be diagnosed by recovery of the organism from the sputum and by a specific serological complement fixation reaction.

3. The organism responds to treatment with tetracycline and occasionally penicillin. Oxytetracycline in a dose of 1 to 2 g daily is the recommended treatment, begun as early as possible in the course of the illness.

INVESTIGATION OF PNEUMONIA

The earliest essential investigation is clinical and bacteriological examination of the *sputum.* The appearance of the sputum may give some clue to the causative organism, for example, the 'rusty' sputum of pneumococcal pneumonia or the red-currant jelly appearance sometimes seen in Klebsiella infections, but early bacteriological studies are the most useful guide to the choice of antibiotic therapy. Not only the organisms but also its sensitivities should be sought.

Suspicion of viral, rickettsial or mycoplasmal pneumonia should lead to microbiological investigation. Paired sera taken at the beginning of the illness and during the convalescent phase may demonstrate a rise in antibody titre to one of the suspected infective agents by complement-fixation techniques, but in most cases the diagnosis is obtained only after the patient has recovered from the acute illness. Although isolation and early identification of these organisms is possible by methods such as tissue culture, fluorescent antibody techniques, and electron microscopy, these procedures are too laborious for routine use in infections so generally benign.

The *chest radiograph* is useful in confirming the nature of the underlying pathology (for example, bronchial carcinoma, the presence of cavitation, coincidental pulmonary collapse) and in defining the extent of the pneumonia and of complications such as pleural effusion. It is invaluable in plotting the course of the disease through the stages of resolution and is essential as a check for complete resolution in the exclusion of bronchial carcinoma as an underlying cause of the acute infection. Lateral views of the chest should not be omitted, and tomography may sometimes be necessary to elucidate the nature of a persistent shadow.

The *blood count* usually shows an acute polymorphonuclear leucocytosis in bacterial pneumonia, with a leucocyte count ranging from 15,000 to 30,000 per mm^3. Persistence of the leucocytosis may be an indication of abscess formation or of empyema. Haemolytic anaemia may be associated with cold agglutinins in *Mycoplasma pneumoniae* infections. In severely ill patients a positive blood culture may be obtained.

In the severely ill cyanosed patient respiratory failure with carbon dioxide retention may develop, usually in those with chronic ventilation:perfusion inequality due to longstanding airways obstruction. Measurement of the *arterial carbon dioxide tension* in such cases gives a useful guide to the progression of respiratory failure and is an important preliminary to initiating assisted ventilation.

An *electrocardiogram* may be indicated when underlying heart disease is suspected, particularly cor pulmonale due to chronic airways obstruction. The presence of chronic cardiac disease has an important bearing on prognosis and is an indication for watchfulness in case of developing cardiac failure or arrhythmias.

MANAGEMENT

Although antibiotic therapy has altered the whole course of treatment in the bacterial pneumonias it is common experience in hospital practice that successful treatment requires considerably more

care than simple choice of an antibiotic, especially among those patients whose illness is complicated by age or underlying disease. Choice of antibiotic and general aspects of management are considered separately in the following paragraphs.

Antibiotic Therapy. In the early stages of treatment, before bacteriological data is available, the choice of antibiotic depends upon:

1. Clinical assessment of the acute illness: does it have, for example, the clinical characteristics of pneumococcal or *Klebsiella* pneumonia? If so, the antibiotic can be selected from those known to be effective against that particular organism.

2. A history of chronic lung disease, implying a likelihood of infection with untypical and possibly antibiotic-resistant organisms. If so, a wide-spectrum antibiotic or one that is effective against penicillin-resistant organisms may be indicated.

3. Knowledge of previous and presumably unsuccessful antibiotic therapy that has already been prescribed. Provided a reasonable trial of the antibiotic has been given it would seem sensible to change treatment to an alternative drug.

Apart from these major factors, consideration should be given to the possibility of sensitivity reactions, the relative cost of different antibiotics and the route of administration since, in severe infections, it is usually preferable to give the antibiotic parentally to ensure adequate blood and tissue levels.

In general terms, intramuscular benzylpenicillin is the treatment of first choice in primary bacterial pneumonia since the pneumococcus is the likeliest infecting organism. A history of underlying chronic infection such as bronchitis or bronchiectasis indicates the need for an antibiotic with a broader spectrum of activity such as ampicillin by intramuscular injection, or amoxycillin, tetracycline or co-trimoxazole by mouth. If infection with penicillin-resistant staphylococci is suspected a combination of benzylpenicillin with one of the penicillinase-resistant penicillins (methicillin or cloxacillin parenterally, or flucloxacillin by mouth) should be used. *Klebsiella* infections are probably best treated with a combination of streptomycin with another drug such as oxytetracyline, co-trimoxazole or one of the cephalosporins, but as a general rule it is probably advisable to reserve streptomycin for the treatment of tuberculosis.

In view of the fact that the tetracyclines are effective in pneumonia due to *Mycoplasma pneumoniae, Chlamydia* infection or *Rickettsia burneti,* a clinical diagnosis of these conditions is an indication for

treatment with oxytetracycline 500 mg 6-hourly until the fever subsides. A reduced dose can be continued thereafter until all radiological signs have disappeared. Tables 13.2 and 13.3 show the effectiveness, dose schedules and contra-indications of the various antibiotics at present most widely used in the treatment of pneumonia.

The antibiotic regimen should be changed if the clinical response is unsatisfactory, but not solely on the grounds of laboratory evidence of resistance of the organism. If a change is indicated sputum or blood culture may suggest the correct alternative choice, based on the

Table 13.2

Antibacterial Chemotherapy

Micro-organism	*Drug of Choice*	*Other Effective Agents*
Streptococcus pneumoniae Streptococcus pyogenes	Penicillin	Erythromycin Oxytetracycline Cephalosporins
Staphylococcus pyogenes (a) Penicillin sensitive (b) Penicillin resistant	Penicillin Methicillin or Cloxacillin with Penicillin	Cephalosporins Fusidic acid Erythromycin Lincomycin Clindamycin
Klebsiella pneumoniae	Streptomycin with Oxytetracycline	Cephalosporins Chloramphenicol
Haemophilus influenzae	Oxytetracycline	Co-trimoxazole Ampicillin Chloramphenicol
Escherichia coli	According to sputum sensitivities	Oxytetracycline Cephalosporins Carbenicillin Kanamycin
Proteus mirabilis	According to sputum sensitivities	Cephalosporins Ampicillin Carbenicillin Kanamycin Chloramphenicol
Pseudomonas aeruginosa	According to sputum sensitivities	Colistin Gentamycin with Carbenicillin
Mycoplasma pneumoniae	Oxytetracycline	
Rickettsia burneti	Oxytetracycline	
Chlamydia group	Oxytetracycline	

Table 13.3

Dose Schedules and Toxic Effects of Antibacterial Agents

Antibacterial Agent	Dose Schedule (Adults)			Toxic Effects and Contra-indications
	Oral	Intramuscular	Intravenous	
Ampicillin	500 mg 6-hourly*	500 mg 6-hourly	—	Penicillin hypersensitivity
Carbenicillin	—	—	20–30 g in 24 hours	Penicillin hypersensitivity
Cephaloridine	—	0.5–1 g 6-hourly	4–12 g in 24 hours	Hypersensitivity, nephrotoxicity in large doses
Cephalexin	250–500 mg 6-hourly	—	—	Severe bone marrow depression
Chloramphenicol	500 mg 6-hourly	—	—	Occasional diarrhoea and skin rashes
Clindamycin	150–300 mg 6-hourly	—	—	Penicillin hypersensitivity
Cloxacillin	0.5 g 4–6 hourly†	250 mg 6-hourly	—	Nephrotoxic and neurotoxic
Colistin	—	1–2 mega units 8-hourly	—	Drug rashes
Co-trimoxazole	2 tablets twice daily	—	—	Haematological effects due to folate deficiency, sulphonamide hypersensitivity, skin rashes. Avoid in pregnancy
Erythromycin	250–500 mg 6-hourly	—	1–2 g in 24 hours	
Fusidic acid	0.5 g 6-hourly	—	—	
Gentamicin	—	80 mg 8–12 hourly	—	Ototoxic
Kanamycin	—	500 mg 12-hourly	—	Nephrotoxic and ototoxic
Lincomycin	500 mg 8-hourly	300–600 mg 12-hourly	600 mg 8–12 hourly	Diarrhoea
Methicillin	—	1 g 4-hourly	—	Penicillin hypersensitivity
Oxytetracycline	250–500 mg 6-hourly	250 mg 12-hourly	—	Gastro-intestinal effects; pruritus; avoid in pregnancy or in children under 9 years because of damage to developing teeth and bones; avoid in renal failure
Penicillin	Phenoxymethylpenicillin 250 mg 6-hourly	Benzylpenicillin 300–600 mg 6-hourly	Benzylpenicillin 1,200–2,400 mg in 24 hours	Hypersensitivity: fatal anaphylaxis, fever, urticaria, systemic reactions, contact dermatitis
Streptomycin	—	0.5 g 12-hourly	—	Ototoxic

* Amoxycillin (250–500 mg 6-hourly) is better absorbed than ampicillin.

apparent sensitivity of the organism shown on culture. Treatment should be continued for several days after the infection has subsided, and for longer periods up to two weeks in patients with chronic underlying disease such as cystic fibrosis of the lungs.

Supportive Treatment. General supportive management should include rest in bed, preferably in hospital if the infection is at all severe. The patient should be encouraged to eat what he fancies and an adequate fluid intake should be maintained, especially because hyperventilation, vomiting and sweating are liable to lead to dehydration. A record of fluid intake and output must be kept. Hyperpyrexia requires cooling by tepid sponging and the use of fans.

Pleuritic pain should be relieved by analgesics given in adequate dosage as frequently as required. Sometimes pethidine or morphine are required because of the severity of the pain, but respiratory depressants such as morphine should be prescribed warily in patients who show signs of respiratory failure since respiratory depression will be further enhanced. Morphine is also likely to lower the systemic blood pressure and may aggravate peripheral circulatory failure.

Exhausting cough may be suppressed when it is painful and unproductive, using Codeine Linctus BP, but when airways obstruction due to bronchial secretions is contributing to dyspnoea and respiratory embarrassment coughing should be encouraged in association with regular physiotherapy and postural drainage. Nitrazepam 5 mg may be used to encourage sleep.

Cyanosis should be treated by oxygen inhalation by oronasal mask; if arterial carbon dioxide tension is normal or low it is probably safe to give a high oxygen concentration (i.e. up to 60% oxygen) provided that careful watch is kept on the patient's state of consciousness and on the arterial carbon dioxide tension. If there is any suspicion of respiratory failure with carbon dioxide retention the concentration of oxygen administered should be low (24 to 28%) and it should be given by means of a mask that does not increase airway dead space (i.e. Venturi mask).

Congestive heart failure may be managed by digitalisation and the use of oral or intravenous diuretic therapy. To obtain a rapid diuretic response frusemide may be given intravenously (40 mg), followed by a daily or twice daily oral diuretic such as bendrofluazide (2·5 to 10 mg daily) or chlorothiazide (0·5 to 2 g daily). Potassium supplements are necessary.

COMPLICATIONS OF PNEUMONIA

Pleurisy

Pleurisy is not a diagnosis but a set of symptoms and signs that

indicate there is inflammation of the pleural membranes. It is characterised by localised chest pain which is sharp and severe, and aggravated by respiratory movements or by external pressure over the inflamed area. When the diaphragmatic pleura is affected the pain may be referred to the tip of the shoulder, or to the upper abdomen from pleurisy affecting the lower lobes. The characteristic signs are rapid, shallow respirations and a pleural friction rub but in many cases these are soon replaced by the signs of pleural effusion as inflammatory exudate accumulates in the pleural space. 'Dry' pleurisy, i.e. pleurisy without clinical or radiological evidence of effusion, is usually due to underlying lung disease such as pneumonia, bronchiectasis, lung cancer, or infarction, but may also occur as a result of external injury to the chest wall, occasionally in rheumatoid arthritis, and in infections with Coxsackie B virus (epidemic pleurodynia or Bornholm disease) although a small pleural effusion is sometimes seen in these conditions.

Bornholm disease is a benign infection occurring in minor epidemics that are commonest in the summer months. It is characterised by sudden attacks of pleuritic and myalgic pain in the thorax and abdomen which are aggravated by movement and may be severe enough to cause considerable prostration and anxiety. The pain often comes and goes inexplicably and may be associated with mild upper respiratory symptoms such as nasal congestion and sore throat, slight fever, and malaise. The diagnosis can be established by demonstrating a rising titre of complement-fixing antibodies in paired sera. The illness usually lasts for five or six days and then subsides without sequelae, its main importance lying in the need to differentiate it from other more serious thoracic or abdominal disorders. Pericarditis is an occasional complication.

Pleural Effusion

A pleural effusion is the usual sequel to pleural inflammation, inflammatory exudate accumulating in the pleural space in sufficient quantity to be seen on the chest radiograph or to be detected clinically. Pleural effusions may also be due to transudation of extra-cellular fluid and to accumulation of pus, blood, or chyle. When it occurs as a complication of pneumonia it commonly consists of a yellow serous fluid with the high protein content characteristic of an exudate (more than 3 g/100 ml). Pleural effusions secondary to pneumonia are usually reabsorbed as the underlying infection subsides, but large effusions occasionally cause ventilatory embarrassment during the acute phase of the illness and require aspiration. If the effusion appears to be persisting in spite of progressive recovery from

the pneumonia, aspiration is indicated to prevent subsequent pleural fibrosis and restrictive impairment of ventilation.

The clinical signs and differential diagnosis of pleural effusion are further discussed on page 111.

Empyema

An empyema is a pleural effusion that contains pus, due to infection of the pleural cavity from the lung or occasionally from penetrating injury of the chest wall. Less commonly, infection of the pleura may arise by blood stream or lymphatic spread, or through the diaphragm from abdominal disease such as subphrenic abscess. Usually there is evidence of bacterial pneumonia which has extended to involve the visceral pleura, often with the formation of lung abscess; this may discharge into a bronchus and into the pleural space, resulting in a bronchopleural fistula and pyopneumothorax. Bronchiectasis and bronchial neoplasms are also frequent causes of infection extending into the pleural space.

CLINICAL PRESENTATION

The diagnosis of empyema should be considered in any patient with pleural effusion due to primary or secondary bacterial pneumonia whose recovery is delayed or interrupted by an exacerbation of toxic symptoms, especially high swinging fever and prostration. Rigors and pleuritic pain may occur, and in longstanding cases, loss of weight. In contrast, the onset of symptoms due to empyema resulting from more chronic lung disease such as tuberculosis or actinomycosis, bronchiectasis, lung abscess, or carcinoma may be insidious and difficult to define, especially when random antibiotic therapy has reduced but not terminated the infection. Cough, purulent sputum and chest pain occur, associated with symptoms of pyogenic infection, such as fever, malaise, anorexia, sweating, rigors, palpitation, fatigue and anaemia. Apart from non-specific signs of infection such as pyrexia and tachycardia, digital clubbing may develop within two to three weeks, while the local signs in the chest are similar to those of a pleural effusion. In chronic empyema the chest wall is flattened and the ribs crowded over the affected area. Occasionally, a sinus may be seen on the chest wall overlying the empyema, where it has discharged to the exterior ('empyema necessitas'), while inward rupture through the lung to a bronchus may result in the expectoration of a large quantity of blood-stained purulent sputum and the formation of a bronchopleural fistula. A polymorphonuclear leucocytosis of 20,000 cells/mm^3 or more is a usual accompaniment of empyema.

The chest radiograph shows a homogeneous opacity sometimes

similar to that of pleural effusion but often localised by adhesions. In chronic cases the dense fibrosis associated with the infection leads to shift of the mediastinum to the affected side, crowding of the ribs and elevation of the diaphragm. A fluid level indicates that air is also present in the pleural cavity, due either to a bronchopleural fistula or as a result of trauma to the thoracic cage.

DIAGNOSIS

The diagnosis is usually established by aspiration of the fluid, which should be cultured in order to discover the infecting organism and its sensitivities, although the pus is frequently sterile. In the past, the pneumococcus and haemolytic streptococcus were commonly responsible for the majority of cases, but resistant staphylococcal, *H. influenzae* and *Klebsiella* infections now play an increasingly prominent part in the pathogenesis of empyema. Actinomycosis is a rare cause and tubercle bacilli should always be sought by direct microscopy and culture. Since lung infection is the commonest cause of empyema the sputum should also be cultured.

TREATMENT

The treatment of empyema in the *acute* stage depends on the use of the appropriate antibiotic, as indicated by the sensitivity of bacterial culture obtained from an aspirate or from a sputum sample. In the early exudative stage of the disease thin pus should be aspirated as often as is necessary to obliterate the empyema space and keep the lung fully inflated, but continuous drainage to a water seal may be necessary if the fluid re-accumulates very rapidly. As the exudate becomes fibrino-purulent the empyema tends to become loculated and the lung stiffened by pleural thickening and fibrosis; at this stage closed intercostal drainage with suction is indicated. When the empyema becomes *chronic* the exudate and the walls of the empyema cavity become fibrosed, loculation is characteristic and the affected portion of collapsed lung becomes fixed by pleural fibrosis. Rib resection and open drainage may be necessary to achieve healing, but where this fails thoracotomy and decortication of the lung with removal of the empyema sac are indicated, allowing the lung to re-expand to obliterate the dead space.

LUNG ABSCESS

A lung abscess is a cavitating lesion due to accumulation of pus and necrosis of tissue in an area of lung infected by pyogenic organisms, and is thus distinguished aetiologically from necrosis in a malignant

tumour or tuberculous cavitation, although these diagnoses demand automatic consideration when lung abscess is suspected.

The usual *causes* of lung abscess are:

1. Aspiration of infected material during unconsciousness or sleep.
2. Pneumonia, particularly due to *Klebsiella pneumoniae*, haemolytic streptococcus and staphylococcus.

Other less common causes are septic necrosis of a pulmonary infarct, septic embolisation of the lung in pyaemia, fungal infections such as actinomycosis, nocardiosis and coccidioidomycosis, amoebic abscess, and secondarily infected congenital or hydatid cysts.

CLINICAL PRESENTATION

Lung abscess should be included in the differential diagnosis of any febrile illness associated with cough, purulent sputum, haemoptysis and chest pain which either occurs as an exacerbation of symptoms or as a delay to recovery in a patient with bacterial pneumonia, or else follows by a period of a few days an episode of unconsciousness. An enquiry should be made into a history of recent anaesthesia (especially for dental surgery), unconsciousness, alcoholism or drug addiction that might suggest an abscess had arisen as a result of aspiration of infected material at a time when the cough reflex was depressed or absent. In addition, laryngeal palsy or oesophageal obstruction may result in 'spill over' of infected saliva or ingested food into the airways especially during sleep, and a history of such abnormalities should be sought. Evidence of pre-existing respiratory tract infection is often obtained, such as sinusitis, dental sepsis, and chronic bronchitis.

The *symptoms* of lung abscess are fever, malaise, a cough productive of purulent and often blood-stained sputum, and pleuritic or aching chest pain. The sudden production of copious amounts of offensive sputum during the illness suggests that the abscess has discharged into a bronchus, and clarifies the diagnosis. The local *signs* are usually not those typical of cavitation but merely localised impairment of percussion note with crepitations and possibly a pleural friction rub. The signs of an effusion may be present. Clubbing of the digits often develops after a few weeks in chronic lung abscess.

INVESTIGATION

In the initial stages of a lung abscess the *chest radiograph* shows an opaque shadow which only later develops a cavity when the abscess discharges into a bronchus; at this stage a fluid level is seen. The site of the abscess may give an indication of its aetiology since aspiration usually occurs with the patient lying on his back or his side so that

infected material tends to find its way into the dependent bronchi, i.e. those leading to the apical segment of the lower lobe of the right lung or to the axillary part of the posterior segment of an upper lobe. Tuberculous cavities are likely to be adjacent to areas of recognisable tuberculous infiltration, but the possibility of a necrotic carcinomatous cavity occurring in such an area should not be neglected, particularly if the abscess fails to resolve in spite of adequate antituberculous therapy. Calcification in the wall of an abscess favours a diagnosis of tuberculosis.

Culture of the *sputum* in order to ascertain the nature and sensitivity of the infecting organism is a necessary preliminary to effective antibiotic therapy. It should also be examined for tubercle bacilli and for malignant cells. Where the abscess is due to actinomycosis typical 'sulphur granules' may be visible in the sputum; ova and cysts should be sought when amoebic abscess is suspected. The *blood count* usually shows a polymorphonuclear leucocytosis of 15 to 30,000 cells/mm^3, and a normocytic normochromic anaemia may develop if the abscess becomes chronic.

TREATMENT

The initial treatment is with an antibiotic that is effective against the organisms concerned, for example, benzylpenicillin intramuscularly in a dose of 1·2 to 6 g daily or more to ensure adequate tissue levels. Treatment should be continued until a satisfactory response is obtained, usually 4 to 6 weeks. The response to treatment should be gauged by the daily reduction in sputum volume and diminution in size of the abscess as judged by serial chest X-rays. Drainage of a cavity should be encouraged by physiotherapy and carefully orientated postural drainage. When an abscess fails to resolve bronchoscopy is necessary to exclude the possibility of a malignant aetiology, or to remove obstructive slough. Surgical removal of the affected lobe is indicated if the abscess persists despite adequate antibiotics and physiotherapy.

14

Pulmonary Tuberculosis

Incidence

Although the incidence of tuberculosis has been declining steadily in the developed countries, especially since effective chemotherapeutic agents became available, the disease remains one of the world's most important causes of ill-health and death.

Human disease can be caused by three types of mycobacteria, the human, the bovine, and the avian strains of which the last named is a rare cause of pulmonary tuberculosis, producing a chronic, indolent infection that is very difficult to treat because the organisms tend to be resistant to the antibiotics at present available. Bovine tuberculosis has been almost eradicated in many developed countries, including the United Kingdom, so that the virtual sole source of infection in these countries is the reservoir of human carriers.

FACTORS INFLUENCING DEVELOPMENT OF THE DISEASE

The factors affecting the development of active tuberculosis are:

1. The size of the infecting dose. The importance of this factor is illustrated by the observation that the incidence of active tuberculosis among child contacts of patients with positive sputum on direct smear was 17 per cent, compared with only 2·6 per cent for contacts of those whose sputum was only positive on culture, and 0·9 per cent for contacts of culture negative patients.

2. Virulence of the infecting organism. Certain strains, particularly those from South India, appear to have diminished virulence.

3. The acquisition of resistance either by prior infection or by BCG vaccination.

4. Environmental factors that lower resistance, including malnutrition, poor and overcrowded housing, alcoholism, heavy smoking, corticosteroid therapy, and certain occupations such as those leading to silicosis.

5. Certain other coincidental diseases, including diabetes mellitus, the pneumoconioses, and following partial gastrectomy.

6. Racial characteristics. Tuberculosis is more prone to develop among populations not previously exposed to the disease.

In all developed countries where treatment and prevention of tuberculosis is actively undertaken there has been a tendency for the incidence of the disease and its mortality to decline steeply among the younger age groups of both sexes in the past twenty years, but this decline has been much less marked among the elderly, particularly among men.

In the first five years of life primary infection is especially likely to be complicated by haematogenous spread of the disease, resulting in miliary tuberculosis, tuberculous meningitis or involvement of bones and joints. Thereafter the incidence of serious disease declines until puberty, but during adolescence and early adult life the likelihood of progressive pulmonary tuberculosis increases, although the advent of effective chemotherapy and BCG vaccination has very markedly reduced the morbidity and mortality in this age group. The relative increase in incidence of the disease among the middle-aged and elderly, particularly in men, is attributed to persistence of infection contracted at a time when the prevalence of the disease was high and treatment and preventive measures inadequate, to higher susceptibility to infection among the earlier generation, and to the deleterious effects of cigarette smoking and alcohol.

Pathology

Mycobacterium tuberculosis may be recognised in a sputum smear as a rod-shaped organism stained pink with Ziehl-Neelsen stain. It is relatively specific for the tubercle bacillus since the organism retains the stain despite washing with alcohol and acid solution. It is slow-growing but may be cultured either in Lowenstein-Jensen medium or by inoculation of a guinea-pig in which it produces a fatal infection within six weeks.

The tissue response to infection with *Mycobacterium tuberculosis* consists of a chronic granulomatous lesion, at the centre of which lie the bacilli surrounded by a greater or lesser amount of necrotic material consisting of dead tissue and leucocytes, and having an appearance somewhat similar to creamy cheese, which has given to the process of its formation the name of 'caseation'. The necrotic area is surrounded by large mononuclear macrophages known as epitheloid cells, some of which coalesce to form multinucleate giant cells (Langhan's cells). Around the zone of epithelioid and giant cells is a rim of lymphocytes interspersed with fibroblasts which form a zone of fibrous tissue between the tubercle and the normal tissues of the lung. Longstanding lesions tend to become calcified. This basic pattern of pathological response is common to tuberculous foci developing in any tissue although factors such as the severity and virulence of the

infection and the resistance of the host may modify some features of the reaction.

PRIMARY FOCUS AND PRIMARY COMPLEX

In patients who have not previously been subjected to tuberculous infection the initial invasion of the lung causes a typical tuberculous reaction in any lung lobe but usually somewhere in the periphery of the lung fields. This primary focus is quickly followed by spread of infection via the lymphatics to the hilar lymph nodes where a further tuberculous inflammatory reaction is set up, the combination of peripheral pulmonary focus and hilar lymphadenopathy being known as the primary complex. The subsequent behaviour of the infection depends on the interplay between host resistance and the size and virulence of the infection; in favourable circumstances both primary focus and hilar gland infection become walled off by fibrous tissue with phagocytosis and destruction of the tubercle bacilli followed by calcification, leaving nothing but a few flecks of calcium in the hilum and the subpleural region of the lung to give radiological evidence of past tuberculous infection.

Where containment of the infection is less effective there may be spread from the primary focus to the pleural cavity causing *pleural effusion* or even occasionally *tuberculous empyema*. The primary focus may progress and break down, causing *cavitation* and discharge of infected material into the airways whence it may be inhaled to distant parts of the lung; more commonly, however, cavitation is taken to be a sign of postprimary infection. *Haematogenous spread* of the primary infection is due to invasion of the pulmonary veins, whence the bacilli are borne to distant organs such as the meninges, kidneys, and joints, or it may be due to lymphatic spread of infection to the superior vena cava resulting in *miliary spread* of the disease to the lungs and sometimes to other organs such as the spleen, kidneys, and liver. Hilar lymphadenopathy may cause *airways obstruction and emphysema* by external pressure upon a bronchus, and necrosis of an infected lymph node may be followed by discharge of caseous material into a bronchus, leading to *tuberculous bronchopneumonia*. The association of segmental or lobar consolidation or collapse with hilar gland enlargement is known as *epituberculosis,* a relatively benign complication of the primary infection in which a localised monocytic or polymorphonuclear exudate in the affected lobe or segment is followed by a rapid hypersensitivity reaction and gradual resolution of the infection. Spread of the disease along the submucosal lymphatics of the bronchi produces a series of tubercles and sometimes ulceration of the bronchial mucosa. Involvement of the bronchial vessels by the inflammatory process leads to impairment of

the blood supply to the bronchial walls, resulting in destructive changes and subsequent *bronchiectasis*.

POSTPRIMARY TUBERCULOSIS

In the majority of cases primary infection is followed by resolution both of the primary focus and the associated lymph node infection over a period of a few weeks, often with little or no systemic disturbance to the patient. During this period the patient develops hypersensitivity to the tubercle bacillus, demonstrable by a positive tuberculin skin test, which induces increased resistance to subsequent infection. Technically, therefore, any new lesion or any further development of a primary lesion arising after hypersensitivity has occurred is called a postprimary infection.

Postprimary infection may occur:

1. As a progressive primary lesion, spreading in one or other of the ways described above.
2. As a result of reactivation of a primary lesion.
3. Due to subsequent exogenous infection.

Most cases of postprimary tuberculosis result either from progression of a primary lesion or from reactivation of a dormant primary or postprimary lesion. The causes of reactivation of infection include the development of other severe illness, malnutrition, local trauma to quiescent foci, intercurrent lung infection and, of great importance, systemic corticosteroid therapy.

The basic histological lesion is similar to that described in the section on primary tuberculosis. The common sites for postprimary foci are the posterior segment of the upper lobe and the apical segment of the lower lobe, a tendency attributed to the good ventilation but decreased blood flow of these areas. Considerable *fibrosis* occurs in longstanding disease, often associated with *cavity formation* and *bronchiectasis*. Tuberculous bronchopneumonia, empyema and haematogenous spread of infection may complicate postprimary infection in a manner similar to the progressive primary lesion.

Hypersensitivity

During the first few weeks of a primary infection with *Mycobacterium tuberculosis* the patient becomes hypersensitive to a protein moiety of the tubercle bacillus. This hypersensitivity is displayed by oedema (induration) and redness of the skin which follows within 48 to 72 hours the intradermal injection of protein-containing material obtained from tubercle bacilli. The absence of a positive skin reaction

is generally taken to mean that there has been no earlier tuberculous infection, but other causes of a negative response must be excluded:

1. The infection may be so recent that hypersensitivity has not yet developed.

2. The test may have been incorrectly performed, or the antigenic material used may be inactive.

3. The patient may be undergoing treatment with drugs, e.g. systemic corticosteroids, which suppress the normal hypersensitivity reaction.

4. The patient may be concurrently affected by a disease, e.g. sarcoidosis or Hodgkin's disease, which is responsible for suppression of hypersensitivity reactions.

5. Miliary tuberculosis, or severe illness due to widespread tuberculous infection may be associated with a negative response.

TUBERCULIN TESTING

A number of different preparations are available for intradermal injection to detect hypersensitivity. Those most commonly used in the United Kingdom are either Old Tuberculin (OT) which is prepared by evaporation from a filtrate of cultures of *Mycobacterium tuberculosis,* or a purified protein derivative (PPD). The *Mantoux Test* is performed by injecting 0·1 ml of OT intradermally with a fine needle on the anterior surface of the forearm, the test being done in three successive stages using first 1 : 10,000, then 1 : 1,000, and finally 1 : 100 strength solutions of the antigen if the weaker dose fails to give a positive result. The test is read 48 to 72 hours after the injection, a positive result consisting of an area of induration 10 mm or more in diameter. Erythema is of no significance. The gradually increasing concentration of OT is used in order to avoid the development of local necrosis and ulceration which may occur at the site of the injection in patients with marked hypersensitivity associated with active progressive tuberculosis, especially children.

The *Heaf Multipuncture Test* makes use of an instrument actuated by a spring which allows six, short, steel needles, arranged in a circle, to penetrate the skin to a precise depth (2 mm in adults, 1 mm in children). A small drop of tuberculin (either OT or PPD) is placed on the skin of the forearm, which is then penetrated through the drop with the multipuncture instrument. The test may be read from 3 to 6 days later, a positive (Grade III) reaction consisting of a circle of induration spreading outwards from the ring of puncture marks. Less pronounced reactions, probably non-specific, consist of four or more papules localised to the site of the puncture marks (Grade I), or a ring of induration joining together the circle of puncture marks but without

induration of the centre of the ring (Grade II). The *Tuberculin Tine Test* is a somewhat similar multipuncture technique used more widely in the United States.

Tuberculin testing is of limited value in clinical medicine, being used mainly as an indicator of previous and possibly current tuberculous infection in communities where the infection rate is low and where BCG is not used. It is of more value in epidemiological surveys to determine the prevalence of tuberculosis in a community and the need for BCG vaccination.

BCG VACCINATION

Artificial hypersensitivity can be induced by vaccinating tuberculin negative subjects with a non-virulent strain of *Mycobacterium tuberculosis*. (BCG stands for Bacille-Calmette-Guerin, the original strain of non-virulent bacillus which was developed in 1922.) Currently, a freeze-dried vaccine is injected intradermally, producing a papule within four weeks which occasionally ulcerates and may be associated with local lymphadenopathy. The tuberculin test should become positive within three months of vaccination. There is now considerable evidence that a high degree of protection against subsequent tuberculous infection may be obtained by BCG vaccination, which should be given to tuberculin negative school-leavers and students, to contacts, and to those working in professions at special risk such as hospital workers, doctors and dentists, nurses and school teachers. Vaccination is contra-indicated in those showing a positive reaction to the tuberculin test, those vaccinated for smallpox, poliomyelitis or yellow fever in the previous four weeks, and those with pyrexia or dermatitis.

Clinical Features

Pulmonary tuberculosis is a disease of insidious onset often with poorly defined symptoms; a high level of suspicion should therefore be cultivated in order to avoid missing the diagnosis, especially in economically developed countries where the impact of the disease on the community has been so much reduced in the last twenty years. It is particularly important to bear the diagnosis in mind when investigating chronic ill-health or persistent unexplained febrile illness in the middle-aged and elderly.

ASPECTS OF THE HISTORY

Any *history of contact* with the disease, particularly among the patient's family or household should be enquired into, and any *past episode of tuberculosis* in the patient's own history should be noted since the present illness may well be a recrudescence of dormant

infection. Coincidental *diabetes mellitus* or previous *partial gastrectomy* increases the chances of a patient contracting tuberculosis, while prior infection, often unrecognised during its active phase, may be rekindled by *systemic corticosteroid therapy* given for such common conditions as bronchial asthma or rheumatoid arthritis. *Alcoholism* also increases liability to tuberculosis infection.

PRESENTING SYMPTOMS

Active pulmonary tuberculosis often occurs in the absence of recognised symptoms, presenting as a radiological abnormality observed in the course of routine examinations such as mass miniature chest radiograph surveys, employment examinations, or in the investigation of symptoms due to an unrelated illness. Alternatively, the patient may present with non-specific symptoms of general ill-health, particularly among the middle-aged and elderly, and in only a proportion of cases do obvious respiratory symptoms direct attention to pulmonary tuberculosis as a presumptive diagnosis.

Symptoms such as *malaise, anorexia, weight loss,* and failure to thrive in children are common early manifestations of tuberculosis. *Fever* may be irregular, swinging or intermittent, sometimes raised in the morning but settling to normal later in the day, and often associated with *night sweats. Irritability* and *lack of concentration* are occasional complaints, while *dyspepsia* is a common associated symptom.

Persistent *cough, haemoptysis,* and *chest pain* should always bring to mind a possible diagnosis of pulmonary tuberculosis. The pain may be aching in character or of pleuritic type when it is related to tuberculous pleural effusion or empyema. Occasionally, it may indicate the development of a pneumothorax. *Breathlessness* is usually a manifestation of extensive disease but may result from pulmonary collapse due to a pneumothorax or the rapid development of a large pleural effusion. A complaint of *localised wheezing* may be due to bronchial narrowing by tuberculous lymph nodes, while *hoarseness* is an important symptom of laryngeal tuberculosis that occasionally complicates severe pulmonary infection. Tuberculosis should always be considered as a possible cause of *pneumonia,* particularly in those patients who fail to respond to treatment with routine antibiotic therapy or in those who show radiological evidence of tuberculosis elsewhere in the lungs.

The presentation of respiratory symptoms is, of course, often associated with the systemic manifestations described above. The diagnosis is much more elusive when tuberculosis occurs coincidentally with other lung disease such as chronic airways obstruction, bronchiectasis, or diffuse pulmonary fibrosis, when the

symptoms are readily attributable to the non-tuberculous disease. Such cases, occurring most commonly among the high-risk group of elderly, cigarette-smoking men, should be carefully reviewed, particular attention being paid to suggestive fibrotic or cavitating lesions in the chest radiograph and to a thorough search of the sputum for tubercle bacilli.

CLINICAL SIGNS

A *wasted appearance* often associated with *pallor, sweating,* and *tachycardia* gives external evidence of active, progressive disease, but in the early case of pulmonary tuberculosis the patient's external appearance is frequently entirely normal. *Clubbing of the digits* is rather uncommon in pulmonary tuberculosis although a moderate degree of clubbing may occur in longstanding disease. The development of pronounced clubbing should suggest an alternative or coincidental diagnosis, particularly carcinoma of the bronchus.

The *chest signs* vary enormously, depending on the pulmonary manifestations of the disease. Evidence of *apical fibrosis* is common with deviation of the trachea towards the side of the lesion, but the typical signs of *cavitation* are rarely observed unless the cavity is remarkably large or close to the surface of the lung. Early signs of disease are *post-tussive crepitations* heard most commonly at the lung apices, and *localised inspiratory wheezing* may be audible in relation to narrowed bronchi. Signs of *consolidation, pleural effusion* and *pneumothorax* may be manifest.

Evidence of hypersensitivity reactions and of miliary spread of tuberculosis may be observed when making a general examination. In primary tuberculosis erythema nodosum sometimes occurs during the first few weeks, and phlyctenular conjunctivitis is an occasional allergic manifestation which occurs mainly in children within a year of infection. The lesions of *erythema nodosum* occur on the shins as tender, raised, purplish-red swellings that fade gradually over several days in a manner rather similar to a healing bruise. They often appear and disappear in different areas over a period of two or three weeks, and occasionally occur also on the backs of the forearms. Fever, joint pains, and a raised erythrocyte sedimentation rate are commonly associated. *Phlyctenular conjunctivitis* begins with conjunctival irritation, lachrymation, and photophobia, occurring in one or both eyes. The typical lesion is a yellowish, shiny bleb 1 to 3 mm in diameter situated at the limbus and associated with a leash of dilated conjunctival vessels. The reaction lasts for about a week, but may recur.

Miliary spread of tuberculosis is most readily confirmed by examination of the retina, *choroidal tubercles* being recognised as

single or multiple yellowish-white spots which later become pigmented. Miliary lesions of the skin rarely present as macules, papules, or purpuric lesions. Enlargement of the *spleen* may be observed in miliary tuberculosis, particularly in children.

Diagnosis

BACTERIOLOGY

The most important diagnostic evidence is the identification of tubercle bacilli in secretions or exudate. Smears of the sputum should be examined directly for acid-alcohol-fast organisms stained by the method of Ziehl-Neelsen, and cultures should be set up on Lowenstein-Jensen medium and examined at intervals for at least six weeks. A further sample of sputum material should be inoculated into a guinea-pig. If no sputum can be produced, samples of gastric washings obtained early in the morning should be similarly examined, as should specimens of exudate obtained by aspiration of a pleural effusion. Laryngeal swabs may be taken as an alternative to gastric aspiration in patients unable to produce sputum. If haematogenous spread of the infection is suspected early morning specimens of urine should also be examined.

HISTOLOGY

Histological examination of biopsy material in an attempt to identify characteristic tubercles may lead to the diagnosis, particularly in miliary tuberculosis in which the main symptom is often an unexplained pyrexia, and radiological or bacteriological evidence of pulmonary involvement is uncertain. Biopsy of the liver and of the bone marrow may be helpful, and it is important that part of the biopsy material should be cultured as well as submitted to histological examination. Pleural biopsy is an important diagnostic technique in pleural effusion of undetermined cause.

RADIOLOGY OF THE CHEST

Certain characteristics of the chest radiograph favour the diagnosis of tuberculosis. These include *calcification* within a shadow and the appearance of *fibrosis,* suggested by linear shadowing which often radiates to the apices from the hilum, and by distortion of the trachea or fissures. The diagnosis is supported by the occurrence of lesions at the *lung apices* or in the upper zones, especially if these are bilateral, and *cavitation* is characteristic of pulmonary tuberculosis although bronchial carcinoma, lung abscess, and actinomycosis are important considerations in the differential diagnosis. Bilateral apical fibrosis closely simulating the radiological appearance of tuberculosis occurs in

a small percentage of patients with ankylosing spondylitis. Cavitation of the lesions and colonisation with *Aspergillus fumigatus* may occur.

In young people the association of *hilar lymph gland enlargement* with a peripheral shadow may indicate a primary complex, while miliary tuberculosis should always be included in the differential diagnosis of widespread bilateral *miliary shadowing* of the lung fields. Serial radiographs may suggest the diagnosis of tuberculosis when *soft, confluent shadows* fail to resolve on routine therapy given for a presumptive diagnosis of bacterial pneumonia.

Tomography is mainly useful in defining the character of a shadow or a cavity, in detecting calcification in its walls, and in diagnosing cavitation in a solid rounded shadow.

THE BLOOD COUNT

A moderate normocytic anaemia is often seen in active pulmonary tuberculosis. The white blood count is usually normal or low, but a polymorphonuclear leucocytosis is not uncommon in primary tuberculosis and may occasionally occur in postprimary disease. In miliary tuberculosis anaemia is common, sometimes of aplastic type, and a leukaemoid reaction that is difficult to differentiate from a true coincidental leukaemia may occur. Purpura is sometimes observed. The erythrocyte sedimentation rate is often raised in active pulmonary tuberculosis but need not be so; consequently it is an unreliable guide to activity.

THE TUBERCULIN TEST

A negative Mantoux test (using 0·1 ml of 1:100 OT) makes the diagnosis of tuberculosis unlikely, although alternative reasons for the negative response should always be considered (page 183).

THERAPEUTIC TRIAL

In patients in whom the diagnosis of tuberculosis is strongly suspected but histological, bacteriological, or definite radiological evidence is absent, it is sometimes justifiable to test the presumptive diagnosis by giving a therapeutic trial of antituberculosis chemotherapy. This situation most often arises in middle-aged or elderly patients with a history of chronic febrile illness for which no cause has been found despite thorough investigation. In the face of continued deterioration such patients should be treated with full doses of para-aminosalicylic acid (PAS) and isonicotinic acid hydrazide (isoniazid) since these agents are specific in the treatment of tuberculosis. Streptomycin should not be given initially since its spectrum of activity is very much wider. Tuberculous infections would be expected to respond to PAS

and isoniazid within two weeks: failure of response after four weeks' treatment suggests that the infection is due to some other cause.

Complications

Local spread from a pulmonary locus of infection may lead to *tuberculous pleural effusion*, usually because of rupture into the pleural cavity of a subpleural caseous nodule which may be representative of either primary or postprimary disease. The effusion is exudative, usually straw-coloured although occasionally blood-stained, and contains lymphocytes and tubercle bacilli. Pleural biopsy may reveal typical tubercles on histological examination. Such effusions become purulent when pleural infection is extensive, resulting in *tuberculous empyema*. Spread of infection to the larynx occasionally occurs when tubercle bacilli are being coughed up in large quantities due to severe pulmonary disease. The major symptoms of tuberculous laryngitis are hoarseness and pain on swallowing.

Progressive pulmonary tuberculosis leads to permanent lung damage due to distortion of the lung parenchyma and airways by fibrosis, bronchial narrowing, bronchiectasis with secondary bacterial infection and obstructive emphysema. Pleural fibrosis may also occur. These changes inevitably lead to some degree of uneven distribution of ventilation and perfusion, sometimes severe enough to cause *respiratory failure*. The destruction of part of the pulmonary vascular bed combined with vascular changes induced by hypoxia lead to pulmonary hypertension and *cor pulmonale* in longstanding cases.

Haematogenous spread of the disease often arises from breakdown of a pulmonary lesion, causing either *miliary tuberculosis* or a secondary focus of infection in a distant organ. *Tuberculous meningitis,* disease of *bones and joints, renal tuberculosis* and *tuberculous epididymitis* should be excluded by examination and investigation.

Secondary amyloidosis is a rare complication of longstanding pulmonary tuberculosis, usually associated with bronchiectasis or tuberculous empyema. Renal amyloidosis is manifested by heavy proteinuria and hypoproteinaemia, and enlargement of the liver and spleen may occur.

Treatment

Before the advent of chemotherapy about half the patients who contracted tuberculosis subsequently died of it; now, almost all ought to recover. Success in treatment depends on the use of appropriate drugs in effective dosage for long enough to eradicate the infection. It is therefore of cardinal importance that any doctor undertaking the

management of a patient with pulmonary tuberculosis should understand the requirements of *effective* drug therapy, both in order to achieve a successful result in the treatment of that patient and to prevent him from harbouring drug-resistant bacilli which might cause resistant infection in other individuals.

INDICATIONS FOR CHEMOTHERAPY

Chemotherapy should be given to patients with positive sputum or from whom tubercle bacilli have been obtained from any source. Radiological evidence of active tuberculosis should also be treated, proof of activity sometimes depending on periodic review of the patient's chest radiograph and sputum culture. Chemotherapy is occasionally indicated for patients in whom the clinical presentation and radiological features are highly suggestive of the disease without there being positive bacteriological proof: such treatment is in the nature of a clinical trial and should begin with isoniazid and PAS only, since these drugs act specifically against the tubercle bacillus.

EFFECTIVE DRUGS

None of the drugs available for the treatment of tuberculosis is without important side-effects which must be taken into account when choosing the most appropriate therapeutic regimen for a particular patient.

Streptomycin must be given by intramuscular injection in a dosage related to age and to the patient's renal function. It damages the eighth cranial nerve, causing impairment of vestibular function which presents with giddiness and slight unsteadiness but progresses to severe vertigo with vomiting and nystagmus if treatment is continued. Deafness is rare. Such complications are most likely to occur in middle-aged or elderly patients and in those with impaired renal function. Allergic rashes and fever may occur.

Isoniazid is a cheap and highly effective oral drug with relatively few side-effects when given in the usual adult dose of 200 to 300 mg daily. The rate of acetylation of this drug after absorption varies in individuals, depending upon genetically determined differences in the amount of drug-metabolising enzymes. Slow acetylators accumulate high plasma concentrations of isoniazid and are more liable to toxic complications of which the most important is peripheral neuritis, preventable by giving pyridoxine. Acute hepatic necrosis occasionally occurs in patients who have been taking the drug for some time without apparent ill effects. Other uncommon side-effects are sleeplessness, impaired memory and an increased liability to epilepsy. Hypersensitivity reactions are rare.

Sodium aminosalicylate (PAS) is given by mouth, and causes gastro-intestinal irritation presenting as nausea, vomiting or diarrhoea which may be severe enough to warrant a change of drug. The usual adult dose is 6 g twice daily. Hypersensitivity reactions are not uncommon and, rarely, PAS interferes with thyroxine production to cause goitre and hypothyroidism.

Ethambutol is an effective agent that is readily absorbed from the gastro-intestinal tract and is given in a dose of 25 mg per kg body weight for the first two months of treatment, and 15 mg per kg thereafter. At this level of dosage the toxicity is low, although in a small proportion of cases it causes retrobulbar neuritis leading to diminished visual acuity, constriction of the visual fields, and impairment of colour vision. Patients should be instructed to report such symptoms immediately, and the drug stopped. Hypersensitivity reactions occur occasionally, and ethambutol should be used cautiously if renal function is impaired.

Rifampicin is a highly effective drug taken by mouth in a dose of 10 mg per kg body weight up to a maximum of 600 mg per day. It causes a brownish-red discoloration of urine, tears and sputum and may interfere with bilirubin excretion and cause a transient elevation of serum transaminases. Liver function should therefore be monitored during the early weeks of treatment. Rifampicin may cause purpura and thrombocytopenia, and sometimes gastro-intestinal symptoms.

Thioacetazone is an effective companion drug to isoniazid and is widely used in developing countries because of its relative cheapness. It causes nausea, vomiting, giddiness, jaundice and agranulocytosis, but the incidence of these side-effects is low when the recognised dose of 150 mg daily is not exceeded.

Reserve Drugs. These drugs are generally more toxic and less effective than the standard drugs, and are therefore used mainly in patients infected with organisms resistant to these drugs or when treatment with the standard drugs has failed. They include ethionamide and prothionamide, pyrazinamide, cycloserine and the antibiotics kanamycin, capreomycin and viomycin.

Drug Resistance. Because of spontaneous mutation, any culture of tubercle bacilli contains a small proportion of naturally-occurring drug-resistant organisms, some resistant to streptomycin, some to isoiazid, and so on. Treatment with one drug alone results in multiplication of the bacilli resistant to that drug by natural selection, and this tendency is enhanced if the dose of the drug used is inadequate. As a result, two- and three-drug schedules have been devised on the basis of extensive controlled clinical trials. Failure to follow this principle of using effective drugs in combination in adequate dosage leads not only to failure of therapy in individual cases but also to the

potentially more serious danger of introducing resistant organisms into the community.

The following traditional standard regimen is of proven efficacy in eradicating all but a tiny minority of infections. It is likely to be superseded in the near future, however, by drug combinations which include the powerful bactericidal agent rifampicin, enabling shorter but equally effective regimens to be introduced.

Traditional standard regimen for previously untreated patients:

1. Initial triple therapy, for 12 weeks or until the results of sensitivity tests on pre-treatment sputum samples are known:

   Streptomycin: 1 g daily for patients under 40 years.
   1 g 3 times a week (or 0·75 g daily) for patients of 40 years or more.
   Isoniazid: 150 mg twice daily.
   PAS: 6 g twice daily.

2. Continuation therapy, with 2 drugs of known efficacy based on the sensitivity tests:

   Isoniazid: 150 mg twice daily.
   PAS: 6 g twice daily.

The duration of treatment should not be less than one year and in most cases should continue for 18 months. In advanced disease or in the presence of a residual cavity two years of treatment is necessary.

As an alternative form of continuation therapy a regimen consisting of streptomycin 1 g plus isoniazid 15 mg per kg body weight, can be given twice weekly under supervision. This is particularly useful for patients who cannot be relied upon to take their oral drugs regularly, but it is necessary to give pyridoxine 10 mg with each dose to avoid side-effects from the large dose of isoniazid.

Modifications of Standard Regimen. Ethambutol may be used in conjunction with isoniazid for patients who are intolerant of PAS although its effectiveness in extensive cavitated disease is not sufficiently established to allow it wholly to supplant PAS in the standard regimen. Rifampicin may be substituted for streptomycin but is much more expensive. Thioacetazone in a single daily dose of 150 mg is used as an alternative to PAS in developing countries where its cheapness is an important consideration.

Recent trials of 6-month treatment regimens consisting of daily administration of streptomycin 1 g intramuscularly, isoniazid 300 mg

by mouth and either rifampicin 450 to 600 mg by mouth or pyrazinamide 2 g by mouth, have been compared with a standard 18-month regimen, without a significant increase in relapse rate being observed in these short-course regimens. If substantiated, these findings will prove a major advance in antituberculosis therapy.

MANAGEMENT

In the foregoing paragraphs the emphasis has been placed on the need for meticulous care in the choice and combination of antituberculosis drugs according to proven regimens of treatment. The responsible physician must also ensure, however, that the chosen course is effective in eradicating the disease, that the patient actually takes the drugs, that spread of the infection to others does not occur once the diagnosis is made, that toxic and hypersensitivity reactions to the drugs are recognised and dealt with, and that the patient's personal life and occupation are disrupted as little as possible during the period of therapy. These conflicting factors require careful judgement and forethought according to the needs of each individual.

Surveillance During Therapy. During chemotherapy the patient's sputum should be examined quantitatively at monthly intervals to determine the number of bacilli present in the smear. If treatment is effective, progressive dimunition in the number of organisms should be observed, and smears normally become negative within three months even in extensive disease. A fall followed by a rise in the number of tubercle bacilli, or the presence of heavily positive smears at three months suggest either that the patient is not taking his drugs or that the organisms are resistant.

A careful history should be obtained from the patient to assess his reliability in taking his current therapy and to determine any earlier treatment with antituberculosis drugs that has been undisclosed. This information may give some guide to the likelihood of resistance having arisen during previous therapy, particularly if it was of short duration or consisted of only one drug or an unsatisfactory combination of drugs. Resistance may be confirmed by drug resistance tests carried out on subcultures from sputum samples, although such tests take two or three months to complete.

If drug resistance is suspected in a patient on standard chemotherapy it is probably best to withhold treatment until sufficient information is available to enable an effective drug combination to be chosen, rather than making indiscriminate additions to the initial regimen. Special care is necessary in the surveillance of patients known to be infected with resistant organisms.

Supervision of Chemotherapy. During the first two or three months

of treatment hospital care is necessary for certain categories of patients. These include:

1. Patients who are seriously ill.
2. Those with positive sputum smears who have susceptible contacts at home, especially BCG negative children.
3. Those who are considered to be unreliable in taking their drugs.
4. Those infected with resistant organisms.

Patients who do not come into these categories may be treated at home provided that adequate services are available for domiciliary supervision. Continuation of normal occupation and reasonable activities should be allowed unless this entails contact with susceptible individuals, particularly children.

The advantages of domiciliary treatment are the saving in hospital expenses and the avoidance of disruption to the patient's life. Nevertheless, some physicians prefer to admit all patients during the initial stage of treatment to ensure regular drug-taking during the early phase when hypersensitivity reactions to the drugs are most liable to occur and when irregular drug-taking is most likely to lead to resistance. Domiciliary therapy demands careful supervision, including out-patient attendances, monitoring of drug-taking by home visits and interrogation of the patient, and painstaking explanations to him and his family of the need for persistence to the end of the course of therapy.

Hypersensitivity reactions are an occasional complication of treatment with all the antituberculosis drugs, usually occurring within the first five weeks of treatment. Such reactions usually present with fever, pruritus and rashes but more serious manifestations such as paraesthesiae, headaches, enlargement of liver, spleen and lymph nodes, jaundice, transient pulmonary infiltrations, eosinophilia, encephalopathy and bone marrow depression may occur. These allergic manifestations nearly always disappear if the drugs are stopped immediately but corticosteroids may be necessary in the treatment of severe reactions. After identifying the offending drug by giving small test doses of each drug individually, desensitisation may be carried out by giving gradually increasing doses over a period of two or three days. Treatment with at least two effective drugs should be restarted as soon as possible to prevent the emergence of resistance.

Corticosteroid Drugs. Corticosteroids are valuable in the treatment of patients desperately ill with tuberculosis and in the control of severe hypersensitivity reactions. They do not increase the rate of sputum conversion or affect the degree of pulmonary damage following tuberculosis infection, and are dangerous if used in conjunction with ineffective antituberculosis drugs, since clinical deterioration is then

likely. Corticosteroids should not therefore be used routinely in the treatment of pulmonary tuberculosis.

Surgery. There is a general indication for surgery only in those patients in whom chemotherapy has failed because of hypersensitivity or resistance, but the extent of lung involvement in such cases is often too great to permit operation. Occasional indications include lobectomy for persistent cavitation if complications are troublesome.

Follow-up of Treated Patients. In the past, it has been customary to arrange periodic chest radiography for five years or longer in order to identify reactivation of the disease. Recent evidence indicates that relapse is very infrequent in patients who have reliably taken a full course of combined chemotherapy, and long term follow-up is therefore falling out of favour.

15

Fungal Infections of the Lungs

Incidence

Although fungal infections of the lungs are relatively uncommon, awareness of their clinical presentation and of the conditions under which they are likely to occur should lead to recognition or at least suspicion of such an infection, and hence to the appropriate investigations. The pulmonary mycoses usually encountered in the British Isles are aspergillosis, candidiasis, actinomycosis, nocardiosis, and cryptococcosis, but increasing travel has also brought occasional cases of histoplasmosis, coccidioidomycosis and blastomycosis from overseas.

The majority of systemic fungal infections in the United Kingdom are 'opportunist', i.e. they occur as a result of suppression or impairment of the patient's defence mechanisms against infection. A pulmonary mycosis is therefore particularly likely in chronic debilitating disease, in malnutrition, in diseases affecting the reticulo-endothelial system such as Hodgkin's disease, leukaemia and multiple myeloma, in sarcoidosis and tuberculosis, and in conditions treated with long-term antibiotics, corticosteroids or immunosuppressive therapy. The possibility of a fungal aetiology should also be considered in pulmonary disease which presents as an atypical pneumonia, as a lung abscess or as a chronic bronchopulmonary infection which has persisted in spite of adequate therapy. Travel within the endemic areas of North or South America, Asia or Africa may be the main indication for suspecting one of the rarer pulmonary fungal infections.

Aspergillosis

This disease is the commonest of the pulmonary mycoses in the British Isles and is usually due to infection with *Aspergillus fumigatus,* although other aspergillus species may be responsible. The organism is a widespread saprophyte in nature, occurring as a filamentous fungus which produces airborne spores. Infection is by inhalation.

Allergic bronchopulmonary aspergillosis is the commonest manifestation of the disease, due to Types I and III allergic respiratory reactions to the fungus (page 116). It is characterised by asthma, chronic cough with sputum, obstruction of the proximal bronchi with mucous plugs containing growing hyphae of *Aspergillus fumigatus,* and the development of bronchiectasis and fibrosis distal to these obstructions. Eosinophilia of blood and sputum and recurring radiographic shadows due to pulmonary collapse and con-solidation are typical findings, calling for the differentiation of allergic pulmonary aspergillosis from other causes of pulmonary eosinophilia such as drug hypersensitivity (page 271), parasitic infestation and pulmonary polyarteritis nodosa (page 256). Diagnosis depends on culturing *Aspergillus fumigatus* from the sputum and on demonstrating immediate skin sensitivity to prick testing with aspergillus extracts. Serum precipitins are found in 70 per cent of cases. Airway obstruction can be demonstrated by tests of ventilatory function and transfer factor (T_L,CO) is often decreased.

Allergic bronchopulmonary aspergillosis may continue for many years with episodes of pulmonary infiltration and wheezing which require symptomatic bronchodilator therapy. Specific antifungal treatment consists of an aerosol preparation of natamycin, given two to three times daily in a dose of 2·5 mg in 2·5 per cent suspension diluted in an alkaline agent. Oral nystatin and inhalation of nystatin, brilliant green and hydroxystilbamidine may be valuable. In severe bronchopulmonary infections or when the infection is disseminated, intravenous amphotericin B is used.

Aspergilloma is due to colonisation by the fungus of a bulla or tuberculous cavity, or of lung tissue damaged by disease such as sarcoidosis, pneumoconiosis or malignancy. The patient presents with fever, weight loss and deterioration in health, sometimes associated with asthma indicative of hypersensitivity to the organism. Purulent and sometimes blood-stained sputum is produced. The chest X-ray shows an opaque mass which almost completely fills the cavity, leaving a crescentic rim or 'halo' of air between the mycelial mass and the wall of the cavity. Tomography may be useful in defining this appearance. Precipitating antibody to aspergillus antigens is present in the majority of cases of aspergilloma.

Surgical resection of an aspergilloma is indicated when the diagnosis is in doubt, when there is persistent haemoptysis or when systemic fungal invasion is likely because of lowered resistance. Resolution of the infection may sometimes be achieved by the relatively minor procedure of evacuating the cavity through a small local thoracotomy, followed by direct irrigation of the cavity with natamycin. In many cases treatment is unnecessary and aspergilloma

cavities sometimes empty spontaneously without therapy. Discriminating use of corticosteroid therapy has proved beneficial in some patients with aspergilloma who can be shown to have positive hypersensitivity reactions to the organism and who have failed to respond to antibiotics and antifungal agents.

Aspergillus species may cause disseminated infection in patients whose natural immunity is diminished by chronic debilitating diseases or by therapy with immunosuppressive and corticosteroid drugs. *Extrinsic allergic alveolitis* (page 227) caused by a Type III, immune-complex reaction in the peripheral gas-exchanging lung tissues has been ascribed to *Aspergillus fumigatus* and *clavatus* hypersensitivity in malt workers.

Candidiasis

Bronchopulmonary infection with *Candida albicans* is rare, occurring as a result of severe underlying disease or because of long-term antibiotic or corticosteroid therapy. *Bronchial candidiasis* presents with cough and scanty mucoid sputum which sometimes has a milky appearance. The finding of *Candida albicans* in the sputum is not diagnostic since the organism is found occasionally in the sputum of healthy individuals and more commonly in hospital patients, but repeated or heavy cultures are of greater significance. *Pulmonary candidiasis* is a more severe illness of cough, fever, haemoptysis, dyspnoea, and chest pain, sometimes associated with consolidation and pleural effusion. Treatment is with nystatin, given in aerosol form every 4 to 6 hours, combined with amphotericin B therapy when there is involvement of other organs. 5-fluorocytosine has also been used in the treatment of invasive *Candida* infections.

Actinomycosis

This disease is due to a branching filamentous Gram-positive organism, *Actinomyces israelii,* which produces a chronic granulomatous reaction with the formation of pus. It is anaerobic but is sometimes found in the oral cavity as a saprophyte located in the tonsils or in the roots of carious teeth, causing infection in the cervico-facial region as a result of direct trauma such as dental extraction, and in the lungs and abdomen by swallowing or aspiration of the organism. It causes a local, slowly-developing inflammatory reaction which develops into an abscess, the infection tending to extend through tissue barriers with the formation of sinuses.

The *pulmonary form of the disease* presents insidiously with cough, irregular fever, and malaise. Purulent and often blood-stained sputum is produced as pulmonary suppuration develops, and involvement of

the pleura causes pleuritic pain and often empyema which may progress to abscess and sinus formation in the chest wall. Complications include extension to the mediastinum and to the thoracic spine. Chest radiographs show irregular shadowing or homogeneous opacities resembling consolidation or pleural effusion, and extension of the infection to the tissues of the thoracic wall causes periostitis with new bone formation and thickening of the ribs. The diagnosis depends on bacteriological examination of the pus, which contains 'sulphur granules', actually colonies of the organism in which peripheral 'clubs' can be distinguished by Ziehl-Neelsen's stain.

Treatment is with penicillin in doses of 10 to 12 million units daily, and may be necessary for at least six months. Alternative antibiotics may be given on the basis of sensitivity if the response to penicillin is unsatisfactory. Surgery is only indicated in the treatment of severe resulting lung damage such as bronchiectasis or local fibrosis.

Nocardiosis

Nocardia asteroides is an aerobic organism in contrast to *Actinomyces israelii* but producing a similar disease which shows a rather greater tendency to disseminate widely, both in the lungs and in other organs such as the brain. It occurs as a soil saprophyte and is therefore more liable to affect agricultural workers through tissue damage or by inhalation. Infection is particularly associated with other diseases or therapy that impair the patient's immune mechanism. The mortality is high, long-sustained therapy with high doses of sulphadimidine being the treatment of choice.

Cryptococcosis (Torulosis)

Cryptococcus neoformans is a yeast that is present in soil, in pigeon droppings and, occasionally, even in healthy individuals, tending to cause disease in patients whose susceptibility to infection is enhanced by an underlying illness such as leukaemia or Hodgkin's disease, or by systemic corticosteroid therapy. The most usual presentation is a subacute meningo-encephalitis which commonly leads to death within a few months. Infection of the respiratory tract presents as a mild self-limiting influenza-like illness or as atypical pneumonia with fever, productive cough, haemoptysis, and pleuritic pain. The chest X-ray may show a solitary shadow similar in appearance to a tumour or lung abscess, a diffuse pulmonary infiltration, or miliary mottling. Diagnosis depends on demonstrating the organism in the sputum by smear and culture.

Amphotericin B is the only effective form of *treatment*, given intratrathecally as well as intravenously when the central nervous

system is involved. Occasional well-localised lung lesions may be suitable for surgical excision.

Histoplasmosis

This disease is caused by *Histoplasma capsulatum,* a soil saprophyte which parasitises the reticulo-endothelial system. The fungus is widely endemic in America, its spores being inhaled in dust to cause a benign pulmonary infection that is usually asymptomatic but may be recognised retrospectively on the chest radiograph as dense round pulmonary opacities and hilar gland enlargement which later become calcified. In less than 1 per cent of cases the disease becomes progressive; there are generalised symptoms of fever, malaise, sweating, loss of weight, and chest pain, often with muco-cutaneous granulomatous lesions around the mouth, hepatosplenomegaly, involvement of the adrenal glands, anaemia, and leukopenia. The chest radiograph may show pulmonary infiltrates associated with hilar gland enlargement, calcified foci often associated with fibrosis and cavitation, and sometimes miliary calcification. It is often difficult to distinguish between the radiographic appearances of pulmonary tuberculosis and histoplasmosis, although in the latter condition the lesions are less liable to be predominantly in the upper zones of the lungs.

Diagnosis depends on the clinical and radiographic presentation, confirmed by a positive histoplasmin skin test and by a rising titre to complement-fixing antibodies in the patient's serum. The organism may be demonstrated in smears of the patient's sputum. Progressive infection is likely to be opportunist, and tends to occur particularly in children and the aged and in patients debilitated by other diseases. Amphotericin B given intravenously is the only effective form of treatment in the progressive pulmonary or acute disseminated forms of the disease.

Coccidioidomycosis

The organism, *Coccidioides immitis,* occurs in the soil in arid areas of North and South America, especially in a particular area of California where the illness it causes is known as San Joaquin Valley Fever. The spores are inhaled with dust into the lungs where they multiply, causing a disease that may present in its primary form, or subsequently as a progressive infection. It affects all ages, but the progressive infection is commoner in males of dark-skinned races.

The *primary infection* of coccioidomycosis is usually asymptomatic, but in about 40 per cent of those infected it presents as a subacute respiratory infection similar to a viral pneumonia, with slight fever, cough, chest pain, headache, sore throat and,

occasionally, blood-stained sputum. Joint pains and skin lesions such as erythema nodosum or erythema multiforme may occur. The chest radiograph may show segmental or diffuse shadowing, hilar lymph gland enlargement, and pleural effusions. The coccidioidin skin test becomes positive about four weeks after infection, and there is a polymorphonuclear leucocytosis. The majority of primary infections clear up completely but cavitation occurs occasionally, and persists.

Progressive infection develops in 1 in a 1,000 cases of primary coccidioidomycosis, with weight loss, malaise, fever, and pulmonary signs. Granulomatous reactions may occur in other organs such as the brain, meninges, bones, and skin. The chest radiograph shows cavitation, solid rounded shadows, hilar lymph node enlargement and diffuse miliary shadowing, all of which may be difficult to distinguish from tuberculosis or pulmonary malignancy. Diagnosis is confirmed by the coccidioidin skin test (analogous to the Mantoux reaction), by finding a rising titre of complement fixing antibodies in the serum, and by identifying the organism in sputum smears. Progressive disease must be treated with amphotericin B, but the great majority of patients with primary infection recover spontaneously.

Treatment with Amphotericin B

This drug is active against all the serious pulmonary mycoses. It is poorly absorbed from the gut and has therefore to be given intravenously. A total of 1 g of the drug given over a period of one month is the minimal acceptable schedule of treatment, and up to 5 g appears to be unlikely to cause irreversible renal damage. Higher doses may cause permanent impairment of renal function and regular examination of the urine is essential throughout the period of treatment, preferably with serial estimations of creatinine clearance. A suggested regimen is an initial dose of 10 mg of amphotericin B on the first day, 25 mg on the second, and 50 mg on each subsequent day, in 1,000 ml 5 per cent glucose over a 6 to 8 hour period. 10 mg of heparin are added to reduce the likelihood of venous thrombosis. Alternatively, the initial dose may be 1·0 mg of the drug, increasing by daily increments of 5 mg until a dose of 0·5 to 1·5 mg/kg/day is reached. To avoid precipitation of the amphoteric antibiotic, salts such as sodium chloride and procaine hydrochloride should not be introduced into the infusion fluid.

Side effects, which include nausea, anorexia, vomiting, fever, chills, headache, and malaise, may determine the rate of increase and the optimal daily dose of the drug. Chlorpromazine may be given to reduce the incidence of side effects.

16

Sarcoidosis

Sarcoidosis is a systemic disease of unknown aetiology that occurs throughout the world but appears to have an increased incidence in northern Europe, among American negroes and among West Indian and Irish immigrants to Great Britain. The overall prevalence is similar in men and women and in Great Britain the disease affects about 20 per 100,000 population. It occurs at any age but most commonly presents between the ages of twenty and forty years.

The manifestations of sarcoidosis are extremely diverse for at one time or another almost every organ or tissue of the body has been described as the site of involvement by the disease. In this account the emphasis is placed on intrathoracic sarcoidosis, for hilar lymphadenopathy and pulmonary involvement are the commonest forms of the disease, and pulmonary sarcoidosis is an important cause of disablement and death due to respiratory and cardiac failure.

Aetiology

The cause of sarcoidosis remains unknown. The hypothesis that has provoked most controversy is that sarcoidosis is an atypical form of reaction to infection with *Mycobacterium tuberculosis*; this argument is based on some morphological points of similarity between the sarcoid granuloma and the tubercle, and the occasional observation of overt tuberculosis occurring in patients with sarcoidosis, and vice versa. On the other hand, the almost invariable absence of tubercle bacilli in sarcoid lesions, the loss of tuberculin sensitivity that occurs in two-thirds of patients with sarcoidosis, differences in prevalence of the two diseases regarding geographical distribution and social conditions, and the lack of therapeutic response of sarcoidosis to antituberculous drugs in contrast to the effectiveness of corticosteroid drugs used alone, are all points that favour independent aetiologies.

Many organisms, including fungi, mycobacteria and protozoa, provoke an inflammatory reaction similar to the sarcoid granuloma but none has yet been shown to cause the disease. The hypothesis that pine pollen is the causative agent, based on epidemiological surveys in

the south-eastern United States and on the ability of this agent to produce granulomatous lesions of the skin, has not been substantiated by inhalation or ingestion tests or by world-wide epidemiological studies.

Immunology

Depression of the delayed type of hypersensitivity response is characteristic of sarcoidosis, occurring in two-thirds of cases. It is not limited to the tuberculin test, which is the one most commonly used in clinical practice, but is also evident when cutaneous tests are made with other antigens including *Candida albicans,* pertussis, and mumps. In contrast, other types of hypersensitivity reaction, such as the immediate, Type I reaction or the Type II reaction that occurs, for example in mismatched blood transfusion, are unaffected.

This depression of delayed-type hypersensitivity is by no means unique to sarcoidosis, for it occurs in reticuloses such as Hodgkin's disease, in uraemic or cachetic patients, in the newborn and elderly, in patients receiving irradiation or immunosuppressive therapy, and in thymectomised individuals. Other causes of a negative tuberculin test are discussed on page 183.

Pathology

THE SARCOID GRANULOMA

The granuloma of sarcoidosis consists of a group of large macrophages, known as epithelioid cells, and a few multinucleate giant cells surrounded by a scanty rim of lymphocytes. The giant cells are similar to the Langhan's type seen in tuberculosis, having about 30 nuclei arranged peripherally. Within the giant and epithelioid cells three types of inclusion body may be observed: the Schaumann body, the asteroid body, and the residual body. These inclusion bodies are not diagnostic of sarcoidosis, for they occur in other granulomatous conditions such as chronic berylliosis, Crohn's disease and, occasionally, in tuberculosis.

Necrosis is rare in sarcoid granulomas, and when present is small in amount. The lesion eventually heals with the formation of a collagenous scar, calcification being uncommon in healed granulomas, in contrast to tuberculosis.

DISTRIBUTION

Sarcoid granulomas of these uniform characteristics occur in almost any organ. The disease is usually widely disseminated although clinically one or two systems only may be apparently affected. The sites most frequently involved are the skin, lungs, lymph nodes, liver,

spleen, bones, eyes, and parotid gland. Both the central and peripheral nervous systems are occasionally affected.

Lymph node involvement may be widespread, but more frequently affects a single group of glands, hilar lymphadenopathy being particularly common. In the lungs the sarcoid granulomas may vary greatly in size from small multiple nodules less than half a centimetre in diameter to large conglomerate lesions, 2 or more centimetres across, consisting of fused nodules. When pulmonary fibrosis develops it is usually of patchy distribution and rarely diffuse. Some degree of disruption of lung tissue results from the fibrosis, causing localised distortion of the bronchi and a little secondary emphysema, but these changes do not appear to cause a significant degree of airways obstruction.

Functional Disorder

The effect of these pathological changes on pulmonary function varies considerably from patient to patient, and often appears inconsistent with the clinical and radiological findings of the individual case. In general, patients with hilar lymphadenopathy but radiologically normal lungs sometimes show evidence of reduced lung volumes and impaired maximum voluntary ventilation, with some reduction in transfer factor for carbon monoxide. Those with radiological evidence of lung parenchymal infiltration show similar changes more constantly and to a greater degree, but it is in patients with established pulmonary fibrosis that the typical restrictive pattern of dysfunction is found, with reduction in all lung volumes, a normal RV/TLC ratio, reduced pulmonary compliance and reduced transfer factor for carbon monoxide, the arterial blood being desaturated with normal or low levels of arterial carbon dioxide tension. Airways obstruction is not characteristic of sarcoidosis.

Clinical Presentation

ERYTHEMA NODOSUM

Erythema nodosum is a benign self-limiting condition which in the United Kingdom is associated most commonly with sarcoidosis or with streptococcal infection. It is also occasionally seen in tuberculosis, as a complication of treatment with a wide variety of drugs, particularly sulphonamides, and in association with various other infections that include coccidioidomycosis, histoplasmosis, and leprosy.

It occurs most commonly in young adult women, presenting most often in the spring; the lesions are red, hot and shiny, occurring as painful swellings on the shins and less frequently on the calves, knees,

buttocks, and forearms. Their appearance is associated with swinging fever, arthralgia and malaise which commonly precede or accompany the onset of erythema nodosum and last for a few days. The skin lesions themselves may persist for two or three weeks (range one to twenty weeks), gradually becoming less painful and changing from dusky red to blue and yellow as they subside, in the manner of a healing bruise. In sarcoidosis this syndrome is associated with hilar lymphadenopathy, sometimes with clinical evidence of disseminated sarcoid lesions elsewhere.

PULMONARY SARCOIDOSIS

Pulmonary sarcoidosis usually presents in one of three ways:

1. Chance detection on routine chest radiography.

2. Detected in the investigation of non-respiratory symptoms or signs which are referable to sarcoidosis, e.g. erythema nodosum or ocular involvement.

3. With non-specific symptoms of a sub-acute respiratory illness such as *cough,* slight *chest pain,* minimal *exertional dyspnoea, malaise* or *fever.*

The first two of these three modes of onset are by far the commonest, indicating that the onset and course of pulmonary sarcoidosis are usually benign and clinically unobtrusive.

In a small proportion of cases pulmonary sarcoidosis progresses beyond the stages of hilar lymph node involvement and minor pulmonary infiltration which are relatively symptomless; once sarcoid infiltration has become extensive or pulmonary fibrosis begins to develop the major presenting features are progressive dyspnoea on exertion and cough with a little mucoid sputum. Direct questioning of such patients may reveal a transient illness such as iritis, arthralgia or skin eruption several years previously which passed unrecognised at the time but indicated in retrospect the onset of sarcoidosis. Rarely, a patient may present with the symptoms of advanced disease due to widespread pulmonary fibrosis; disabling dyspnoea is the main complaint, complicated by symptoms of congestive cardiac failure. Haemoptysis and chest pain sometimes occur at this stage of the disease, the latter occasionally due to spontaneous pneumothorax.

The clinical signs in the chest vary according to the stage of the disease; in the early symptomless stage they are usually absent altogether, but scattered crepitations may be heard when pulmonary infiltration is extensive, becoming more diffuse and prominent as pulmonary fibrosis develops. Digital clubbing occurs rarely in longstanding fibrotic disease.

EXTRAPULMONARY SARCOIDOSIS

Symptoms due to sarcoid involvement of extrathoracic organs and tissues often draw attention to unsuspected pulmonary disease. Although such manifestations are extremely diverse, certain tissues appear to be particularly prone to sarcoidosis, the most common presentation being *erythema nodosum with hilar lymphadenopathy* described above. Other important manifestations include:

1. *Lymph Node Involvement.* This usually affects a single group of nodes, often in the neck or mediastinum; generalised lymphadenopathy is less common. The individual nodes may be barely palpable, or increased to 3 or 4 centimetres in diameter, being separate, fairly firm, mobile and seldom tender. In many respects they resemble the enlarged nodes of Hodgkin's disease.

2. *Ocular Involvement.* Bilateral iritis and uveitis are the commonest abnormalities but sarcoid granulomas may also involve the lachrymal glands, the eyelids, the conjunctiva, the sclera and the choroid and retina. Some disturbance of vision is usually complained of, occasionally progressing to blindness although usually the lesions heal over a period of months or even years. Sarcoidosis of the eyes is commonly associated with lesions elsewhere, notably in the lungs.

3. *Uveo-parotid Fever.* This syndrome is characterised by a mild febrile illness associated with uveitis and bilateral parotid swelling, often accompanied by unilateral or bilateral facial palsy. There may be a prodromal period of several days or weeks during which lassitude, fever, gastro-intestinal symptoms, skin eruptions, joint pains and ill-defined cerebral symptoms are noticed, the first distinctive sign being parotid gland enlargement. Other manifestations of disseminated sarcoidosis including lymphatic and pulmonary involvement often occur. The course of the syndrome is rather irregular but the symptoms usually subside over weeks or months although the ocular abnormalities seem particularly liable to relapse or recur.

4. *Skin Eruptions.* The three commonest types of skin manifestation are: (*a*) discrete nodules up to a centimetre in diameter, yellowish in colour with a dry scaly surface, occurring mainly on the face, shoulders and arms; (*b*) large lobulated nodules of purplish colour, occurring on the nose or about the joints of the hands or feet; and (*c*) large flat patches with a granular or scaly surface occurring principally on the extremities or trunk. Sarcoidosis of the skin is always associated with other manifestations of the disease.

The *liver* and *spleen* are commonly involved in disseminated sarcoidosis. Less common manifestations include *bone involvement,* usually of the digits where intraosseous granulomas cause distortion of the bones and characteristic cystic lesions that are apparent

radiologically; *hypercalcaemia,* which is not necessarily associated with bone lesions, and may lead to renal calculi, nephrocalcinosis and renal insufficiency; involvement of the central and peripheral *nervous system,* causing a wide variety of neurological abnormalities including pituitary involvement leading to *diabetes insipidus*; and rarely, involvement of the heart and of the kidneys.

Investigations

CHEST RADIOGRAPH

Sarcoidosis is often first diagnosed from changes observed on the chest radiograph. *Enlargement of the hilar lymph nodes* is rarely massive and is commonly rather symmetrical. There is a well-defined outer border to the shadows except when associated lung infiltrations are present. All the groups of lymph nodes in the hilar region tend to be involved, particularly those situated at the major divisions of the main bronchi. *Pulmonary sarcoid infiltration,* which may or may not be associated with hilar gland enlargement, causes nodular radiographic shadows up to 5 mm in diameter; alternatively, a 'ground glass' appearance may be observed, due to large numbers of minute shadows less than 1 mm in diameter. The infiltration is bilateral, appearing diffusely throughout the lung fields or in the upper and mid zones. Occasionally, large shadows due to patches of infiltration may be observed in the upper zones. *Pulmonary fibrosis* is indicated by the appearance of linear streaks radiating into the lung fields from the hila, associated later with distortion of the hilar shadows and condensations of fibrous tissue spreading horizontally into the lower parts of the upper zones of both lungs.

KVEIM-SILTZBACH TEST

The Kveim-Siltzbach test is a specific skin test for sarcoidosis which is positive in three-quarters of patients with active disease. The antigen, prepared from human sarcoid spleen, is injected intracutaneously into the flexor surface of the forearm. A biopsy of the site should be taken four to six weeks after the injection whether or not there is an obvious papule; the finding of a typical sarcoid granuloma in the biopsy indicates a positive diagnosis of generalised sarcoidosis.

There is no evidence that false positive reactions occur, but false negative reactions are most likely in chronic disease or when activity has subsided.

TISSUE BIOPSY

The Kveim-Siltzbach test is one way of obtaining histological proof of the diagnosis. Biopsy of other tissues that appear clinically to be

involved by disease is equally valuable, the most readily accessible being the lymph nodes and skin. In the absence of obvious superficial disease the diagnosis may sometimes be clinched by expectant biopsy of the liver or of a scalene lymph node since these tissues are especially liable to be incidentally involved in disseminated sarcoidosis. Occasionally, mediastinoscopy and biopsy or lung biopsy are indicated.

MANTOUX TEST

This test is negative in two-thirds of people with sarcoidosis. A positive test weighs slightly against the diagnosis.

OTHER INVESTIGATIONS

Hyperglobulinaemia is a common accompaniment of sarcoidosis, increase in the γ and $\alpha2$ globulins being the most usual. The erythrocyte sedimentation rate is often accelerated in active disease, levels of 50 to 100 mm in the first hour (Westergren method) being typical.

Characteristic lesions may be observed in the *radiograph of the hands and feet,* usually in the phalanges or metacarpal and metatarsal bones. Lace-like thinning or longitudinal streaking occurs in the medulla, but the most typical appearance is that of round or elongated 'punched-out' areas. Destructive changes with mutilation of the terminal phalanges occur in the advanced stages of the disease.

Hypercalcaemia is present in a small proportion of cases, not necessarily associated with radiographic evidence of bone lesions or of serum phosphorus or alkaline phosphatase abnormalities. Hypercalciuria also occasionally occurs.

Course and Complications

The majority of patients with pulmonary sarcoidosis show a remarkable lack of incapacitating symptoms. Patients whose illness presents with erythema nodosum have a particularly good prognosis. Those with radiological evidence of hilar lymphadenopathy alone have a 60 per cent chance of complete radiographic clearing within a year, while a minority go on to develop bilateral pulmonary infiltration. Those patients who show pulmonary infiltration with or without hilar lymph node enlargement have a 50 per cent chance of improving spontaneously in about one year; if the infiltration persists for more than two years it is unlikely to remit spontaneously, but even so, in more than half such patients the infiltration remains static or only progresses very slowly, leading to pulmonary fibrosis and significant dyspnoea after at least five years. In the remainder, the pulmonary infiltration develops into massive fibrosis, causing steady

deterioration of exercise tolerance associated with such complications as secondary infection, bronchiectasis and spontaneous pneumothorax. Pulmonary hypertension leading to cor pulmonale is the commonest cause of death in patients with progressive disease.

Treatment

In the early stages of sarcoidosis the symptoms of fever and arthralgia which accompany erythema nodosum and hilar lymphadenopathy can be controlled with anti-inflammatory agents such as aspirin, oxyphenbutazone 100 mg three times daily or indomethacin 25 mg three times daily. The dosage should be reduced gradually and the drug discontinued when it is found that withdrawal does not produce recurrence of symptoms.

Spontaneous remission occurs commonly in sarcoidosis, particularly in patients presenting with erythema nodosum and in those with hilar lymph node enlargement with or without pulmonary infiltration of less than two years duration. Corticosteroids should be withheld from such patients, but they should be followed radiographically, clinically, and functionally at regular intervals.

The main indications for corticosteroid treatment are:

1. Progressive pulmonary disease, indicated by increasing dyspnoea, progressive impairment of pulmonary function (e.g. carbon monoxide transfer factor) and radiographic deterioration, from serial observations made over a period of 3 to 6 months.
2. Hypercalcaemia, to prevent nephrocalcinosis and corneal band opacity due to metastatic calcification.
3. Uveitis.
4. Involvement of the heart or central nervous system.
5. Severe skin lesions.

Treatment with prednisolone should be started in a dose of 20 to 40 mg daily by mouth in divided doses, and gradually reduced to a maintenance dose of about 10 mg daily. It may need to be continued for at least a year, and withdrawal must be undertaken cautiously for fear of relapse.

Where corticosteroids are contra-indicated chloroquin may be used to suppress skin lesions or pulmonary infiltrations, but its use is severely limited by the risk of serious side-effects, especially retinal degeneration.

17

Diffuse Fibrosing Alveolitis

Widespread involvement of the lungs by fibrosis which particularly affects the alveolar walls produces a typical clinical picture and functional disturbance characterised by increasing breathlessness on exertion and progressive reduction in lung volumes and impairment of gas transfer (T_L,CO). This pattern of illness may be the end-result in a number of diseases of diverse aetiology which may be grouped as follows:

1. Pulmonary granulomas; e.g. sarcoidosis, extrinsic allergic alveolitis, berylliosis.

2. Pulmonary exudates; e.g. reaction to cytotoxic agents such as busulphan or to ganglion blocking agents such as hexamethonium; recurrent inhalation of gastric contents or mineral oils in hiatus hernia; possible immunologically-induced reactions in conditions such as systemic lupus erythematosus and idiopathic pulmonary haemosiderosis.

3. Pneumoconiosis due to inorganic dust; e.g. silica, coal-dust and asbestos.

4. Disorders of unknown aetiology; e.g. the Hamman-Rich syndrome and cryptogenic fibrosing alveolitis.

The description of diffuse fibrosing alveolitis which follows relates primarily to the cryptogenic form of the disease (chronic diffuse interstitial pulmonary fibrosis) and to the Hamman-Rich syndrome (acute diffuse interstitial pulmonary fibrosis).

Pathology

MORPHOLOGICAL APPEARANCES

Cryptogenic fibrosing alveolitis is characterised by inflammatory changes in the periphery of the lung beyond the terminal bronchiole, with two main histological features:

1. Cellular thickening of the alveolar septa with lymphocytic infiltration and a tendency to fibrosis.

2. Large mononuclear cells, originating as Type II pneumocytes, in the alveolar spaces.

Other changes in the alveoli such as hyaline membrane, organisation of exudate and the presence of eosinophils have been described, but they appear to be infrequent and associated more with the acute, rapidly progressive type of interstitial fibrosis of the lungs, known as the Hamman-Rich syndrome. Lymphoid follicles in the periphery of the lungs are an additional feature that occurs in a proportion of cases.

The relative predominance of each of these features varies from case to case, but in one series of lung biopsies it appeared that there was an inverse relationship between the degree of alveolar wall thickening and the number of large granular mononuclear cells in the alveolar spaces, and that the likelihood of a response to corticosteroid therapy was greatest among those patients whose biopsies showed predominant cellular changes with the least thickening of the alveolar walls. The condition known as 'desquamative interstitial pneumonia' shows many of the histological features of the more cellular type of cryptogenic fibrosing alveolitis, and may be a variant of this disease.

The type of histological pattern observed at lung biopsy seems to be unrelated to the duration of the clinical symptoms, but radiological studies have shown that as time goes on mottled shadows are seen in the late stages of the disease, giving the appearances of 'honeycomb lung'. Histologically, the fibrous tissue in the affected areas of honeycomb lung is condensed, leaving cyst-like air spaces in place of the gas-exchanging part of the bronchopulmonary tree; these spaces are lined by hypertrophied bronchial epithelium, occasionally in several layers. Smooth muscle hyperplasia of the lung is sometimes an associated feature.

FUNCTIONAL PATHOLOGY

Widespread interstitial changes in the lung cause the characteristic restrictive pattern of lung function. All lung volumes are reduced but airway resistance is normal. (FEV1 is often lower than normal because of the general reduction in lung volumes, but the FEV1/FVC ratio is normal and sometimes unusually high.) Lung compliance is reduced and the resting lung volume (FRC) is lower than normal; the work of breathing is increased by the abnormal 'stiffness' of the lungs, and the patient usually adopts a rapid, shallow pattern of respiration. Transfer factor for carbon monoxide (T_L,CO) is reduced early in the course of the disease, and provides a useful index of progress in response to therapy.

The main cause of impaired gas exchange is thought to be uneven distribution of ventilation and perfusion; tests of inspired gas distribution often show that it is very uneven, and perfusion of the alveolar capillaries is disrupted by fibrosis of the interstitial tissues. The unevenness of ventilation is ascribed to non-uniformity of compliance of different alveolar units due to variation in the degree of fibrosis in different parts of the lungs. Whether diffusion limitation of oxygen (i.e. 'alveolar-capillary block') due to thickening of the alveolar-capillary membrane contributes significantly to the impairment of gas exchange remains an open question; the rate of diffusion of oxygen is so high that thickening of the membrane would not be expected to affect oxygen uptake, but there is some recent experimental data suggesting that impaired diffusion, *when it is distributed unevenly in relation to blood flow,* may cause arterial hypoxaemia in the absence of significant ventilation/perfusion inequality. In some patients there is an increase in venous-to-arterial shunt which makes a further contribution to arterial hypoxaemia.

Cyanosis at rest is encountered in advanced disease, but a moderate degree of arterial oxygen desaturation (85 to 90%) is quite common even in the early stages; however, it is characteristic of these patients that they become further desaturated and more deeply cyanosed on exercise. Carbon dioxide retention is not a feature unless there is concomitant airways obstruction, and the arterial carbon dioxide tension is usually normal or low.

Pulmonary hypertension sometimes occurs in longstanding disease, and is attributed to the obstructive and obliterative changes in the pulmonary capillary bed. Right ventricular enlargement and cor pulmonale are late complications.

Clinical Features

Cryptogenic fibrosing alveolitis is an uncommon condition that affects both sexes equally, usually occurring after middle age, although it is occasionally encountered in younger people. The four patients described by Hamman and Rich were all under the age of forty but their illness was somewhat atypical in that it came on acutely and followed a rapid, downhill course lasting no longer than four months. Very rarely it affects more than one member of the same family, suggesting that there can be an inherited predisposition to the disease.

The onset of the illness is usually insidious, causing gradually increasing *dyspnoea on exertion*. There is a *cough* which is dry or productive only of a little mucoid sputum, although slight haemoptysis occasionally occurs. *Clubbing* of the fingers is common

and often so pronounced that the patient himself complains of it. Cyanosis, increased by exertion, is characteristic of advanced disease. Clinical examination reveals a rapid respiratory rate (sometimes 30 to 40 breaths a minute) with diminished chest expansion. Widespread fine crepitations are audible on auscultation, most marked at the lung bases but often extending upwards to a variable level. They are typically limited to the end of inspiration and may disappear when the patient bends forward. Signs of congestive heart failure and pulmonary hypertension may be encountered in the late stages of the disease.

The course of fibrosing alveolitis is variable. The subacute form (Hamman-Rich syndrome) is rare, coming on abruptly with fever and dyspnoea and progressing rapidly to death from right ventricular failure within a few months. In the middle-aged or elderly patient the disease follows a chronic course, the rate at which it progresses tending to vary inversely with age of onset. Often it appears to become stationary for a time but most commonly the pulmonary changes slowly advance, leading to increasing dyspnoea and, ultimately, pulmonary hypertension after several years. Intercurrent bronchial infections are quite common and may aggravate the impairment of gas exchange by causing airways obstruction.

Aetiology

The aetiology of cryptogenic fibrosing alveolitis is unknown. The association of similar lung changes in some of the collagen diseases, particularly rheumatoid arthritis and scleroderma, and the finding of antinuclear factor, non-organ specific complement-fixing antibodies and rheumatoid factor in a high proportion of patients with fibrosing alveolitis have led to the hypothesis that the pulmonary changes have an autoimmune basis. It has been further suggested that the lung disease may depend upon the presence both of circulating autoantibodies and an external provoking agent such as a viral or bacterial infection or inhaled dust particles, but at present these ideas are largely speculative.

Diagnosis and Investigations

In determining the cause of diffuse pulmonary fibrosis a wide range of alternative possibilities may have to be considered, the diagnosis usually being suggested by a combination of clinical and radiological features. The *subacute form* of fibrosing alveolitis presents quite different diagnostic problems from the commoner chronic type of disease. The patient presents with fever, dyspnoea and patchy radiological shadows which are sometimes confluent and more

extensive in the lower zones. The alternative diagnoses which may have to be considered include:

1. Bronchopneumonia.
2. Left ventricular failure.
3. Pulmonary infiltration with eosinophilia.
4. Multiple pulmonary emboli.
5. Alveolar cell carcinoma.
6. Drug sensitivity to busulphan, chlorambucil or hexamethonium.
7. Poisoning with the weedkiller, Paraquat.

The *chronic form* of the disease usually presents with severe dyspnoea associated with diffuse mottling on the chest radiograph, although in the early case the lung fields may appear normal. Usually, however, there is a fine mottled shadowing, sometimes giving a 'ground glass' or stippled appearance involving predominantly the bases of the lungs, and proceeding over the years to produce a coarse mottling that may extend to involve the whole of both lung fields. In the late stages a honeycomb type of shadow may be seen at the lung bases, due to condensation of fibrous tissue around cystic spaces. Shrinkage of the lungs due to fibrosis may cause elevation of the diaphragm. The differential diagnoses suggested by this clinical and radiological presentation include:

1. Pulmonary fibrosis due to inhalation of organic and inorganic dusts.
2. Sarcoidosis.
3. Rheumatoid arthritis, systemic lupus erythematosus and diffuse sclerosis (scleroderma).
4. Other causes of honeycomb lung, e.g. tuberous sclerosis and eosinophilic granuloma.
5. Lymphangitis carcinomatosa.

The diagnosis of cryptogenic fibrosing alveolitis must often be reached by exclusion. As part of a careful history and clinical examination, particular attention should be paid to occupational exposure to dust or toxic fumes, and details of recent drug therapy should be obtained. It is often useful to carry out the following series of tests as a routine:

Sputum: Smear and culture for tubercle bacilli;
Microscopy, for eosinophils and asbestos bodies;
Cytological examination, for malignant cells.
Blood: Full blood count and differential white cell count, including eosinophils;
Rheumatoid factor, anti-nuclear factor, LE cells.
Kveim-Siltzbach test, for sarcoidosis.

If a diagnosis cannot be reached by any of the methods mentioned above it is necessary to carry out *lung biopsy*. This investigation is hazardous to the severely dyspnoeic patient since thoracotomy and open lung biopsy at best automatically lead to some temporary impairment of pulmonary function, while trephine biopsy carries the risk of pneumothorax and pulmonary bleeding, and should not therefore be performed unless full thoracic surgical cover is readily available. Occasional instances of death due to pulmonary bleeding following trephine biopsy have been described.

Apart from the risk of complications it may be argued that the lung sample obtained by trephine biopsy may well be unrepresentative of the lung changes as a whole and may therefore fail to give diagnostic information or sufficient evidence of the state of activity of the lesion. On the other hand, corticosteroid treatment, which is the most likely to be effective in cryptogenic fibrosing alveolitis, carries inherent risks that tend to contra-indicate this form of therapy in the absence of a definite diagnosis. The decision to carry out lung biopsy and the method of its performance must therefore depend on a careful assessment of the individual case.

Treatment

Corticosteroids are the only form of therapy likely to affect the course of the disease. They should certainly be used in the subacute form of the disease which tends to progress rapidly, and in which steroid therapy is likely to show its most dramatic effect, although only in a minority of cases. In chronic fibrosing alveolitis the response to steroids is very variable, although clinical improvement and radiological clearing of the lung fields is sometimes seen. If the disease is progressing a trial of prednisolone should be given, starting with 20 to 40 mg daily and observing the effect by serial measurement of lung volumes, transfer factor, and arterial oxygen tension. Steroids should be given for a limited trial period and then either withdrawn or continued in a low maintenance dose, depending on the results of objective tests of pulmonary function. Some patients require large doses to be continued indefinitely, becoming severely dyspnoeic when the dose is reduced beyond a certain level so that they gradually become subject to the complications of steroid overdosage such as osteoporosis and vertebral collapse.

18

Occupational Lung Disease

The Occupational History

The lungs are readily damaged by the inhalation of dusts or poisonous gases and fumes, the type of pathological reaction varying according to the nature and quantity of toxic material inhaled. In general terms there are four types of reaction:

1. Acute pulmonary oedema, coming on within a few minutes or at most a few hours after exposure.

2. Destructive changes to the lung parenchyma, eventually causing pulmonary emphysema and chronic airways obstruction.

3. Pulmonary fibrosis, developing slowly over many years to produce a restrictive type of disorder.

4. Malignant disease of the lungs or pleura, occurring many years after exposure.

The symptoms and signs of these reactions are by no means specific for disease of industrial origin but occur frequently among common conditions of quite different aetiology; for example, left ventricular failure, chronic bronchitis, or sarcoidosis. The clue to the aetiology lies in the patient's occupational history which must be probed in detail whenever the clinical or radiological features of the disease are suggestive. The history should include:

1. Details of *all* occupations since the patient left school, with the duration of each.

2. An account of the actual industrial task in which the patient is engaged, with enquiry into the presence of dust, gases or fumes in the environment, whether resulting from the patient's own occupation or from those of nearby workers.

3. The patient's observations on the time relationship between exposure to his occupational environment and the onset of any symptoms.

Diagnosis of an industrial disease may have important financial implications for the patient since he may thereby benefit under the British Industrial Injuries Act, and this advantage must not be lost by default.

Acute Lung Irritants

Certain highly toxic products, including gases, metallic fumes, and a few metallic dusts may be inhaled accidentally by workers engaged in their commercial production, or may incidentally contaminate the environment of a worker occupied in a task such as arc-welding. The effect of inhaling such substances depends mainly on the concentration, causing successively tightness in the throat and a hoarse voice, cough and wheezing, and acute pulmonary oedema with cyanosis and severe dyspnoea. An acute chemical pneumonia sometimes occurs, due to outpouring of protein-rich exudate into the alveoli as a result of intense pulmonary inflammation. The rate of development and extent of the pathological reaction varies somewhat according to the nature of the inhaled poison.

IRRITANT GASES

Ammonia, Oxides of Sulphur, Chlorine. Accidental inhalation of these gases causes acute irritation of the upper respiratory tract with sneezing and coughing, and pulmonary oedema. When recovery occurs there may be residual bronchial damage leading to chronic airways obstruction. It is possible that the release of sulphur dioxide into the atmosphere by the burning of coal, coke and oil plays a part in the pathogenesis of chronic bronchitis.

Oxides of Nitrogen. Nitrogen dioxide (NO_2) and tetroxide (N_2O_4) are dangerous pulmonary irritants that may cause only tightness in the chest or cough at the time of exposure, but induce severe pulmonary oedema and bronchopneumonia after a delay of a few hours. When not immediately fatal the acute illness may be followed by obliterative bronchiolitis some weeks later, and sometimes subsequent bronchiolar fibrosis.

Nitrogen dioxide inhalation is an occupational hazard in the shipbuilding industry, where oxyacetylene burners are used in confined spaces for heating metal, in mining or tunnelling when the gas is released by combustion of explosives, and in farming, when it is produced by the fermentation of silage causing toxic levels of the gas to accumulate in the silos—'silo-fillers disease'.

IRRITANT METALS

Cadmium, when inhaled acutely, causes a severe chemical pneumonia with high mortality, requiring prompt treatment with oxygen,

corticosteroids, and a prophylactic broad-spectrum antibiotic. Tracheostomy may be indicated. Chronic inhalation causes destruction of the lung parenchyma leading to severe emphysema. The metal has many industrial uses; for example, as an alloy with copper in cables and wires, in the preparation of pigments, in pesticides, and as an electrode material in alkaline electric batteries. Welders engaged in cutting scrap metal may be exposed to high concentrations of cadmium oxide fumes.

Magnesium dust or fume may be inhaled by workers engaged in the production of this metal when used in the steel industry, in the dry battery industry, for glass colouring, and for the production of potassium permanganate. Inhalation causes a severe, acute pneumonia, due to chemical irritation of the lungs by manganese dioxide fume.

Vanadium causes mild upper and lower respiratory tract irritation in men exposed either in plants processing vanadium ore for alloying with steel, or in situations where they may breathe the ash or soot of burned fuel oil that contains a high concentration of vanadium.

Zinc is used in galvanising and forms an ingredient of brass. Welding, melting or casting of brass or galvanised iron produces zinc fume which causes symptoms some hours after exposure. The acute pulmonary irritation of zinc fume may cause an illness ranging from mild cough to acute pulmonary oedema: 'metal fume fever' is an accompanying systemic upset similar to the symptoms of acute influenza and attributed to the circulation of protein breakdown products of dead pulmonary leucocytes.

ARC WELDING

Welding is performed at extremely high temperatures that cause vaporisation of many of the component materials involved. These materials include the metal to be welded, the atmospheric gases, and the surface coating of the electrodes and of the metals. As a result, many irritant gases and fumes may accumulate in the welder's immediate environment, including ozone, nitrogen dioxide, iron, cadmium, manganese, and zinc. If the work is prolonged and undertaken in a confined space, toxic concentrations of these substances may produce both acute and chronic effects on the lungs, and it is not uncommon for symptoms and signs of chronic respiratory disease, usually of the obstructive type, to be found among welders. Nevertheless, the term 'arc-welder's lung' does not denote a specific pathological entity and is better avoided.

Diseases due to Inorganic Dust

The pulmonary diseases that result from the inhalation of dust, both

organic and inorganic, are known collectively as the pneumoconioses. In most of these diseases the pathological process leads to pulmonary fibrosis coming on after many years of exposure and causing the characteristic clinical and functional picture of restrictive lung disease sometimes secondarily associated with chronic airways obstruction. The inorganic materials that most commonly produce this type of disease are silica, coal dust, asbestos, and the dust of various metals.

SILICOSIS

The association of pulmonary fibrosis with the inhalation of fine dust into the lungs was gradually recognised in a number of industries in Great Britain in the eighteenth and nineteenth centuries. The condition arises from work in the manufacture of pottery, metal grinding, sandstone dressing and quarrying, boiler-scaling, mining, and certain tasks in iron foundries, all occupations that result in the inhalation of fine particles of silica in high concentration over a lengthy period of the working life. Other forms of silica that may induce pulmonary fibrosis include kaolin (China clay) and talc.

Pathogenesis. Deposition of dust particles in the alveoli depends on their size, the larger particles of more than 10 microns in diameter being deposited by sedimentation in the upper air passages while the very small particles of 0·01 microns or less are deposited by diffusion on the bronchial epithelium. Only a small proportion of dust particles of intermediate size is deposited in the alveoli and an even smaller percentage is retained, because much of the dust is gathered in by alveolar macrophages and excreted by ciliary action, while some finds its way into lymph vessels and accumulates in the lymphatic tissue.

The cause of lung fibrosis in silicosis is uncertain. The theory that silica dust particles dissolve to form free silicic acid which, in turn, stimulates collagen formation has become less acceptable, largely because the degree of fibrosis that can be produced experimentally appears to be unrelated to the varying solubility of different forms of silica. Two alternative biological theories as yet unproven are either that the reaction to silica is an immunological one, or that fibrosis develops as the result of phospholipid release from dead, dust-laden macrophages.

Pathology. Dust tends to accumulate at the level of the respiratory bronchioles, where a fibroblastic reaction occurs and eventually progresses to form islets of acellular fibrous tissue which is often hyaline and arranged in a whorled manner. Increasing exposure to silica dust leads to the enlargement of existing nodules and the development of new ones, so that scattered discrete lesions occur throughout the lung measuring up to 5 mm in diameter and being somewhat larger and more numerous in the upper than in the lower

parts. This form of the disease is known as *simple silicosis*, and causes relatively few symptoms; more prolonged exposure to the dust leads to extensive fibrosis which involves and obliterates the bronchi and blood vessels. This stage of the disease is called *massive fibrosis*, and is complicated by secondary emphysema and often by tuberculous infection.

The functional effect of these changes is to produce a restrictive pattern of lung disorder due to the fibrosis, with some degree of airway obstruction due to secondary emphysema. Gas exchange is affected adversely because of resulting uneven distribution of ventilation and perfusion.

Clinical Features. Silicosis is a chronic condition of insidious onset occurring in individuals who have been exposed to the dust for many years. The diagnosis is suggested by the occupational history in a patient presenting with *progressive dyspnoea* on exertion, associated with *unproductive cough* and *recurrent bronchitis. Haemoptysis* occurs occasionally, but is more frequent in those cases complicated by *tuberculosis*; the *sputum* should always be examined for tubercle bacilli, especially when rapid deterioration is associated with weight loss, cachexia, and fever. The clinical signs may reflect predominant fibrotic changes with restricted chest expansion and scattered fine crepitations, or may be more characteristic of airways obstruction with wheezing and prolonged expiration, depending on the stage of the disease. *Cor pulmonale* may develop in advanced disease.

The *chest radiograph* characteristically shows diffuse or nodular lesions throughout both lung fields, classically more pronounced in the upper parts of the lungs. In massive fibrosis, dense shadows, which may be cavitated, are seen against this background. Calcification commonly occurs in the hilar lymph nodes.

COALWORKERS' PNEUMOCONIOSIS

Like silicosis, coalworkers' pneumoconiosis is due to the deposition of coal dust in the lungs, and produces two forms or stages of disease: *simple pneumoconiosis*, in which the lungs become clogged with dust leading to a small amount of irregularly disposed fibrosis which causes few if any symptoms; and *progressive massive fibrosis* (PMF) which develops in a small proportion of patients with simple pneumoconiosis because of further exposure to inhaled dust, and leads to serious progressive disease. The duration of exposure to dust among coal miners before symptoms due to progressive massive fibrosis appear is likely to be at least ten years, but the attack rate of PMF seems to be much greater in some coal-fields (e.g. South Wales) than in others, and is also greater among those exposed to dust at an

early age. Once present, the lesions of PMF continue to develop even though further exposure to coal dust is avoided.

Pathogenesis. Deposition of coal dust in the lungs occurs in a similar manner to the deposition of silica particles described above. The dust accumulates in the region of the respiratory bronchioles, along the lymphatics and in the hilar lymph nodes. The stimulus to fibrous tissue formation in these areas appears to come from the coal dust itself, and is not related to the small amount of silica present in most coal dust samples, although a high concentration of silica in the inhaled dust has been shown experimentally to produce a greater degree of fibrosis than either coal dust or silica dust alone.

Although simple pneumoconiosis predisposes to progressive massive fibrosis the factors that promote this change in a small proportion of pneumoconiotic individuals are undetermined. It is no longer believed that tuberculous infection plays any part, but it seems possible that the deposition of fibrous tissue may be part of an immune mechanism. This hypothesis seems particularly relevant in *Caplan's syndrome*, a form of massive fibrosis in which the pulmonary lesions have the histological characteristics of rheumatoid nodules, and the condition is associated clinically and immuno-logically with rheumatoid arthritis (page 251).

Pathology. The simple dust lesion of coalworkers consists of a sleeve of dust and a little fibrous tissue disposed around the respiratory bronchioles. Dilatation of these small airways occurs secondarily, resulting in focal emphysema of centrilobular distribution; this emphysematous change is much more characteristic of coalworkers' pneumoconiosis than of silicosis.

The massive lesions of coalworkers occur mainly in the upper parts of the lung, consisting of dust irregularly mingled with bundles of coarse, hyaline collagen fibres. Blood vessels and air passages may be obliterated by fibrous tissue, and cavitation may occur within these massive lesions, due either to necrosis following vascular obliteration or to tuberculous infection. The lesions associated with rheumatoid arthritis are discrete, rounded nodules which occur in the periphery of the lung fields, usually appearing in crops. Histologically they show concentric bands of collagen separated by lines of dust and surrounded by a zone of palisaded histiocytes similar to the appearance in subcutaneous rheumatoid nodules. The discrete lesions are usually 1 to 2 cm in diameter, but commonly coalesce to form larger fibrotic areas. Necrosis may occur within the rheumatoid nodules, leaving thin-walled cavities.

Functional Disorder. Simple pneumoconiosis causes little disturbance of lung function, but in progressive massive fibrosis there is considerable reduction in ventilatory capacity and, later, gross

unevenness of gas distribution due to secondary airway obstruction. Gas exchange is affected mainly by uneven distribution of ventilation and perfusion.

Clinical Features. Simple pneumoconiosis may be observed in the chest radiograph of coalworkers who are quite free of respiratory symptoms, but it appears to have no adverse effect on pulmonary function, or to alter life expectation significantly. Coincidental chronic bronchitis in such patients may cause symptoms of cough and breathlessness which lead to considerable anxiety among men who are aware that their chest radiography is abnormal, especially if they have acquaintances suffering from the massive form of the disease. Reassurance and a thorough explanation of the differences between simple pneumoconiosis and progressive massive fibrosis may be effective in relieving symptoms, although any coincidental bronchitis should obviously be vigorously treated.

When the lesions of progressive massive fibrosis first appear, usually ten to twenty years after beginning work at the coal-face, they cause no symptoms, but *exertional dyspnoea* is usually the earliest and comes on very insidiously. *Cough* with *mucoid sputum* is common, and there is an increasing tendency to acute exacerbations of *bronchitis* in the winters. Slight *haemoptysis* is common, and *melanoptysis*, the coughing up of jet black fluid in fairly large quantities, occurs in advanced disease. It is due to rupture into a bronchus of the dust-stained, liquified contents of a massive lesion. *Chest pain* frequently occurs in the late stages of the disease, usually diffuse, dull and aching in quality. The clinical signs may suggest both bronchitic and fibrotic changes.

Investigations should include examination of the sputum for tubercle bacilli, since tuberculosis frequently complicates the massive form of the disease. The *chest radiograph* in simple pneumoconiosis shows tiny opacities scattered throughout the lung fields, and the severity of the disease may be classified according to the extent of the opacities. The radiological changes of progressive massive fibrosis consist of one or more irregular opacities situated in the peripheral parts of the upper lobes, against the background miliary opacities of simple pneumoconiosis. Cavitation may be observed.

Course and Management. Simple pneumoconiosis of mild degree, with a small number of radiological opacities in an area not greater than one third of both lung fields, carries a 1 per cent risk of developing PMF, but this risk increases to about 30 per cent when there are profuse opacities covering the whole of the lung fields. Once PMF is established nothing can be done to halt the disease itself, but the complications of chronic bronchitis and tuberculosis are amenable

to treatment. Death may be due to tuberculosis, respiratory failure, or cor pulmonale.

ASBESTOSIS

Asbestos is the name given to a group of silicate minerals that have the important commercial properties of heat-resistance and a fibrous structure, the type most widely used in industry being chrysotile. It is used in a wide range of commercial products which include textiles, roofing materials, pipes, floor and ceiling tiles, brake linings and gaskets for cars, and insulating materials. As a result, the consumption of asbestos has increased dramatically in the past twenty years.

Exposure to asbestos is greatest among men engaged in extracting the material from the ground by quarrying or mining, in those handling the raw material, and in a small group of workers in secondary industries who are engaged in sawing or milling asbestos components. Less serious but significant exposure occurs among those occupied in the manufacture of asbestos-containing products, in workers such as pipe laggers or plumbers who handle these materials, and among maintenance and demolition workers both in the building and ship-building industries in which heavy environmental contamination is likely to occur when insulating material is stripped and replaced. Under such conditions intermittent exposure may affect workers in allied occupations such as maintenance engineers, electricians, painters, and joiners.

Exposure to asbestos predisposes to three types of lung pathology: diffuse pulmonary fibrosis, bronchial carcinoma, and mesothelioma of the pleura. The latter conditions are discussed in Chapter 19.

Pathogenesis. Asbestos dust is inhaled into the lungs, the particles consisting of bundles of fibres of which the majority are less than 20 microns in length. The larger fibres lodge in the terminal bronchioles and penetrate the tissues where they are surrounded by macrophages. Some are coated with a protein iron complex which resembles clear amber and stains positively for iron. These bodies are about 70 microns long and 2 microns thick, having slightly bulbous ends which give the *asbestos body* its characteristic appearance. The significance of the asbestos bodies in relation to pulmonary fibrosis is uncertain, but their presence in sputum at least provides evidence of previous asbestos exposure. Smaller fibres may deposit in the alveoli where they are taken up by macrophages which coalesce to form giant cells at the centre of a granulomatous reaction.

The sharp needles of asbestos are liable to penetrate the tissues and may be carried to distant parts of the body. They also migrate towards the subpleural tissue and tend to accumulate there, setting up an

inflammatory reaction that is responsible for the fibrous plaques and pleural adhesions characteristic of asbestosis.

Pathology. Diffuse fibrosis occurs around the terminal bronchioles and spreads into the alveolar walls, causing shrinkage and rigidity of the lung tissue. This contraction leads to widening and distortion of the terminal airways which become lined with bronchial epithelium, forming the characteristic cystic change of honeycomb lung. The visceral and parietal pleura become adherent in some areas, and fibrocartilaginous plaques form on the parietal pleura, particularly over the diaphragm and in the mid-zone laterally and in front. In older persons the plaques become calcified and radiologically visible.

The *functional effect* of these changes is to produce a typically restrictive form of disability with reduction in all lung volumes but maintenance of normal air flow. Tests of carbon monoxide transfer are impaired and gas exchange is affected by uneven distribution of ventilation and perfusion. Pulmonary compliance is abnormally low.

Clinical Features. A history of prolonged exposure to asbestos dust is an essential feature of asbestosis, not less than seven years in the dustiest occupations and usually twenty years or more. The patient must be questioned closely about his occupation since asbestos exposure may be only a coincidental aspect of his trade. The onset of symptoms is insidious, usually increasing *breathlessness on exertion* and *cough* with a little mucoid sputum. *Tightness in the chest* or poorly localised *chest pain* are relatively late symptoms. Clinical examination may reveal *asbestos warts* on the hands, subcutaneous nodules due to a granulomatous reaction where asbestos fibres have entered the skin through cuts or abrasions. *Clubbing of the fingers* occurs frequently. When pulmonary fibrosis is fully developed chest expansion may appear restricted and *fine crepitations* are heard on auscultation, most marked at the lung bases and occurring at the end of full inspiration.

The disease may be complicated by tuberculosis, chronic airways obstruction, respiratory insufficiency, and cor pulmonale. Bronchial carcinoma is likely to occur in the sixth decade or later, especially in patients exposed to the additional hazard of cigarette smoking. Mesothelioma of the pleura is a late complication, but may occur in individuals whose exposure to asbestos has been slight or even unrecognised.

Diagnosis. The diagnosis of asbestosis depends greatly upon the history of exposure, and on clinical and physiological evidence of restrictive lung disease. The *chest radiograph* in the fully developed case of pulmonary fibrosis shows fine mottled shadows which are most prominent in the lower parts of the lung fields, but in patients

who have received lesser degrees of exposure it is more common to see only radiological evidence of pleural thickening and linear streaks or patches of dense shadowing where pleural plaques have become calcified. The finding of *asbestos bodies in the sputum* is indicative of exposure to the dust, but provides no evidence of lung damage.

Prevention of disease due to asbestos can be achieved only by maintaining dust concentrations at a low level by ventilation and dust suppression. Where exposure to dust in high concentration is unavoidable, workers in the area should be segregated and should wear masks and protective clothing.

Management. Once the diagnosis of asbestosis has been established the patient should be removed from exposure to the dust. Corticosteroid therapy may be given a trial in progressive disease, although its effectiveness is doubtful and it should not be continued unless there is objective radiological and physiological evidence of improvement.

PNEUMOCONIOSIS DUE TO METAL INHALATION

A number of metals may be deposited in the lungs as a result of occupational exposure to fumes or dust. They include:

1. *Iron* (Siderosis). This causes generalised reticular and nodular shadows on the chest radiograph of silver polishers (who use rouge, an iron oxide powder), arc-welders, and haematite miners. The iron deposition does not cause pulmonary fibrosis or symptoms, although haematite miners may get concurrent silicosis (sidero-silicosis) which produces a disease similar in all respects to that caused by the inhalation of other silicotic dusts.

2. *Beryllium* (Berylliosis) causes an acute chemical pneumonia in workers exposed to heavy concentrations of dust during the process of extracting beryllium from its ores. Prolonged exposure, which occurred among workers in the fluorescent lighting industry when beryllium was used to coat the inner surface of the tubes, causes a chronic granulomatous inflammation histologically similar to sarcoidosis, with generalised lung fibrosis and a restrictive pattern of functional disorder.

3. *Aluminium* (Aluminosis) is a rare cause of pulmonary fibrosis and restrictive lung disease among those engaged in the manufacture of explosives; for example, in the fireworks industry.

4. *Tin* (Stannosis) causes radiological opacities of reticular or nodular pattern throughout the lung fields without any pulmonary fibrosis or functional disability.

Table 18.1

Extrinsic Allergic Alveolitis

Disease	Occupation	Dust Exposure	Precipitins Present Against
Farmer's lung	Dairy farmers, cattle-breeders	Mouldy hay	Thermophilic actinomycetes *Micropolyspora faeni*. *Thermoactinomyces vulgaris*
Bagassosis	Handling sugar-cane bagasse (in the manufacture of paper, cardboard, etc.)	Mouldy sugar-cane bagasse	*T. vulgaris*
Mushroom worker's lung	Handling mushroom compost, or mushroom-picking	Mushroom compost dust	*T. vulgaris*
Maple-bark pneumonitis	Maple-bark strippers	Mouldy maple bark	*Cryptostroma (Coniosporum) corticale*
Malt worker's lung	Distillery or brewery workers	Mouldy barley, malt dust	*Aspergillus clavatus* and *A. fumigatus*
Bird fancier's lung	Pigeon breeders, parrot and budgerigar fanciers, chicken farmers	Pigeon, budgerigar, parrot, hen droppings	Serum protein, and droppings
Pituitary snuff-taker's lung	Patients with diabetes insipidus	Heterologous pituitary powder	Serum protein, pituitary antigens
Wheat weevil disease	Mill workers	Infested wheat flour	*Sitophilus granarius*
Suberosis	Cork workers	Mouldy oak-bark, cork dust	Mouldy cork dust
'New Guinea lung'	New Guinea natives	Mouldy thatch dust	Thatch of huts
Sequoiosis	Timber workers	Mouldy sawdust	*Graphium* *Aureobrasidium pullulans*

Diseases due to Organic Dust

EXTRINSIC ALLERGIC ALVEOLITIS

Inhaled organic dusts cause different pulmonary allergic diseases, depending partly on the site of the antigen-antibody reaction. The asthmatic type of response (page 116) occurs in the bronchi and is mediated either by IgE (the Type I, immediate reaction), or by precipitin antibodies (the Type III, immune-complex reaction), or occasionally by both types of reaction in succession (the dual response). Alternatively, the Type III, immune-complex reaction may occur in the alveoli, resulting in allergic alveolitis or bronchiolo-alveolitis. Here the circulating precipitin antibodies react with inhaled antigen leading to extracellular phagocytosis of antigen-antibody aggregates, followed by destruction of the phagocytes and release of lysosomal enzymes. These, in turn, cause extracellular digestion and tissue damage coming on several hours after exposure to the antigen. In atopic subjects a dual response sometimes occurs, i.e. an immediate, Type I reaction characterised by bronchoconstriction, followed several hours later by the systemic manifestations of the Type III response.

The *clinical syndromes* produced by this allergic alveolar reaction are known collectively as *extrinsic allergic alveolitis* although at present they are generally recognised by names descriptive of their occupational or antigenic origin (Table 18.1).

The *clinical features* typically consist of:

1. Acute episodes of fever, headache, chills and malaise, coming on four or five hours after exposure to the antigen, and lasting for about 24 hours.

2. Cough and dyspnoea, with basal pulmonary crepitations.

3. With repeated exposure, a restrictive type of pulmonary disability due to pulmonary fibrosis, leading to chronic exertional dyspnoea, cyanosis and ultimately cor pulmonale.

In some cases the onset of the disease is more insidious, producing gradually increasing dyspnoea without the acute episodes; this pattern of disease is attributed to persistent exposure to low concentrations of the antigen, rather than to intermittent episodes of intensive exposure. In a proportion of cases, which varies with the type of antigen, a rapid asthmatic attack occurs in response to the antigen, followed by the systemic response four or five hours later.

The *pathological changes* consist of a polymorphonuclear exudate in the lung parenchyma, followed by a predominantly mononuclear infiltration. An epithelioid cell granulomatous reaction occurs and diffuse pulmonary fibrosis develops subsequently. These

morphological changes lead to a restrictive type of *functional disability,* with diminution in lung volumes, and a decrease in lung compliance and in carbon monoxide transfer factor. A significant proportion of patients with chronic disease show evidence of airways obstruction which is not reversed by isoprenaline inhalation.

The *investigation* of extrinsic allergic alveolitis should include examination of the serum for *precipitins* against extracts of the suspected antigens. A Type III response is obtained a few hours after injecting the offending antigen into the skin, and inhalation tests will precipitate a typical febrile systemic reaction. The *chest radiograph* usually shows diffuse miliary shadowing during the acute stage of the illness, followed in chronic cases by diffuse fibrosis and 'honeycomb' changes affecting particularly the upper lobes.

Management of the condition depends primarily on removal of the offending antigen from the patient's environment, and this may sometimes require a change of employment. Corticosteroid therapy may result in dramatic improvement in the acute or subacute case.

BYSSINOSIS

In contrast to the primarily alveolar reaction produced by the various organic dusts that cause extrinsic allergic alveolitis, the pathological reaction in byssinosis occurs in the bronchi, producing chronic airways obstruction. Byssinosis is an occupational disease of the cotton, flax, and hemp industries, causing illness in two-thirds of the workers engaged in the dustiest tasks associated with cleaning and combing out the raw vegetable fibre, and among those who are occupied in stripping and maintaining the machines that carry out these processes.

Clinical Features. The illness comes on after many years exposure to the dust, with the typical syndrome of 'Monday Fever': following the week-end break the worker returns to the dusty atmosphere of the mill and after a few hours develops a characteristic sense of tightness in the chest, sometimes combined with cough, which lasts throughout the day but subsides for the remainder of the week. As time goes on the symptoms persist for longer and, finally, progress to permanent dyspnoea, often with cough and sputum, which is similar in all respects to chronic bronchitis and emphysema as it occurs in the general population. Respiratory failure, pulmonary hypertension, and cor pulmonale occur in the late stages of the disease.

The *pathogenesis* of the condition is uncertain; the slow onset of symptoms and gradual recovery in spite of the continued presence of dust appears uncharacteristic of an immediate Type I hypersensitivity. It has been suggested that the symptoms may be due to a Type III reaction affecting the bronchi rather than the alveoli, in

which the amount of precipitins is limited so that a single vigorous reaction could make the subject refractory to repeated exposure on successive days until the amount rose again when exposure ceased during the following week-end.

An alternative hypothesis is based on recent evidence that histamine release is stimulated by inhalation of aqueous extracts of cotton, flax and hemp. It is suggested that the initial bronchoconstrictor effect of histamine causes a typical 'Monday Fever' syndrome which subsides as histamine reserves are depleted by persistent exposure during the working week. There is at present no satisfactory explanation for the ultimate development of permanent airways obstruction.

The *chest radiograph* shows no features typical of the disease, and diagnosis depends on the occupational clinical history associated with the functional changes of obstructive airways disease, a decline in FEV1 on Mondays being characteristic among workers engaged in the dustier occupations of the cotton and flax mills.

Management. Periodic checks of pulmonary function enable those workers with early signs of byssinosis to be singled out and transferred to less dusty occupations. Treatment of fully developed byssinosis is similar to that of other forms of chronic bronchitis and emphysema.

19

Malignant Disease
of the Lungs

The lungs are commonly the site of primary and metastatic cancer. The mode of presentation varies widely, from acute respiratory symptoms and signs to vague systemic manifestations of insidious onset, unsuggestive of lung cancer except to the most suspicious clinician. Early diagnosis and successful management depend on a wide knowledge of the clinical manifestations, radiological changes and surgical problems that occur in all types of pulmonary malignant disease.

CARCINOMA OF THE BRONCHUS

The commonest intrapulmonary neoplasm is carcinoma of the bronchus. It is also the most frequent type of primary malignant disease in males both in North America and in England and Wales, and its incidence is increasing steadily in both sexes. In 1942 the death rate due to malignant disease of the lower respiratory tract (the bulk of which was carcinoma of the bronchus) among men in England and Wales was 265 per million, compared with 1086 per million in 1972. The corresponding figures for women were 53 and 236 deaths per million population in 1942 and 1972 respectively. Recently the rate of increase in women has risen more rapidly than in men. It is a disease of middle and old age, being rare before the age of forty and reaching its peak incidence in the late fifties, the subsequent decline after that age being due to the increasing death toll from other causes.

Epidemiology

This startling increase in the incidence of bronchial carcinoma can be largely attributed to three factors: *air pollution, industrial hazards,* and *cigarette smoking*. The role of *air pollution* is the least well defined of the three, being based on the observation that the disease is more frequent in urban than in rural populations by a ratio of about 2 : 1. Extracts of atmospheric dust from city air have been shown to

be carcinogenic to mice when injected subcutaneously, and it seems reasonable to suppose that such atmospheric contamination is due to exhaust fumes from motor vehicles, industrial waste fumes, and smoke from domestic fires.

Of the various *industrial hazards* the most important is undoubtedly asbestos. This material is widely used in the building and ship-building industries, in operations such as pipe-lagging, sound proofing, and roofing. Although the workers actually handling the material face the greatest hazard, others who are working in the same area and breathing the same dust-laden atmosphere are also at risk. It has been estimated that the death rate from lung cancer in asbestos workers exposed for more than twenty years is about ten times that of the general population, although measures taken to suppress dust in factories has reduced the hazard considerably. The risk is enhanced by cigarette smoking. Other industries associated with increased risk of lung cancer are the gas industry, the chromate industry, the horticultural use of arsenical sprays, and the mining of iron ore. Miners involved in the extraction of radioactive ores from Schneeberg and Joachimstal in Czechoslovakia also have a high incidence of lung cancer, and a similar high incidence has been observed among men engaged in fluorspar mining in Newfoundland where the mineshafts are contaminated with water containing radon.

In 1950 the results of several studies both in North America and in the United Kingdom showed an association between *lung cancer and smoking,* especially of cigarettes. These studies were retrospective, but were followed by three large prospective studies which showed that there was an increased death rate from all causes among cigarette smokers when compared with non-smokers, that the disease most likely to develop among cigarette smokers was bronchial carcinoma, and that the risk of developing bronchial carcinoma was directly related to the daily consumption of cigarettes. Among men who smoke more than 25 cigarettes a day the risk of developing lung cancer is more than twenty times that for non-smokers, but it decreases in proportion to the length of time that smoking has been given up. There appears to be a relatively low risk of lung cancer in pipe and cigar smokers, probably two or three times the risk to non-smokers.

Although smoking clearly plays a major part in the increasing incidence of lung cancer, there are many indications that it is by no means the only factor. Attempts to produce lung cancer in experimental animals by inhalation of tobacco smoke have been universally unsuccessful, and its occurrence among cigarette smokers varies considerably in different parts of the world, as, for example, in South Africa where lung cancer is uncommon although the

consumption of cigarettes is extremely high. Among migrants from the United Kingdom to New Zealand the incidence of bronchial carcinoma is significantly higher than among the local people in spite of similar smoking habits, suggesting that the migrants have already sustained some form of carcinogenic lung damage before leaving England. Among workers exposed to asbestos the risk of lung cancer is enormously enhanced if the individual is also a cigarette smoker. These facts suggest that carcinoma may be due to a variety of influences upon the lung including chronic infection, smoking, industrial products, and air pollution, each predisposing to cancer but being even more liable to induce the disease when combined with one or more of the others. Nevertheless, cigarette smoking is undoubtedly the single most important cause of lung cancer.

Cell Types

The three histological types of tumour that make up more than 95 per cent of all cases of carcinoma of the lung can be broadly divided into the *squamous-cell* carcinoma (55%), the *anaplastic* (large cell and small cell) type, which includes the *oat-cell* carcinoma (35%), and the *adenocarcinoma* (10%). Both squamous and oat-cell cancer are at least ten times commoner in men than in women and both are increasing in incidence. In contrast, the rise in incidence of adenocarcinoma has been much slower, and it does not appear to be closely related to cigarette smoking. Adenocarcinoma is much more evenly distributed between the sexes, being only twice as common in men as in women.

The site of origin and the degree of differentiation of a tumour are important as a guide to prognosis and to management. In general, surgery is most likely to be successful in the treatment of peripherally placed, well-differentiated tumours. *Squamous-cell carcinoma* is often well-differentiated but occurs mainly in the larger bronchi, tending to spread by local invasion or by metastasis to local lymph nodes, although distant metastases via the lymphatics or blood stream are liable to occur from poorly differentiated tumours. Squamous cell cancer often presents with the manifestations of bronchial obstruction and is liable to central necrosis, producing a malignant lung abscess. The life expectancy in this tumour is greater than in other forms of lung cancer because its rate of spread is often slow.

The *oat-cell carcinoma* usually arises centrally but spreads rapidly both locally and by distant metastasis, so that the prognosis in this type is poor. Systemic manifestations of bronchial carcinoma such as the endocrine syndromes and neuromyopathies are most frequently associated with oat-cell tumours.

The majority of *adenocarcinomas* are situated in the periphery of

the lung, and consequently the tumour may be clinically silent until symptoms are caused by distant metastases. In some cases they are associated with pulmonary scars or fibrosis. *Alveolar cell carcinoma* is a rare form of adenocarcinoma in which the tumour spreads directly through the airways to fill wide areas of the lung with well-differentiated, mucus-secreting tumour cells.

Clinical Features

Although the symptoms and signs of carcinoma of the bronchus are numerous the common modes of presentation fall into a few well-defined groups: (1) non-specific, (2) respiratory, (3) due to local spread, and (4) due to distant metastases. In a certain number of patients the diagnosis is first suspected because of an abnormality detected on a routine chest radiograph, and in a few, perhaps 2 per cent of the total, the presentation is due to some unusual systemic manifestation such as an endocrine syndrome or a neuromyopathy.

NON-SPECIFIC MANIFESTATIONS

About 15 per cent of patients present with non-specific symptoms such as *weakness, loss of weight, tiredness, anorexia* and *fever,* all of which are frequent in the late stages of the disease but which may also be an important early indication of bronchial carcinoma. Investigation of such symptoms should always include chest radiography.

Clubbing of the fingers and toes is an important clinical sign because of its common association with carcinoma of the bronchus, sometimes when the tumour is too small to be detected on a chest radiograph. Rapid development of clubbing is rather suggestive of bronchial carcinoma, its more gradual progression being associated with chronic conditions such as pulmonary fibrosis or hepatic cirrhosis. Following excision of an underlying bronchial carcinoma clubbing regresses slowly to normal over a period of several months. Occasionally, it may be associated with thickening of the soft tissue of the face and scalp, and it nearly always accompanies hypertrophic pulmonary osteoarthropathy.

The syndrome of acute arthritis of the wrists and ankles, clubbing of the digits and radiological evidence of periostitis of the long bones, known as *hypertrophic pulmonary osteoarthropathy,* is a rare feature of bronchial carcinoma. Periostitis is seen as a thin, irregular layer of new bone laid down symmetrically at the ends of the long bones nearest to the wrist and ankle joints which are swollen, warm and tender. The underlying tumour, which is usually squamous cell carcinoma or pleural mesothelioma, is frequently small and often situated in the periphery of the lung fields. *Gynaecomastia* is occasionally seen in conjunction with hypertrophic pulmonary

osteoarthropathy and some patients may have the clinical appearance of acromegaly with spatulate hands and radiological tufting of the terminal phalanges. It seems likely that breast development is stimulated by a hormonal substance originating from the tumour cells, probably gonadotropin. The severe joint symptoms of hypertrophic pulmonary osteoarthropathy are rapidly relieved by excision of the primary tumour, and if this is too extensive for resection, denervation of the lung root or section of the vagus nerve on the side of the lesion is sufficient to relieve the arthritis completely. Alternatively, the symptoms may sometimes be relieved with corticosteroids.

RESPIRATORY MANIFESTATIONS

The commonest respiratory manifestations are *cough, failure of chest infection to resolve, haemoptysis, dyspnoea,* and *chest pain. Cough* is a presenting symptom in about 40 per cent of patients with bronchial carcinoma, being due to encroachment of the tumour upon a bronchus. It is at first dry and spasmodic but subsequently mucus is produced and infection is liable to occur distal to the narrowed bronchial segment so that the sputum may become muco-purulent. Since many patients who develop lung cancer are habitual cigarette smokers they tend also to suffer from chronic bronchitis with long-standing productive cough. In such patients a worsening of the cough, perhaps becoming more paroxysmal in nature, or the appearance of blood streaks in the sputum may indicate the presence of carcinoma.

An acute febrile illness, often described as influenza from which the patient makes only a slow recovery, may be the outward sign of infection caused by bronchial carcinoma. Sometimes cough, fever and pleuritic pain may herald the onset of pneumonia distal to an obstructed bronchus, and failure of resolution or recurrence of such an infection should lead to a search for an underlying neoplasm.

Haemoptysis occurs at some time in their illness in more than 50 per cent of patients with bronchial carcinoma, and is a presenting symptom in about 5 per cent. It is due to ulceration of the bronchial mucosa overlying the tumour, and is increased by the presence of infection. Usually, the sputum is bloodstreaked or contains small clots of blood, massive haemorrhage being rare. Haemoptysis is an important symptom because it should always initiate extensive investigation and may lead to early diagnosis and successful treatment.

Dyspnoea is a common symptom but not usually a disabling one unless it is due mainly to underlying chronic airways obstruction. It may be due to collapse or consolidation of lung parenchyma distal to the obstructed bronchus, or to pleural effusion; in the latter case great symptomatic relief may be achieved by aspiration. Occasionally,

dyspnoea may be suddenly aggravated by occlusion of a major bronchus, or by the development of lobar pneumonia.

Chest pain may occur in various forms but commonly as an ache or discomfort, worse at night and relieved by change of posture or by activity. It is intermittent, annoying rather than severe, and unaffected by cough. In contrast, pleuritic pain due to pleural involvement by the tumour or to secondary pneumonia or pulmonary infarction is sharp, severe, and aggravated by coughing or deep breathing. Extension of the tumour to the bones of the thoracic cage generally causes severe aching pain and localised tenderness. In the late stages of the disease pain may become a severe, constant, and progressive symptom, very difficult to relieve.

Wheezing and stridor due to narrowing of a large bronchus or the trachea are less common symptoms of bronchial carcinoma, but when present they suggest that the tumour is likely to be inoperable. Production of very large quantities of clear, watery sputum, often without other symptoms, suggests the diagnosis of alveolar cell carcinoma and should lead to careful cytological examination of the sputum for malignant cells.

Examination of the chest may reveal the signs of consolidation, pulmonary collapse or pleural effusion, and localised wheezing heard on auscultation and unaffected by cough may suggest narrowing of a bronchus due to tumour. Rarely the signs of pneumothorax may be found, due to necrosis of the pleura following malignant infiltration.

MANIFESTATIONS DUE TO LOCAL EXTENSION

About 5 per cent of patients with bronchial carcinoma present with the clinical features of *superior vena caval obstruction. Hoarseness* of the voice and a 'bovine' cough are due to adductor paralysis of the vocal cords resulting from spread of the tumour to involve the left recurrent laryngeal nerve. An *apical carcinoma* may involve the lower part of the brachial plexus, leading to pain around the shoulder joint and in the arm with sensory impairment along the ulnar border of the forearm and hand and the development of muscular weakness and wasting. If the cervical sympathetic nerves are involved the patient will show the characteristic features of *Horner's syndrome*: ptosis, meiosis, enophthalmos, loss of the cilio-spinal reflex and reduced sweating on the affected side of the face. The axillary vessels may become obstructed, resulting in loss of the peripheral pulses or oedema of the arm, and erosion of a rib will cause local pain and bony tenderness.

Spread of the tumour to involve the oesophagus results in oesophageal obstruction and dysphagia. Cardiovascular abnormalities may arise from direct involvement of the heart and

pericardium, resulting in cardiac arrhythmias or signs of pericardial effusion and congestive heart failure.

METASTATIC MANIFESTATIONS

Evidence of metastatic deposits may be an important guide to the clinician in deciding the appropriate method of treatment since, in general, surgery is contra-indicated in the presence of extrathoracic metastases. The distant organs most commonly affected are the brain, bones, liver, and adrenal glands. About 3 per cent of patients with bronchial carcinoma present because of symptoms from cerebral metastases. The commonest presenting manifestations are personality change, hemiplegia, and epilepsy, but symptoms of raised intracranial pressure and of cerebellar disorder are also frequently encountered.

Bone metastases present with pain and tenderness at the site of the deposit. Liver involvement may present with jaundice, a complaint of pain or discomfort in the right hypochondrium or with tenderness on palpation over the liver. The liver itself may feel enlarged, firm, and irregular, umbilication of the nodules being occasionally palpable when the metastases are rapidly growing and necrotic. Malignant ascites may occur, and rectal examination may reveal deposits in the recto-vesical pouch. Adrenal involvement is a common post-mortem finding but clinical evidence of hypoadrenalism is comparatively rare, presenting as malaise, muscular weakness, hypotension and the typical pigmentation of the skin and buccal mucosa.

Spread of bronchial carcinoma to cervical lymph nodes occurs commonly. Lymph node involvement is also frequent in the mediastinum, the supraclavicular and axillary nodes and in the abdomen.

UNCOMMON SYSTEMIC MANIFESTATIONS

Although the systemic features of bronchial carcinoma are relatively rare they are important because they may indicate the presence of a hitherto unsuspected neoplasm.

Thrombophlebitis migrans. Recurrent thrombophlebitis, sometimes referred to as thrombophlebitis migrans, may be an indication of underlying bronchial carcinoma although it is classically associated with cancer of the pancreas and stomach. It is difficult to control with anticoagulant therapy and often involves the superficial veins with little inflammatory reaction, unusual sites such as the veins of the neck, axillae or arms being sometimes affected.

Endocrine Group. The endocrine manifestations of bronchial carcinoma are due to secretion by the tumour cells of biologically-active peptides which are similar to the hormones normally secreted by certain endocrine tissues. *Cushing's syndrome* is due to tumour

secretion of an ACTH-like polypeptide which may produce a clinical presentation similar in most respects to that caused by hyperactivity of the pituitary or adrenal glands, although its occurrence in a middle-aged man would suggest an underlying bronchial neoplasm. More often, however, the presentation is primarily a biochemical one, being characterised by a severe hypokalaemic alkalosis with vague symptoms of muscle weakness, lethargy, and fatigue. Occasionally the patient may suffer from mental symptoms such as severe depression due to the high level of circulating corticosteroids, and gross dependent oedema due to sodium retention is often a troublesome complaint in the later stages. Although the syndrome may regress if the tumour, usually an oat-cell carcinoma, is excised, the course of this complication of bronchial carcinoma is usually a rapidly progressive one with a prognosis of only a few weeks. The syndrome may be confirmed biochemically by demonstrating raised urinary levels of 17-hydroxy and 17-ketogenic steroids and raised plasma cortisol levels with loss of the normal diurnal variation.

The clinical syndrome due to *inappropriate secretion of antidiuretic hormone* (ADH) is characterised by anorexia, nausea and vomiting, restlessness or lethargy, mental confusion or irritability, and generalised muscular weakness. Body temperature may be subnormal and the relaxation phase of tendon reflexes may be sluggish, simulating myxoedema. The symptoms are ascribed to water intoxication and hyponatraemia resulting from excessive secretion of ADH by tumour cells, usually of the oat-cell type, and the striking biochemical findings are a low serum sodium level, sometimes as low as 107 m Eq/litre, usually associated with hypochloraemia, normal or low serum potassium and a low serum urea, often in the region of 5 to 10 mg/100 ml. In spite of the hyponatraemia the kidneys excrete large amounts of sodium with the result that urine osmolality exceeds that of plasma. Restriction of fluid intake to less than 1 litre a day is the most successful way of treating the hyponatraemia. Occasionally, a proximal renal tubular defect due to potassium depletion may be demonstrated in such patients by the detection of glycosuria, amino-aciduria and increased urinary phosphate excretion.

Although *hypercalcaemia* due to widespread bone metastases is a not uncommon feature of various types of malignant disease it may also occur in association with carcinoma arising in a number of organs, including the lung, without any evidence of bone secondaries. It seems likely that biologically-active material similar to parathyroid hormone is secreted by the tumour, usually a squamous cell carcinoma of the lung. The syndrome may be suggested by a chance finding of raised serum calcium level or may present with the symptoms and signs of hypercalcaemia: muscular weakness and hyporeflexia, lethargy and

drowsiness, anorexia, nausea or vomiting, constipation, urinary frequency, and dehydration and sometimes mental confusion. Changes characteristic of hypercalcaemia may be seen in the electrocardiogram. These findings are indistinguishable from those of primary hyperparathyroidism although a reduction in the hypercalcaemia in response to cortisone treatment and the absence of typical radiological changes would tend to exclude that diagnosis.

The *carcinoid syndrome* may sometimes be produced by bronchial oat-cell carcinoma, but usually results from bronchial adenomata of the carcinoid type and is considered on page 244.

The *nephrotic syndrome* may rarely be associated with extrarenal malignancy including oat-cell carcinoma of the lung. The renal lesion is attributed to immune-complex deposition at the glomerular basement membrane, either as a result of specific antigen production by the tumour or due to antibody formation against nuclear antigen released by tumour necrosis.

Neuromuscular Syndromes. Although neuromuscular disorders may be linked with a wide variety of malignant tumours, in more than half the association is with carcinoma of the lung, most commonly an oat-cell tumour. They are unrelated to metastases in the central nervous system but their cause is unknown, although it has been suggested that the tumour may produce some substance that affects nervous tissue or that an autoimmune process is responsible for the degenerative changes. The neurological features often precede the discovery of the primary tumour although occasionally they may develop some time after apparently successful surgical treatment. Degenerative changes may affect any part of the central nervous system but in general they tend to produce neurological changes that follow one of several well-recognised patterns, although mixtures of these patterns commonly occur.

The commonest presentation is a combination of neurological and myopathic manifestations. The *myopathic syndrome* consists of a proximal muscular weakness of subacute onset affecting the limb girdles and trunk, often associated with ptosis, bulbar paresis, loss of reflexes and peripheral neuropathy. Fluctuation and even spontaneous remission of the muscle weakness may occur and sometimes a myasthenic element is apparent. A *myasthenic syndrome* characterised by increased fatiguability mainly affecting the proximal muscles is rarely associated with carcinoma of the lung. It differs from classical myasthenia gravis in that symptoms of ocular and bulbar involvement are uncommon and the response to anticholinergic drugs such as neostigmine is poor.

The next most common pattern is a *peripheral neuropathy* with both motor and sensory abnormalities, characterised by limb pains

and dysaesthesiae, posterior column loss leading to ataxia, muscle wasting and weakness and loss of tendon reflexes. Often there is a concurrent myopathy. This syndrome tends to run a progressive course for up to a year without remissions, dementia being a frequent complication. Pure sensory loss is a much less common variety of the syndrome.

The syndrome of *subacute cerebellar degeneration* presents with typical signs of bilateral cerebellar disease including vertigo, ataxia, dysarthria and signs of progressive bulbar involvement. Dementia is common and the condition follows a relentless, fairly rapid course. This disorder is sometimes associated with muscular weakness and peripheral neuropathy.

Among the other neurological syndromes associated with carcinoma of the bronchus are included *limbic encephalitis,* characterised by anxiety or depression, disturbance of affect and loss of recent memory progressing to global dementia; *encephalomyelitis* affecting the brain stem and spinal cord with such signs as ophthalmoplegia, pupillary changes, cerebellar disturbances, bulbar palsy and muscle wasting and weakness; and a pattern simulating *motor neurone disease* but with a more benign and prolonged course than occurs in the classical syndrome.

Skin Disorders. Two uncommon skin disorders, dermatomyositis and acanthosis nigricans, are often associated with various underlying neoplasms, including bronchial carcinoma, in patients over forty. *Dermatomyositis* presents as a pinkish-purple, raised rash over the face, especially the forehead and cheeks, the backs of the hands and fingers, and on the trunk. A lilac suffusion of the upper eyelids is pathognomonic. It is associated with muscular weakness and tenderness, particularly of the hips and shoulders, and may regress if the primary tumour is excised. *Acanthosis nigricans* consists of a dark brown, velvety, elevated rash affecting the trunk particularly in the axillae, skin folds and groins, and sometimes occurring in the mouth and around the umbilicus and anus. Its presence is associated with some form of malignancy in virtually every case occurring over the age of forty.

Investigations

Chest Radiology. Support for a clinical diagnosis of bronchial carcinoma is obtained most readily by radiological examination of the chest. Postero-anterior and lateral films may demonstrate a shadow which can be more precisely investigated by tomography or bronchography. Any previous radiographs should be compared with the current one, since the new appearance or increase in size of a solitary peripheral lung shadow would support the diagnosis. Solid

shadows due to carcinoma may be well defined but usually have slightly fuzzy margins, and breakdown of the centre of a carcinoma produces a ragged thick-walled abscess cavity. The presence of calcium within a shadow makes the diagnosis of carcinoma unlikely.

Evidence of collapse of a lobe or segment indicates bronchial obstruction which may be due to carcinoma. Shadows due to lobar or segmental consolidation should be carefully reviewed to confirm complete resolution; failure to resolve is highly suggestive of an underlying neoplasm, and when the infective element has been treated with antibiotics it is often possible to see the underlying neoplastic mass. Tomography is of value in defining the outline of the major bronchi since any narrowing of or protrusion into the lumen of a bronchus is suggestive of a neoplasm. Bronchography may be used to give similar information.

Enlargement of one hilum is suggestive of carcinoma, and elevation of a paralysed lobe of the diaphragm due to hilar involvement of the phrenic nerve may be a related finding. The bony shadows of the thoracic cage should be examined carefully to exclude the presence of secondary deposits or of malignant erosion from a neighbouring tumour.

Cytological Examination of the Sputum. The discovery of malignant cells in the sputum is the simplest way of making a histological diagnosis. About 80 per cent of cases of lung carcinoma can be diagnosed by cytological examination of three specimens of sputum, the percentage rising if more specimens from each patient are examined.

Bronchoscopy. Since tissue diagnosis of carcinoma of the bronchus is of the first importance in determining prognosis and management, bronchoscopy and bronchial biopsy should be performed in all suspected cases in which sputum examination has proved negative. The procedure enables a diagnosis to be made in about 60 per cent of cases, either on the basis of successful biopsy or on the grounds of suspicious narrowing or distortion of the bronchial tree, and allows the operability of a tumour to be assessed. Lesions in the periphery of the lung fields cannot be visualised, and the rigid bronchoscope allows only limited inspection of the upper lobe bronchi with the aid of a right-angled telescope.

The recent introduction of the *fibreoptic bronchoscope* has increased the range of bronchoscopy because the thin (5 mm) flexible instrument permits deeper exploration of the segmental bronchi to subsegmental level with the facility for obtaining tissue samples or material for cytological examination. The instrument can be readily passed via the nose, using local anaesthesia, with little risk or discomfort to the patient.

Tissue Biopsy. Occasionally it may be possible to obtain a histological diagnosis by biopsy of a lymph node which appears to be clinically abnormal, or by biopsy of the pleura in patients with pleural effusion, using a special biopsy needle. Cytological examination of a pleural aspirate may also demonstrate neoplastic cells.

The other investigations that should be carried out serve only to support the diagnosis of bronchial carcinoma or to exclude other possible diagnoses. Examination of the blood may show a moderate normocytic, normochromic anaemia or widespread depression of all cell types due to disseminated bone metastases. A polymorphonuclear leucocytosis may occur, provoked either by the neoplasm or by a related pulmonary infection. Biochemical abnormalities in the serum may reflect one or other of the endocrine manifestations mentioned above, or may be due to metastases in the liver, bones, or adrenals. The sputum should be examined, not only for malignant cells but also for evidence of tuberculosis, bacterial or fungal infection of the lungs.

There remains a small number of cases in which the diagnosis cannot be made unequivocally except at thoracotomy.

Treatment

Untreated bronchial carcinoma leads to death in the majority of cases within two years of diagnosis. At present the treatment that offers the best chance of a cure is surgery, but only about 50 per cent of all cases appear suitable for operation on clinical grounds, and about half these are found to be inoperable at bronchoscopy or on thoracotomy. Of the 20 to 25 per cent of patients in whom resection can be carried out, only one third will be alive five years later.

SURGERY

The ideal patient for surgery is one with a small, peripheral pulmonary lesion, without evidence of metastases and with normal respiratory and cardiac function. The operative mortality for lobectomy is about 6 per cent, being doubled if the tumour is extensive enough to require pneumonectomy and increasing also with the age of the patient. The success of operation depends largely on the extent to which the hilum is involved.

Many patients may be excluded from surgery on clinical grounds, either due to age, extensive malignant disease or to inadequate cardiac and respiratory reserve. Evidence of spread of the cancer should be looked for. Signs of local spread to the mediastinum causing superior vena caval obstruction, dysphagia due to oesophageal invasion, or cardiac arrhythmias due to myocardial involvement by the tumour indicate inoperability. Paralysis of the phrenic or recurrent laryngeal nerves, involvement of the brachial plexus or cervical sympathetic

nerves, or direct spread to a rib usually exclude operation, although occasionally a successful resection may be carried out. The finding of a pleural effusion containing malignant cells implies pleural involvement which is inoperable except as a palliative procedure. A bloodstained pleural effusion does not necessarily indicate extension of the growth to the pleura, and is an indication for further investigation. In general, distant metastases exclude operation although brain metastases are occasionally single and have been successfully excised in conjunction with pneumonectomy.

Spread of the tumour to the mediastinum renders it inoperable, and evidence for this should be sought preoperatively to avoid unnecessary thoracotomy. *Bronchoscopy* may reveal signs of proximal extension of the tumour, ulceration of the carina or trachea, or widening and splaying out of the carina, all of which would exclude operation. The diagnosis of oat-cell carcinoma based on bronchial biopsy has been taken by some as an indication of inoperability, on the basis of poor survival figures in patients selected for surgery compared with those selected for radiotherapy. Not all surgeons would agree with this conclusion. *Fluoroscopy* may be useful, not only in diagnosing diaphragmatic paralysis due to phrenic nerve involvement but also in revealing displacement of the barium-filled oesophagus. *Mediastinoscopy* and mediastinal biopsy is being increasingly used to obtain preoperative evidence of mediastinal metastases. A small transverse incision is made just above the suprasternal notch and the upper mediastinum is explored with a finger passed downwards along the front of the trachea. The area can be inspected with a laryngoscope and a biopsy taken from a lymph node or from tumour tissue exposed by the exploration.

Evidence of co-existing respiratory or cardiac disease, including chronic airways obstruction, pulmonary fibrosis or myocardial ischaemia excludes operation in about 4 per cent of cases. Apart from increased operative mortality, chronic pulmonary disease may render an operation unsuccessful because of postoperative respiratory failure due to infection of the remaining lung, intolerable dyspnoea due to loss of lung tissue, or cor pulmonale resulting from diminution of the pulmonary vascular bed. Measurements of lung volumes, airway resistance and arterial blood gas tensions may be useful, but operability is probably best indicated by testing the patient's exercise tolerance. A patient who shows evidence of a severe degree of chronic airways obstruction, or whose arterial carbon dioxide tension is persistently above normal is likely to be unsuitable for surgery.

RADIOTHERAPY

Although surgery appears to be the better method of treatment for operable cases of squamous cell carcinoma, there is evidence from a

controlled clinical trial that radiotherapy gives longer survival than surgery in the treatment of oat-celled carcinoma. In anaplastic lesions other than oat-celled the results of radiotherapy and surgery are similar.

Radical radiotherapy is given when there seems to be a good chance of achieving a 'cure', i.e. survival for three to five years without evidence of recurrence; this means that there should be no evidence of disease outside the chest and that the patient's condition appears good enough to withstand a four-week course of treatment. There is clearly no justification for subjecting a patient with no hope of recovery to the discomforts of high dosage irradiation.

The presence of a pleural effusion containing malignant cells contra-indicates radical radiotherapy since it indicates widespread intrapleural dissemination which would require irradiation of more than half the chest. Chronic bronchitis may be exacerbated by irradiation but is not in itself a contra-indication to this form of treatment. Acute infection should be controlled prior to radiotherapy, and tuberculosis treated with antituberculosis drugs throughout the course of treatment.

The sequelae of radiation therapy include fibrosis of the lung which occasionally leads to severe dyspnoea and even cor pulmonale. Dysphagia due to radiation reaction in the oesophagus is occasionally severe enough to necessitate stopping treatment.

Palliative radiotherapy is of value in the relief of severe and persistent haemoptysis, in relieving pain, especially if it is due to invasion of bone, and sometimes in the relief of bronchial or tracheal obstruction. It is particularly valuable in treating superior vena caval obstruction.

CHEMOTHERAPY

Chemotherapy using cytotoxic agents such as nitrogen mustard or cyclophosphamide is occasionally of value in the palliative treatment of threatened obstruction to the trachea or a large bronchus, or in superior vena caval obstruction, mainly when the tumour is of the anaplastic or oat-cell variety. Combined drug regimes are currently under trial but the most effective schedules of administration have yet to be established. Chemotherapy has a particular place in the treatment of *malignant pleural effusions,* which often reaccumulate very rapidly after aspiration and cause troublesome dyspnoea. It may be possible to avoid frequent aspirations by the instillation of a cytotoxic agent such as mustine hydrochloride (0·4 mg per kg body weight) into the pleural space after it has been aspirated. The dose may be repeated at 3-week intervals if the blood count permits. An alternative drug is quinacrine (mepacrine) hydrochloride in an initial dose of 90 mg, repeated at two to three day intervals in increasing

dosage until about 500 mg has been given. Side effects include fever and pleuritic pain which may limit the size of the dose.

COMBINED TREATMENT

The value of surgery combined with irradiation either before or after operation is still unproven. The combinations of chemotherapy and surgery or chemotherapy and radiotherapy do not appear to prolong survival and result in an increased number of complications and toxic reactions.

SUPPORTIVE TREATMENT

Treatment with antibiotics is often valuable in controlling infections associated with bronchial carcinoma, with relief of symptoms such as productive cough and haemoptysis. There should be no hesitation about the effective use of analgesics to control pain, giving adequate doses of morphine or pethidine as often as is necessary. Much suffering may be due to anxiety and fear, often engendered by the tendency for the medical staff to shy away from conversation with the patient for fear of being asked to discuss the diagnosis. Although it usually seems advisable to withhold full information from the patient, tactful discussions may help him to form his own judgement about his illness without removing the solace of hope. Sedative or tranquillising drugs, e.g. chlorpromazine, may be used to give additional support.

BRONCHIAL ADENOMA

The term bronchial adenoma refers to a group of small bronchial tumours arising in the lower trachea or major bronchi, the most important being the rare *bronchial cylindroma* (adenocystic carcinoma), which has the greater tendency to metastasise, and the *bronchial carcinoid*. They tend to occur at an earlier age than bronchial carcinoma, with an equal incidence between the sexes. Both are relatively slow-growing cancers, inclined to local invasion and late distant metastasis, and both cause local symptoms and signs due to intrabronchial bleeding and obstruction. A small proportion cf bronchial carcinoids cause systemic manifestations due to hormonal secretion by the tumour cells.

Pathology

The bronchial carcinoid is usually a well-differentiated tumour, consisting of uniform small cuboidal cells with granular eosinophilic cytoplasm and round darkly-staining nuclei, arranged in sheets, strands or acini. Argentaffin granules can occasionally be

demonstrated. The cylindroma is probably derived from bronchial glands and has a pleomorphic appearance with small cells of dark staining characteristics arranged in tubular or cylindrical fashion. It tends to infiltrate the bronchial wall, the larger part of its substance often lying outside the bronchus.

Clinical Features

These tumours are highly vascular, and haemoptysis is a common early symptom. Cough due to irritation of the bronchial mucosa is frequent, and obstruction of the bronchus leads to local wheezing and distal infection with the complications of pneumonia, bronchiectasis, lung abscess, and empyema.

The *carcinoid syndrome* is caused by the secretion by the tumour cells of certain biologically active substances which include serotonin, 5-hydroxytryptophan and, possibly, bradykinin-like peptides. The syndrome is characterised by flushing attacks which are more prolonged and severe than in the usual carcinoid syndrome, frequently associated with anxiety and tremulousness, fever, periorbital and facial oedema, increased lachrymation and salivation, rhinorrhoea, explosive diarrhoea, nausea and vomiting, hypotension and oliguria. Left-sided valvular heart lesions occasionally occur, and osteogenic bone metastases are common. Investigation of these patients should include measurement of urinary 5-hydroxy-indoleacetic acid (5-HIAA), although occasionally, severe symptoms may be present in patients showing normal 5-HIAA levels. Symptoms may be relieved by surgical excision of the primary tumour or of hormone-secreting metastases, and there is sometimes a favourable response to corticosteroid therapy.

Treatment

Bronchial cylindroma and carcinoid should be treated by thoracotomy and resection, lobectomy combined with clearance of the hilar lymph nodes being the operation of choice. Endoscopic resection should be avoided unless the patient has too little cardiac or respiratory reserve to withstand thoracotomy.

MESOTHELIOMA OF THE PLEURA

Interest in this tumour has grown since it was recognised that environmental exposure to blue asbestos (crocidolite) plays a major part in its aetiology. The significant history may be difficult to discern, stories such as playing on an asbestos slag heap during childhood or the regular washing of asbestos-contaminated overalls being typical of the inconspicuous nature of the exposure. More commonly the patient

gives an occupational history of contact with asbestos although in about 30 per cent of cases no significant history can be obtained, possibly because the patient has forgotten or has been unaware of past exposure. The mesothelioma occurs in both sexes, the delay between first exposure and death from the tumour being approximately forty years. Other evidence of asbestos exposure such as pulmonary fibrosis or asbestos warts is often absent.

Clinical Features

The symptoms of mesothelioma usually begin gradually with pain or breathlessness. The pain is dull or aching in character, confined to the site of the lesion at first but later radiating to the shoulder or epigastrium. It is usually unaffected by breathing or movement. Breathlessness on exertion is due to the accumulation of fluid in the pleural space and to increasing restriction of lung movement. A large pleural effusion is usually apparent on clinical examination and the underlying tumour may be palpable in the supraclavicular fossa or between the ribs.

Investigations

The radiographic appearance of mesothelioma is that of a large pleural effusion, although thickening of the pleura may be apparent after aspiration of the fluid. Suggestive features of asbestosis may be pulmonary fibrosis or calcified pleural plaques. Rib destruction is late to appear and local lymph node enlargement is rarely apparent.

The pleural fluid should be examined for abnormal cells. It is frequently blood-stained, and mesothelioma-like cells may be identified, but the diagnosis should not be based on this finding alone. Biopsy of the tumour, either through a needle or at thoracotomy, will give confirmation although histological variation in different parts of the tumour may mislead the pathologist into diagnosing chronic inflammatory changes.

Course and Treatment

Patients seldom survive more than two years from the time the diagnosis is established, and neither radical surgery nor radiotherapy will alter the course of the disease. Thoracotomy and pleural biopsy may encourage direct extension of the tumour through the chest wall so that interference is better avoided except to aspirate excessive accumulations of pleural fluid if this is responsible for dyspnoea. Instillation of nitrogen mustard into the pleural space may discourage the rapid accumulation of exudate. Death is usually due to restriction of ventilation or to intercurrent chest infection.

MALIGNANT INVASION OF THE LUNGS

It is not uncommon for the lungs to be involved by malignancy which originates elsewhere, either by direct spread as occurs, for example, in Hodgkin's disease arising in mediastinal lymph nodes, or by blood or lymph-borne metastases from cancer of other organs, e.g. 'cannon-ball' secondaries from carcinoma of the kidney. Although a full account of these several conditions is outside the scope of this book certain specific points are mentioned here because of their importance in differential diagnosis or in management.

Malignant Lymphomas

Both Hodgkin's disease and lymphosarcoma may be confined initially to the lymph nodes of the mediastinum, presenting either with asymptomatic radiographic evidence of mediastinal enlargement or with symptoms of invasion or obstruction of the bronchi, venous obstruction or pleural effusion. Occasionally, there may be infiltration of the lung fields and even abscess formation. A mistaken diagnosis of bronchial carcinoma is likely in such cases and a careful search for lymph node enlargement, skin lesions, hepatosplenomegaly, an abnormal peripheral blood picture, or osteolytic bone lesions should be made if the rate of progress of the disease or the radiographic appearances seem in any way atypical of carcinoma. Occasionally, suggestive symptoms such as intermittent fever or itching of the skin may indicate Hodgkin's disease. Tissue biopsy may be necessary to establish the diagnosis, either by aspiration or excision of a lymph node, by mediastinoscopy, or even occasionally at thoracotomy.

Pulmonary Metastases

Secondary deposits of cancer originating in other organs commonly occur in the lungs because blood-borne microscopic tumour emboli are likely to be enmeshed in the pulmonary capillary bed. Lymph-borne tumour cells from the body may be arrested as they pass through the thoracic duct, or continue with the lymph drainage into the left subclavian vein and then to the right side of the heart and the pulmonary capillaries. Metastases may be single, and difficult to differentiate radiologically from a bronchial carcinoma. Very occasionally excision of a solitary peripheral nodule, especially one arising from carcinoma of the kidney, may be followed by freedom from recurrence for several years, provided that the primary cancer is also operable. Multiple pulmonary metastases are usually fairly easy to diagnose radiologically although the primary site may sometimes be difficult to identify. A patient will often retain surprisingly good lung function despite widespread pulmonary

metastases, symptoms of cough, dyspnoea or chest pain being uncommon until the late stages of the disease.

Lymphangitis carcinomatosa is a rare metastatic complication of cancer which usually originates in the stomach though tumours of the breast, bronchus and elsewhere may occasionally behave in the same way. The tumour spreads from hilar lymph nodes along the lymphatic channels of the lungs, producing a diffuse, finely-nodular radiological shadowing which simulates fibrosing alveolitis or even miliary tuberculosis. Patients with widespread diffuse pulmonary involvement of this sort occasionally present with symptoms of wheezing or dyspnoea that may simulate asthma, and gas exchange may be impaired sufficiently to cause cyanosis. Pulmonary hypertension and congestive heart failure may result from thrombosis and tumour embolisation of the pulmonary vascular bed.

20

Pulmonary Manifestations of Connective Tissue Disorders

It is not surprising that the lungs are occasionally involved in the disease process of connective tissue disorders, for although these conditions show a predilection for certain tissues or organs they are essentially systemic diseases and are likely to affect a wide variety of tissues at one time or another. In clinical practice the outlines between different connective tissue disorders are sometimes ill-defined; for example, patients with rheumatoid arthritis sometimes develop peripheral vascular lesions similar to those of polyarteritis nodosa, while on clinical and immunological grounds the syndromes of rheumatoid arthritis, systemic lupus erythematosus, and systemic sclerosis occasionally overlap one another.

In them all the aetiology is obscure, and attempts to identify external causal agents have been unsuccessful. The diseases themselves are uncommon, excepting only rheumatoid disease, and even here the pulmonary manifestations are a rare complication. They are of interest to the chest physician, because of their relevance to the differential diagnosis of many much commoner respiratory conditions, and because of the interesting aetiological problem they pose.

Rheumatoid Disease

Rheumatoid arthritis is a systemic disease that primarily affects connective tissue. Although widespread lesions occur, the dominant clinical manifestation is inflammation of the joints. The course is variable but tends to be chronic and progressive, leading to the characteristic deformities and disability. The disease affects women three times as frequently as men, most commonly presenting in the fourth decade.

The most characteristic pathological lesions are rheumatoid

synovitis, consisting of focal hyperplasia of synovial lining cells with nodular infiltrations composed of lymphocytes and plasma cells, and the rheumatoid nodule, which has a central zone of fibrinoid material containing nuclear debris indicating cellular necrosis. Around this is a zone of large mononuclear cells arranged in radially orientated rows called palisades, and, more peripherally, a zone of granulation tissue infiltrated by plasma cells. These lesions occur in the walls of vessels, in the periarticular tissue, in serous membranes, beneath the skin and in almost any organ.

Although the pathogenesis of the disease is still uncertain these pathological features suggest that hypersensitivity plays a part in the aetiology. Patients with rheumatoid arthritis often show multiple serological abnormalities, particularly anti-IgG and anti-IgM antibodies known as rheumatoid factors, and antibodies to tissue components such as antinuclear and antithyroid antibodies. These features have focused attention on autoimmune processes in the pathogenesis of rheumatoid arthritis, possibly triggered by some unknown factor such as a viral infection which initiates the inflammatory reactions.

RHEUMATOID LUNG

Not all lung lesions in patients with rheumatoid arthritis are part of the systemic disease; there is some evidence that the common pulmonary complaints such as acute and chronic bronchitis, pneumonia and other respiratory infections occur more frequently in rheumatoid arthritis than in the rest of the population. Nevertheless, there is a range of lung disorders that appears to be aetiologically linked with systemic rheumatoid disease either because of associated arthritis or rheumatoid factor, or because of the histological appearance of the pulmonary lesion.

Pleural effusion is the commonest of such lesions, occurring quite frequently in active rheumatoid arthritis and sometimes preceding its onset. It is commoner in men, and presents as a mild or fleeting pleurisy associated with a small, transient pleural effusion that is sometimes bilateral. It usually disappears within a few months but may become indolent, causing chronic pleural thickening which requires surgical decortication to restore ventilatory function.

The pleural fluid may have characteristics similar to the changes seen in the synovial fluid from rheumatoid joints, namely, a low glucose content, a high level of lactic dehydrogenase, sometimes a high lipid content and rheumatoid factor activity. Pleural biopsy usually shows only fibrosis and non-specific chronic inflammatory thickening, but characteristic rheumatoid necrobiotic nodules on the pleura have been described.

Fibrosing alveolitis occurs occasionally in rheumatoid arthritis, usually coming on within three years of the onset of the joint symptoms but rarely preceding them. The clinical presentation is similar in all respects to that of diffuse fibrosing alveolitis (page 21) excepting only that the majority of patients have rheumatoid arthritis. Circulating rheumatoid factor is present in most cases, but to a somewhat lower titre in patients without joint symptoms.

Histologically the lungs show a diffuse interstitial fibrosis with associated bronchiolitis; honeycomb lung occurs in the advanced stages of the disease. These changes lead to a typical restrictive pattern of lung disorder. Once fibrosis is well developed the chest radiograph shows mottled and reticular shadowing which tends particularly to affect the lower lobes; but the clinical symptoms and signs of fibrosing alveolitis and physiological evidence of lung dysfunction may be manifest long before there is much radiological change.

Rheumatoid nodules are rare, and may occur years before any joint symptoms develop. Histologically they show central necrobiosis surrounded by palisading and plasma cell infiltration similar to that seen in rheumatoid nodules elsewhere. The lesions are 1 to 2 cm in diameter and usually occur in the periphery of the lung fields, most frequently in the upper or mid zones. They may appear successively over the years, first in one lung and then in the other, and may be associated with chronic pleural effusion. They most commonly present as a radiographic abnormality in a patient with rheumatoid arthritis, but occasionally a nodule may cavitate, causing haemoptysis as a presenting symptom.

Caplan's syndrome is characterised by large rounded nodules scattered fairly evenly through the lung fields of workers who are exposed to inhaled dust such as coal dust, silica, and asbestos. Rheumatoid arthritis is usually present, although the lung lesions occasionally precede the onset of arthritic symptoms. Circulating rheumatoid factor is found.

Systemic Lupus Erythematosus

Systemic lupus erythematosus (SLE) is an inflammatory connective tissue disorder that affects different tissues in varying combinations and thus presents clinically in many different ways. It tends to run a chronic irregular course with periods of activity and remission, and it occurs most frequently among women of child-bearing age.

The *pathological changes* are not very specific, consisting of fibrinoid change and cellular infiltration in the walls of blood vessels of the organs involved, and inflammatory changes in serous

membranes. The most characteristic histopathological finding is 'haematoxylin bodies', homogeneous purple masses of altered nuclear material that have been shown to be identical with the inclusion body of the LE cell. Among the pathological lesions of SLE are the verrucous endocarditis of Libman and Sacks, segmental thickening of the basement membrane of the glomerular tuft ('wire-loop' lesion) and periarterial concentric fibrosis of the spleen ('onion-skin' lesion).

The *clinical features* of the illness are very variable. The onset is often insidious, consisting of non-specific constitutional symptoms such as fever, weakness, fatiguability, or weight loss. Classically, there is involvement of multiple tissues, most characteristically producing skin lesions, polyarthritis, myositis, renal damage, inflammation of serous membranes causing pericardial and pleural effusions, and a variety of neurological and psychiatric manifestations. The joints are affected in 90 per cent of patients at some stage in the disease, severe joint pain with little or no objective evidence of arthritis being a common feature. The cutaneous lesions vary greatly, being usually erythematous and occurring on the face, neck, fingertips and palms, or about the elbows. Only a minority show the classical 'butterfly' rash over the face. Focal glomerulonephritis leading to renal failure is the most serious feature of the disease. The heart is commonly affected, pericarditis or myocarditis being the usual manifestations; verrucous endocarditis may affect the mitral, tricuspid, or aortic valves but seldom leads to any functional disturbance. Cardiac involvement is frequently associated with pulmonary manifestations of SLE.

The *LE cell phenomenon* is the classical serological finding in SLE. A typical LE cell is a polymorphonuclear leucocyte filled with a mass of homogeneous material of specific staining characteristics, and it is produced by a serum factor found in patients with SLE, which acts both on nuclei and on active phagocytic cells. An easier and much more sensitive test for SLE is the fluorescent antibody technique for demonstrating antinuclear factor, and failure to find this antibody in untreated patients who are suspected of having SLE makes this diagnosis unlikely. However, antinucleoprotein antibodies are found in other connective tissue disorders, and antibody to deoxyribonucleic acid (DNA) is a more precise indication of SLE.

Hypergammaglobulinaemia is a common finding in SLE and the erythrocyte sedimentation rate is greatly increased. Characteristic haematological changes also occur: haemolytic anaemia is due to a Type II (cytotoxic antibody) sensitivity, and the presence of antileucocyte and antiplatelet antibodies lead to leucopenia and platelet deficiency. Biological false positive tests for syphilis occur.

The *aetiology* of SLE is undetermined, but current theories suggest

either that it is an inherited immunological disorder, or that there is an alteration of immunological function due to a virus infection.

VARIANTS OF SLE

Apart from the classical syndrome described above, SLE may present in several other ways:

1. As a localised, 'presystemic' illness, in which the disease is limited to a single organ or tissue, for example, polyarthralgia or pleural effusion, associated with the characteristic serological changes.

2. Associated with chronic hepatitis, in which serological changes occur and fibrosing alveolitis is found as an uncommon coexisting feature.

3. Associated with other connective tissue diseases such as rheumatoid arthritis and systemic sclerosis, in which the serological features of SLE occur.

4. As a drug-induced disease, due to hypersensitivity to a wide range of drugs including practolol, sulphonamides and isoniazid. The disease is usually reversed by stopping the drug.

PULMONARY MANIFESTATIONS

The commonest form of pulmonary involvement in SLE is *secondary infection,* including bacterial pneumonia, tuberculosis, lung abscess, and opportunist infections with unexpected micro-organisms such as fungi. It is important, therefore, to avoid the error of assuming that a particular pulmonary manifestation is due to SLE when a bacterial agent is responsible. Sometimes, however, the pulmonary illness can be properly attributed to SLE, and there are a number of clinical patterns.

Breathlessness of no obvious cause may occur in about one-third of cases of SLE. Breathing is rapid, often associated with difficulty in taking a deep breath and with orthopnoea. A bilateral aching chest pain is often complained of, but examination reveals no abnormal signs in the chest. The radiological changes are nonspecific but some elevation of one or both lobes of the diaphragm is often seen, associated with sluggish movement on fluoroscopy. Obliteration of the costophrenic angles occurs due to small pleural exudates, and linear shadows suggestive of localised atelectasis are often visible in the lower zones. Pulmonary function studies reveal a restrictive functional defect, with normal air flow and some reduction in carbon monoxide transfer.

Pleurisy is common and is often bilateral. It is usually dry but may be associated with a small to moderate effusion, and is sometimes

accompanied by persistent pleuritic pain which may be very distressing. It may occur in conjunction with pericarditis and is commonly a complication of lupoid pneumonia.

Pneumonia in SLE shows a histological picture characterised by focal necrosis of the alveolar walls, mucinous oedema and hyaline membranes in the alveoli, and areas of interstitial pneumonia and haemorrhage. These changes are variable in extent, producing a wide range of clinical manifestations. In some, the respiratory involvement is the dominant feature of the disease, causing fever, dyspnoea, cyanosis, and tachycardia, associated with diffuse radiological shadowing at the lung bases and progressing to severe respiratory failure. More commonly, patchy involvement of the lungs causing local atalectasis or persistent consolidation may precede or accompany generalised manifestations of SLE, producing such clinical features as cough, pleuritic pain, and localised areas of crepitations. The chest radiograph shows evidence of segmental collapse, patchy consolidation and, rarely, diffuse micronodular infiltration similar to that seen in diffuse fibrosing alveolitis.

Diffuse fibrosing alveolitis occurs rather uncommonly in SLE, but it may be associated with chronic active hepatitis and is sometimes the predominant disorder. In this syndrome the pulmonary features consist of breathlessness on exertion, clubbing of the fingers and widespread crepitations audible on auscultation; liver involvement is characterised by enlargement of the liver and spleen and occasional jaundice.

Systemic Sclerosis

This uncommon chronic illness of unknown aetiology causes characteristic fibrous thickening of the skin (scleroderma) and diffuse sclerosis of various organs including the lungs, heart, gastrointestinal tract, and kidneys. It affects women twice as often as men, usually beginning in early middle age. It appears to be related to other connective tissue disorders, for example SLE, and the occasional finding of hypergammaglobulinaemia and antibodies such as rheumatoid and antinuclear factors have suggested that it may have an autoimmune basis.

The histopathology of the skin shows coarse collagen bundles which lie parallel to the epidermis and extend downwards into the subcutaneous fat. Fibrosis also occurs in the lungs, heart, alimentary tract, muscles and serous membranes. Lesions of the small arteries and arterioles are seen, especially in the kidney where they lead to focal glomerular necrosis or cortical infarction.

The clinical features of scleroderma are often preceded for several years by Raynaud's phenomenon and sometimes excessive sweating

of the palms and soles. In the early stages the fingers are stiff, and gradually the skin on the backs of the fingers becomes waxy, taut, hard and thickened, being bound firmly to the underlying tissues. Similar changes develop elsewhere on the hands and feet, face, neck, and upper chest, leading to a mask-like facial appearance with loss of the normal facial folds and 'pinching' of the mouth. Brownish pigmentation and telangiectases appear in the affected areas, and peripheral arteritis may lead to ulceration and loss of tissue at the tips of the fingers. Subcutaneous calcification may occur in the digits. A subacute polyarthritis may affect the hands, wrists and knees, and muscle weakness and atrophy occur in advanced disease.

Visceral involvement causes oesophageal immobility leading to dysphagia, intestinal malabsorption, myocardial fibrosis which gives rise to cardiac failure and arrhythmias, and renal involvement leading to hypertension and renal failure. The disease usually follows a slowly progressive course over many years.

PULMONARY MANIFESTATIONS

The lungs appear to be involved in the majority of patients with scleroderma. Dyspnoea on exertion is the earliest symptom, often associated with a cough. Sputum occurs mainly as a result of secondary bronchial infection. The most characteristic physical signs are limitation of chest expansion with rapid shallow breathing, associated with scattered fine crepitations most prominent at the lung base.

In the early stages the chest radiograph shows diffuse mottled and reticular shadowing which is most marked in the lower zones. This progresses to diffuse symmetrical pulmonary fibrosis affecting the major part of both lung fields although the apices are usually spared. A honeycomb appearance at the lung bases is commonly described.

The histological changes in the lungs consist of interstitial fibrosis and thickening of the alveolar septa, usually most marked in the lower lobes. As the process advances, large areas of the parenchyma become fibrotic causing the alveoli and alveolar capillaries to be obliterated. The small pulmonary arteries and arterioles become obstructed by intimal proliferation, medial hypertrophy and perivascular fibrosis. Bronchiectasis, bronchial dilatation and cystic changes occur in the late stages of the disease.

The functional abnormality has a typically restrictive pattern, with reduction in all lung volumes, reduced compliance, impaired carbon monoxide transfer but normal gas flow in the airways. Hypoxaemia occurs, probably because of ventilation/perfusion inequality, but carbon dioxide excretion is maintained by increased ventilation of well-ventilated alveoli, and arterial carbon dioxide tension is often low.

Pulmonary hypertension may result from obliteration and narrowing of the pulmonary vascular bed, leading to cor pulmonale.

The complications of systemic sclerosis include aspiration pneumonia, due to spill-over of ingested material into the respiratory tract from the sclerosed oesophagus, and alveolar cell carcinoma, which is said occasionally to affect patients with longstanding pulmonary fibrosis.

Polyarteritis Nodosa

Polyarteritis nodosa is characterised by segmental inflammation and necrosis of medium and small arteries, causing a variety of clinical manifestations according to the site and extent of arterial involvement. It occurs most commonly among males in middle life. Although the aetiology is unknown, hypersensitivity is thought to play a part because of the similarity of the lesions to those occurring in serum sickness, and because the disease occasionally appears to follow treatment with various drugs, including sulphonamides, iodides and penicillin.

The clinical manifestations of polyarteritis nodosa are diverse but may follow one of a number of different patterns:

1. Fever of uncertain origin.
2. Renal involvement, often an acute glomerulonephritis complicated by hypertension and progressive renal failure.
3. Abdominal symptoms, such as pain, vomiting, and bloody diarrhoea, sometimes associated with infarction of the bowel.
4. Central nervous system involvement, including peripheral neuropathy.
5. Muscle and joint pains associated with weight loss.
6. Myocardial infarction and cardiac failure.
7. Asthma and pneumonia.

The onset of the disease is sometimes insidious, sometimes abrupt due to the obstruction of an important vascular supply. Although remissions occasionally occur the course of polyarteritis nodosa is usually progressive, leading to death within a few months.

PULMONARY MANIFESTATIONS

Pulmonary involvement in polyarteritis usually presents either as bronchitis, asthma, or pneumonia. These features frequently appear just before or simultaneously with the onset of the systemic illness, but the asthmatic presentation, particularly, may precede the systemic symptoms by several years. In such cases the asthma is unusually severe and frequent, accompanied by marked eosinophilia in the blood and sputum. Episodes of pneumonia are accompanied by

cough, haemoptysis and pleuritic pain, with localised crepitations indicating areas of consolidation, which may be transient but are sometimes progressive due to necrosis of the affected lung tissue. Digital clubbing may occur.

WEGENER'S GRANULOMATOSIS

This condition is a variant of polyarteritis nodosa, characterised by necrotising, granulomatous lesions of the upper respiratory tract, generalised vasculitis which involves both arteries and veins, especially in the lungs, and focal glomerulonephritis. It affects adults, most commonly presenting with sinusitis or rhinitis, or as subacute pneumonia with cough, haemoptysis and pleuritic pain. Eosinophilia is a common manifestation of the disease, and other features of polyarteritis nodosa frequently accompany or follow the respiratory tract involvement. Death usually occurs within six months, often as a consequence of renal failure, but successful treatment with cytotoxic agents such as chlorambucil has recently been described.

Clinical Implications

Because of their rarity, the connective tissue disorders of the lungs described in this chapter present only occasionally as respiratory problems in clinical practice. Nevertheless, their manifestations mimic the features of many common pulmonary disorders such as pleurisy, pneumonia, pulmonary fibrosis, asthma, and nodular or cavitating lung lesions, and it is therefore important to bear these conditions in mind when considering differential diagnosis, especially when other features of the clinical presentation suggest a systemic rather than a purely pulmonary disease. Suspicion should be aroused by anomalies sometimes disregarded because they cannot be readily explained: inappropriate weight loss or malaise, persistent elevation of the erythrocyte sedimentation rate, recurrent respiratory infections or an unsatisfactory response to antibiotic therapy.

Specific treatment of these disorders is at present limited to the use of corticosteroid drugs. Such therapy is most effective in treating acute manifestations as occur in systemic lupus erythematosus or polyarteritis nodosa, and the current tendency is to give large doses such as 40 to 80 mg of prednisolone daily to control an acute exacerbation, reducing the prednisolone gradually to a maintenance level (preferably about 10 to 15 mg daily) when a response has been obtained. Treatment is continued for several months on a maintenance dose before any attempt is made at gradual withdrawal. In the pulmonary complications of rheumatoid disease and systemic sclerosis the value of corticosteroid therapy is debatable, although some studies seem to have shown a useful effect in the early stages of pulmonary fibrosis.

21

Pulmonary Thromboembolic Disease

By common use, pulmonary embolism has come to mean the impaction in the pulmonary arteries of thrombus originating from the systemic veins, usually those of the iliofemoral system. Very rarely, emboli may arise from extravascular sources, such as fat or air emboli following trauma, or amniotic fluid embolism occurring as a rare complication of labour, but in this account discussion is limited to thromboembolic disease.

The true incidence of pulmonary embolism cannot be determined because of the difficulty of the clinical diagnosis, but the incidence in post-mortem studies of hospital cases varies from 15 to 25 per cent, and clinical recognition of the diagnosis may be achieved before death in less than half. Despite increased understanding of methods of prevention and treatment the incidence of acute pulmonary embolism in hospital has shown an increase in recent years, and the mortality remains constant at about 50 per cent. There is no significant difference between the sexes but the incidence increases considerably over the age of fifty, heart disease and, particularly, congestive heart failure being the most important predisposing cause.

Pathogenesis

The great majority of pulmonary emboli originate from venous thrombosis occurring in the iliofemoral veins. The factors that contribute to the formation of venous thrombosis are venous stasis, trauma to the vein, and abnormalities of coagulation.

VENOUS STASIS

Venous stasis is the single most important cause of venous thrombosis, and can occur in a variety of ways. Among hospital patients venous blood flow is reduced by:

1. Immobilisation, both in bed or while undergoing surgical anaesthesia.

2. Heart failure, due to reduced cardiac output and raised venous pressure.
3. Compression of the calf muscles in bed.

In the ambulant person, venous blood flow is diminished by *obesity,* and by *varicose veins* which drain blood away from the deep veins through which flow against gravity is augmented by muscular contraction. *Inactivity* such as prolonged sitting on journeys will contribute to the stasis. Venous thrombosis in *pregnancy* is attributed to mechanical obstruction of the inferior vena cava and also to hormonally induced venous dilation; the latter mechanism may also be responsible for the increased liability to thrombosis occurring among women taking oestrogen-containing *contraceptive pills*.

VENOUS TRAUMA

Local trauma to the vein wall may arise as a result of a football or similar blunt injury, and a single episode of venous thrombosis may contribute to subsequent recurrence because collateral flow tends to be slower and through more tortuous channels. Thrombophlebitis may be a predisposing factor.

CHANGES IN COAGULATION

Apart from *splenectomy* and *polycythaemia*, the part played by hypercoagulability in the production of pulmonary thromboembolism is poorly determined. Demonstration of increased platelet adhesiveness or fibrinogen turnover is common in thromboembolic disease, but it simply indicates thrombotic activity without necessarily being the cause. It is possible that the increased thrombotic tendency associated with *adenocarcinoma* may be attributed to a change in coagulation.

Pathology

EMBOLISATION

Pulmonary emboli are nearly always multiple and usually lodge in the lower lobes. The majority probably undergo complete lysis within two or three weeks but repeated showers of small and large emboli may occur, leading to severe pulmonary artery obstruction. Some emboli eventually organise and contract to the side of the vessel, leaving a channel that becomes relined with endothelium.

It is uncertain whether the haemodynamic effects of pulmonary embolisation are entirely due to mechanical obstruction by impacted emboli, although undoubtedly this is often the case, or whether vasoconstrictive substances such as 5-hydroxytryptamine (Serotonin)

are liberated from the platelets trapped within the embolus and contribute to the rise in pulmonary arterial pressure.

INFARCTION

Because the lung has a double blood supply through the bronchial and pulmonary arteries infarction does not necessarily follow pulmonary embolisation. The factors that appear to predispose to infarction include obstruction of a very large branch of the pulmonary artery, and pulmonary venous obstruction as in mitral stenosis or left ventricular failure. As in embolisation, pulmonary infarction is commonest in patients past middle age and usually occurs in the lower lobes, multiple infarcts being twice as common as single ones.

When a branch of the pulmonary artery is obstructed the capillary bed becomes congested with blood flowing from patent vessels in the neighbouring lung, and this may be sufficient to prevent necrosis of the affected tissue. If the obstruction is more extensive, capillary damage results in the leakage of oedema fluid and red cells into the ischaemic area, but the rapid establishment of improved circulation from precapillary anastomoses between the bronchial and pulmonary vessels may prevent necrosis of pulmonary tissue, and the lung is gradually restored to normal. Only if the capillary walls necrose, leading to gross haemorrhage and tissue disruption, does complete infarction occur; this is followed by organisation and subsequent fibrous scar formation.

Functional Disturbance

THE HEART

Sudden obstruction to the outflow of the right ventricle by a massive pulmonary embolus causes it to dilate. This leads to an increase in the force of contraction, while release of adrenaline from the adrenal medulla causes a tachycardia which helps to boost cardiac output. Unless the obstruction is rapidly relieved, however, either by fragmentation of the embolus or by its onward propulsion into the wider cross-sectional area of the pulmonary vascular bed, right ventricular output quickly falls away. The clinical signs that indicate this critical situation are wide splitting of the pulmonary second sound because of delayed emptying of the right ventricle, and dilatation of the neck veins due to the rise in right ventricular diastolic pressure.

The left ventricle is starved of blood and stimulated by release of catecholamines so that it empties rapidly into a vasoconstricted systemic circulation, producing a sharply rising but poorly sustained arterial pulse. Pulmonary venous dilation during inspiration reduces left ventricular filling still further, resulting in pulsus paradoxus.

PULMONARY FUNCTION

In the absence of infarction or pulmonary congestion, the effect of embolisation is to produce an area of lung that is ventilated but unperfused. As a result, no gas exchange can take place in this 'compartment', physiological dead space is increased, and there is an abnormally low concentration of carbon dioxide in the expired gas, leading to a raised arterial-alveolar carbon dioxide tension difference. In theory, measurement of physiological dead space and the arterial—end-tidal carbon dioxide tension difference should be useful tests in the diagnosis of pulmonary embolisation; in practice, however, pulmonary congestion and infarction do commonly occur, and all too often underlying chronic airways obstruction or cardiac disease confuse the interpretation of these tests.

Reflex bronchoconstriction occurs in the affected areas, and it has a compensatory effect in reducing the unevenness of ventilation and perfusion caused by vascular obstruction. Nevertheless, considerable arterial hypoxaemia commonly occurs, attributed mainly to venous admixture occurring in parts of the lung which are also affected by reflex bronchoconstriction because they lie adjacent to the embolised areas. In the 20 to 25 per cent of patients who have a patent foramen ovale the high right atrial and low left atrial pressures may contribute to arterial hypoxaemia by causing intracardiac shunting through the defect.

The lung volumes and the rate of gas flow in the airways are normal in uncomplicated pulmonary embolism, but carbon monoxide transfer is commonly diminished due to a reduction in the surface area of the alveolar-capillary membrane available for gas exchange. Hyperventilation is characteristically observed although the mechanism of its production is obscure. It leads to rather low levels of arterial carbon dioxide tension.

Clinical Features

The diagnosis of pulmonary thromboembolism is often extremely difficult, but careful attention to the patient's state of health prior to the illness sometimes provides important clues. The patient should be questioned about any condition that might predispose to venous thrombosis such as chronic heart disease (particularly the symptoms of congestive cardiac failure), a period of immobility such as a long journey or confinement to bed, recent surgical operations, recent pregnancy or parturition, the use of contraceptive pills, injury to the legs or the presence of varicose veins. A history of transient pain or swelling of the legs may indicate an episode of iliofemoral thrombosis, but it should be borne in mind that overt symptoms and signs of deep venous thrombosis are absent in more than 50 per cent of patients

with pulmonary thromboembolism at the time of clinical presentation, although they may become manifest later. Any past incidents of unexplained 'pneumonia' or pleurisy may indicate that the present illness is one of a series of episodes due to recurrent pulmonary thromboemboli.

The clinical presentation of pulmonary embolism can follow one of three patterns: *pulmonary embolism with infarction,* in which the embolus lodges in a more or less peripheral branch of the pulmonary vascular bed, causing infarction of the affected area of lung; *chronic thromboembolic pulmonary hypertension,* caused by minor episodes of embolism which gradually obstruct the pulmonary circulation and lead to obliterative pulmonary hypertension; and *massive pulmonary embolism,* in which a large embolus lodges in the main pulmonary trunk causing acute obstruction to the outflow of the right ventricle.

PULMONARY EMBOLISM WITH INFARCTION

The most characteristic *symptom* of pulmonary infarction is the sudden onset of *pleuritic pain,* usually localised to the site of the lesion but sometimes referred to the tip of the shoulder or to the abdomen. *Dyspnoea* is variable, usually attributable to the chest pain which limits expansion and causes rapid shallow breathing. *Haemoptysis* occurs in about 50 per cent of cases only.

Signs. The patient appears distressed by the pleurisy, and may have a low grade *pyrexia* and moderate *tachycardia.* A *friction rub* may be audible over the infarct, followed subsequently by the signs of a *pleural effusion*; the latter is usually serous but may be blood-stained. The signs of consolidation are usually absent, but crepitations may be heard in the area. *Cyanosis* and slight *icterus* are uncommon accompaniments of pulmonary infarction, usually occurring only in the presence of heart failure.

A *polymorphonuclear leucocytosis* of 15 to 20,000/mm^3 frequently occurs, and the *erythrocyte sedimentation rate* and serum *lactic dehydrogenase* level are increased, but none of these tests is sufficiently specific to assist the diagnosis materially. The *chest radiograph* may show pulmonary opacities resembling pneumonia, linear collapse, pleural shadows indicative of effusion, and elevation of the diaphragm on the affected side. The shadows are frequently bilateral and occur most commonly in the lower zone. *Radioscanning* of the lungs (page 95) with macroaggregates of ^{131}I-labelled human serum albumin is a method of assessing the integrity of the pulmonary vascular bed, and may be of considerable diagnostic value in pulmonary infarction when taken in conjunction with the clinical and radiological findings.

Differential Diagnosis. The diagnosis of pulmonary infarction is

difficult because none of the clinical features or diagnostic tests is specific for the disease, and success depends on careful weighing up of the evidence. Differentiation of the condition from lobar or segmental pneumonia is a recurring problem and it is sometimes necessary to treat a patient for both conditions until the diagnosis becomes clear. Other conditions that have to be considered are bronchial carcinoma, pulmonary tuberculosis, postoperative collapse of the lung, spontaneous pneumothorax, and polyarteritis nodosa.

CHRONIC THROMBOEMBOLIC PULMONARY HYPERTENSION

The *symptoms* of this condition are usually insidious in onset, consisting of *dyspnoea* on exertion, undue *fatigue* and occasional episodes of *chest pain*. Nevertheless, a careful history often reveals past episodes of pleuritic pain or haemoptysis indicative of minor embolic incidents. *Syncope* on exertion and *angina pectoris* may occur because cardiac output is limited by obliteration of the pulmonary vascular bed. There may be a persistent low grade pyrexia.

The *signs* are those of right ventricular strain and pulmonary hypertension. A giant 'a' wave may be seen in the jugular venous pulse, and palpation of the praecordium reveals a right ventricular impulse at the left sternal margin. The second heart sound in the pulmonary area is narrowly split and sometimes single, the pulmonary element being louder than normal. A systolic ejection click may be associated with pulmonary artery dilatation, and a gallop rhythm is occasionally audible over the right ventricle. Signs of congestive heart failure develop as the condition progresses.

The *chest radiograph* shows cardiac enlargement with dilatation of the main pulmonary arteries and rather oligaemic lung fields. *Pulmonary angiography* may show lack of filling of the larger vessels if the condition is a sequel to major pulmonary embolism, but often the larger branches of the pulmonary vascular tree appear relatively normal and filling defects are only apparent by careful study of the smaller peripheral vessels. The *electrocardiograph* shows right axis deviation, *P* pulmonale, tall *R* waves in the right ventricular leads signifying right ventricular hypertrophy, and widespread *T* wave inversion.

MASSIVE PULMONARY EMBOLISM

Symptoms. The commonest symptom of massive pulmonary embolism is sudden *collapse or faintness* due to impairment of cerebral blood flow. *Central* chest pain similar to the pain of myocardial infarction is due to reduction in coronary perfusion. Acute *dyspnoea* occurs frequently and may be the only presenting

symptom, both dyspnoea and faintness being commonly increased when the patient sits up. *Pleuritic pain* and *haemoptysis* sometimes occur at the time of the massive embolic episode or may have been observed in the preceding few days because of initial small pulmonary infarcts.

Signs. The physical signs can be explained by the haemodynamic changes that result from a sudden fall in cardiac output and right ventricular failure. The patient appears gravely dyspnoeic, anxious, pale and slightly cyanosed; the pulse is rapid and small in volume with a sharp upstroke, and the blood pressure is low. Pulsus paradoxus is a sign of serious import. The jugular venous pressure is raised, and auscultation of the heart commonly reveals a gallop rhythm over the right ventricle, due either to loss of right ventricular compliance causing a diastolic filling sound (3rd or protodiastolic sound) or to powerful right atrial contraction producing a 4th or presystolic sound; a combination of these sounds due to shortening of diastole may cause a 'summation' gallop. The pulmonary second sound is often split due to delayed right ventricular ejection, but loud pulmonary valve closure is not a feature of acute massive pulmonary embolism.

Diagnostic Aids. The *electrocardiographic changes* of massive pulmonary embolism are occasionally absent or transient because the circulatory disturbance rapidly rights itself. The changes most commonly seen are sinus tachycardia and low voltage complexes due to reduced stroke output, '$S1$ $Q3$ $T3$' pattern due to coronary insufficiency, T inversion in the right praecordial leads attributable either to hyperventilation or to right ventricular dilatation, and right axis deviation, right bundle branch block, S in $V5$ and P pulmonale due to right ventricular dilatation and failure.

The *chest radiograph* may show evidence of pulmonary infarction due to previous embolic episodes. Occasionally, areas of diminished vascular shadowing due to oligaemia can be distinguished, contrasting with nearby areas of hyperaemia. The pulmonary trunk is typically not dilated. *Pulmonary angiography* has been found useful in confirming the diagnosis in doubtful cases, and in defining the extent of the obstruction. It is a more precise technique than radioscanning, which is often difficult to perform in the acutely dyspnoeic patient.

Among the conditions that should be considered in the *differential diagnosis* of massive pulmonary embolism should be included myocardial infarction, dissecting aneurysm of the aorta, spontaneous pneumothorax, and postoperative pulmonary collapse.

Management

PREVENTION

Iliofemoral thrombosis and its sequel, pulmonary embolism, should be prevented in hospital patients by avoiding venous stasis in the legs,

particularly in those conditions that predispose to venous thrombosis. Early postoperative ambulation should be encouraged, and elderly patients should be confined to bed as little as possible. Regular and frequent leg exercises should be performed by those who are compelled to remain in bed, special attention being paid to patients with heart disease or polycythaemia. Prophylactic oral anticoagulant therapy has been shown to be effective in reducing the incidence of postoperative thromboembolism in elderly patients with fractured hips, and also in obstetric and gynaecological practice. Alternatively, subcutaneous heparin in a low dose of 50 mg (5,000 units) twice daily is a valuable form of prophylactic therapy in hospital, especially for recumbent obese individuals.

If deep venous thrombosis develops it should be treated immediately with anticoagulants, beginning with heparin and an oral anticoagulant such as warfarin simultaneously, and discontinuing the heparin after 48 hours, by which time the warfarin will have become effective. The patient should be kept in bed for about a week to allow the thrombosis to become firmly adherent to the vessel wall. Oral anticoagulation is maintained until the patient has returned to normal activities after discharge from hospital.

PULMONARY INFARCTION

Once the diagnosis of pulmonary infarction has been made heparin should be started simultaneously with an oral anticoagulant, and anticoagulation continued as described for the treatment of deep venous thrombosis. If coincident pulmonary infection is suspected, or if the differential diagnosis between pneumonia and pulmonary infarction is undetermined, a broad spectrum antibiotic such as oxytetracycline or amoxycillin may be given. Pleuritic pain should be relieved with morphine or pethidine.

CHRONIC PULMONARY THROMBOEMBOLISM

Recurrent pulmonary emboli, with or without pulmonary hypertension, should be treated by long-term oral anticoagulant therapy. The prognosis is good in those without raised pulmonary arterial pressure, but in a series of patients with hypertension due to obliteration of the pulmonary vascular bed the mortality was found to be 50 per cent within five years. Where pulmonary hypertension is shown by arteriography to be due to obstruction of the large pulmonary arteries thrombectomy may be considered.

MASSIVE PULMONARY EMBOLISM

The immediate steps to be taken in the treatment of a massive pulmonary embolus are:

1. External cardiac massage.
2. Oxygen by mask or endotracheal intubation.
3. Correction of acidosis.
4. Vasopressor drugs such as isoprenaline, if indicated.
5. Intravenous injection of 150 mg of heparin.

Further management consists of continued therapy with heparin or with streptokinase, the latter drug having the advantage of accelerating the lysis of recurrent pulmonary emboli. After recovery from the acute illness, oral anticoagulant therapy is continued for at least three months and, occasionally, for longer if multiple emboli have occurred.

If the patient deteriorates rapidly during the hours following the initial episode, so that maintenance of an adequate systemic blood pressure becomes impossible, pulmonary embolectomy is probably indicated. The correct selection of patients for this operation, which has a high mortality, is difficult and is best preceded by pulmonary scanning or angiography to confirm the diagnosis provided that the patient's condition is good enough to permit these investigations. The operation is usually carried out by employing cardiopulmonary bypass or hypothermia but some recent successful operative methods have been devised which avoid the need for bypass techniques. The mortality for pulmonary embolectomy varies from 25 to 50 per cent in different series, but appears to be greatest in patients who suffered circulatory arrest prior to operation.

DRUGS USED IN THE TREATMENT OF THROMBOEMBOLISM

Heparin acts by neutralising thrombin, inhibiting the conversion of prothrombin to thrombin and reducing platelet stickiness. It has an immediate effect which lasts for about six hours, and it is best administered by continuous intravenous infusion since subcutaneous or intramuscular injections are likely to lead to painful haematomas. The required dose varies from 100 to 150 mg (10,000 to 15,000 units) every six hours and accurate assessment of dosage requirements is necessary at regular intervals, using the Lee and White method for measuring the clotting time which should be prolonged by therapy to 15 to 30 minutes (normal value 5 to 11 minutes). The anticoagulant effect of heparin can be rapidly reversed with protamine sulphate, given by slow intravenous injection.

Oral anticoagulant drugs include *dicoumarol* and *warfarin sodium*, both of which have a duration of action lasting two to four days, and *phenindione* which has a slightly shorter anticoagulant effect. The latter drug has become less popular than formerly because of its tendency to cause side effects which include agranulocytosis, hepatitis

and nephrotic syndrome, whereas warfarin is less toxic and is currently the drug of choice. These drugs act by inhibition of factor VII and reduction in prothrombin concentration, and their action can be reversed with Vitamin K1.

The loading dose of warfarin is 25 to 30 mg, the effect of this dose being checked 48 hours after the start of treatment and the maintenance dose determined accordingly, usually from 5 to 10 mg daily. The therapeutic level of anticoagulation which is usually aimed for is 2 to $2\frac{1}{2}$ times the control value using the one-stage prothrombin time, or 5 to 15 per cent of normal using the thrombotest.

Streptokinase is a thrombolytic agent that acts upon the complex plasminogen molecule in two ways: in low dose it activates circulating plasminogen with maximum generation of plasmin, producing generalised fibrinolysis and a liability to bleeding; but in high dosage streptokinase causes only a transient increase in plasmin, its main effect on circulating plasminogen being to generate a high level of activator which permeates occluding thrombi and becomes attached to the adsorbed plasminogen within the thrombus, inducing thrombolysis.

Streptokinase is administered by infusion in normal saline into a peripheral vein. A widely used scheme of administration is to give 600,000 units in the first half hour followed by 100,000 units per hour for 72 hours. Previously administered heparin should be neutralised with protamine sulphate before any streptokinase is infused, and a preliminary intramuscular dose of hydrocortisone 100 mg should be given to control febrile hypersensitivity reactions to the streptokinase. Further corticosteroids may be necessary during the course of the infusion. Treatment may be monitored by measuring the thrombin clotting time, aiming for two to four times the control value.

The most important complication of this form of therapy is bleeding, and streptokinase is contra-indicated in the presence of active peptic ulceration, systemic hypertension, cerebrovascular haemorrhage, a known bleeding state, during pregnancy or within ten days of a surgical operation. If bleeding occurs during therapy fresh blood should be given.

22

Drug-induced Lung Disease

The Problem of Drug Toxicity

Almost any drug can cause toxic reactions, and such reactions are often severe enough to cause serious illness and even death. Although many such illnesses are probably not recognised as due to drugs there are several published studies which show that drug reactions may be a major cause for admission in up to 5 per cent of hospital patients. The incidence of reactions among those undergoing treatment in hospital is even higher, affecting between 10 and 18 per cent of patients.

Respiratory disorders attributable to the unwanted effects of drug therapy are commonly encountered, and some have been mentioned briefly in the relevant sections of this book. In this chapter the different types of pulmonary reactions due to drug toxicity are grouped under clinicopathological headings, with a short account of the drug or group of drugs so far known to cause each disorder.

AETIOLOGICAL FACTORS

Dosage. As a general rule the larger the dose of a drug that is administered, the more likely are side-effects to occur. This is either because the required pharmacological action of the drug may be exaggerated at higher dosage to a degree which causes undesirable symptoms, or else because coincidental pharmacological side-effects tend to become increasingly troublesome as the dose is raised. On the other hand, hypersensitivity reactions are not dose related, for they may occur in response to quite small doses of a drug given to sensitive individuals.

Abnormal Metabolism or Excretion. Many drugs are metabolised by the liver to inactive derivatives, or excreted by the kidneys. In the presence of coincidental hepatic or renal disease the plasma concentration of such drugs may increase to toxic levels unless the dosage is modified appropriately. The age of the patient is an important consideration in this respect, for hepatic drug-metabolising enzyme systems may be undeveloped in infants and renal function is frequently impaired in the elderly. A similar problem arises in patients

with respiratory failure since hypoxia slows down the handling of drugs by the liver and kidneys.

Genetic Factors. Genetically-determined variations in drug metabolism may be the cause of differences between individuals in their response to a drug. For example, the rate at which isoniazid is inactivated depends upon a single gene, slow inactivators tending to accumulate higher plasma levels of isoniazid than rapid inactivators and to be consequently more liable to develop peripheral neuritis.

Drug Interactions. The effect one drug may have on the concentration of or the response to another is being increasingly recognised as a major consideration of therapy. The reason for this is the increasing use of multiple drug therapy in the treatment of an individual patient, and the need for considerable precision in adjusting the dose of some drugs to obtain the optimal effect. Drug interactions can be classified into two types:

1. Those that alter the patient's response to a drug without altering its concentration at the receptor site or in the plasma (pharmacodynamic interactions).

2. Those that alter the drug concentration (pharmacokinetic interactions).

An example of a pharmacodynamic interaction is the effect of hypokalaemia induced by a thiazide diuretic such as bendrofluazide upon the myocardial response to digitalis; and of a pharmacokinetic interaction, the effect of a drug such as phenylbutazone in increasing the plasma level of warfarin, because it displaces warfarin from its binding site to albumin. There are several other ways in which pharmacokinetic interactions can occur, including enzyme induction and inhibition and alterations in renal excretion.

Alteration of Immune Mechanisms. Treatment with corticosteroid drugs and immunosuppressive agents is liable to affect the patient's immune response not only to common bacterial and mycobacterial infections, but also to opportunistic infection with micro-organisms which are rarely pathogenic to a normal individual.

Hypersensitivity Reactions. These are the least predictable of drug-induced pulmonary diseases in that they are unrelated to the known toxicity or dosage of the drug, although some, particularly the asthmatic reactions, are perhaps more likely to occur in atopic individuals. Besides asthma they include pulmonary eosinophilia, drug-induced polyarteritis nodosa and systemic lupus erythematosus, and certain forms of pulmonary fibrosis.

THERAPEUTIC ASPECTS OF THE HISTORY

Current Therapy. Bearing in mind the numerous ways in which

different drugs can cause toxic effects it is clearly important to obtain an accurate account of a patient's current therapy when he presents with symptoms and signs of pulmonary illness. All too often he is unaware of the names of the drugs he is taking and has only an uncertain notion of their therapeutic purpose. Reference to hospital records or to the family doctor should be made for the necessary information. Certain types of drug may be used habitually and come to be regarded as being of no particular significance by the patient; direct questions should therefore be asked about sedatives, analgesics and contraceptive tablets. Note should also be taken of drugs that are applied topically since these may be responsible for hypersensitivity reactions; for example, pulmonary eosinophilia has been described following the application of sulphonamide-containing cream to the vagina.

Concurrent Diseases. Because both renal and hepatic disease may prolong or increase the action of a drug by delaying its metabolism or excretion, enquiry should be made for evidence of present or past illnesses that might have led to impaired renal or hepatic function.

History of Atopy. Patients with an allergic history or a family history of allergy may show an increased liability to drug hypersensitivity, sometimes in the form of asthma. Penicillin allergy is an example of this association. However, drug-induced asthma is by no means confined to atopic individuals, and in subjects with aspirin-induced asthma the incidence of atopy is rather low.

Respiratory Failure

In incipient respiratory failure normal levels of arterial oxygen and carbon dioxide tension are maintained initially by hyperventilation which depends partly on voluntary effort and partly on the stimulatory activity of the respiratory centre. Any factor that reduces ventilation in these circumstances will precipitate overt respiratory failure with hypoxaemia and hypercapnia, as may occur when acute infection complicates chronic bronchitis or when bronchial obstruction and physical exhaustion overcome the patient in status asthmaticus. In a similar way the incautious administration of a sedative or hypnotic drug may tip the balance by suppressing the response of the respiratory centre to hypoxia or hypercapnia and allowing ventilation to diminish so that respiratory failure ensues. The dangers of morphine and barbiturates in this situation are well recognised, but even mild sedatives such as nitrazepam are hazardous, and as a general rule all forms of sedation should be avoided when there is a risk of respiratory failure. The restlessness and mental confusion often met with in patients with respiratory failure

are usually a consequence of hypoxia and carbon dioxide retention, and should be treated appropriately with physiotherapy and, if necessary, mechanically-assisted ventilation, *not* with sedatives.

Drug-induced Asthma

Beta-blocking Agents. Patients who are liable to asthma may have an exacerbation of bronchoconstriction if they are treated for cardiovascular disease with a beta-blocking drug such as propranolol or oxprenolol. Practolol has less effect on bronchial beta-receptors but carries a significant risk of causing hyperkeratotic skin lesions and keratoconjunctivitis sicca, and should, therefore, be used with caution.

Paradoxical Effect of Bronchodilators. An allergic broncho-constrictor response to isoprenaline has been described in atopic patients, only relieved by discontinuing all sympathomimetic-amine-containing aerosols.

Hypersensitivity Asthma. A wide variety of drugs may cause a Type I allergic reaction resulting in asthma, urticaria and sometimes anaphylactic shock. They include a number of antibiotics such as the penicillins, streptomycin, tetracycline, erythomycin and neomycin, ethionamide, monoamine oxidase inhibitors, local anaesthetics, mercurials, antisera and vaccines. Serum sickness induced by such drugs as penicillin, streptomycin and sulphonamides may also cause asthma associated with other symptoms such as maculopapular eruptions, fever, urticaria, arthralgia and lymphadenopathy.

Asthma due to aspirin ingestion is the commonest form of drug-induced asthma although the mechanism of its provocation is not clearly understood. It occurs mainly in non-atopic individuals in middle age and is usually preceded by rhinitis and nasal polyposis. The asthmatic attack comes on about half-an-hour after ingesting the drug and is usually severe and prolonged, being often associated with urticaria and laryngeal oedema. It is usually relieved by treatment with corticosteroid drugs. Intolerance to other peripheral analgesics such as indomethacin and paracetamol may be associated.

Acute Exudative Hypersensitivity Reactions

Infiltration of the lungs with inflammatory exudate often containing large numbers of eosinophils, associated with marked eosinophilia of the blood and sputum, may occur in a number of conditions. These include infection with *Aspergillus fumigatus* (page 197), infestation with a variety of parasitic worms, and diseases of uncertain pathogenesis such as polyarteritis nodosa and Wegener's granulomatosis (page 256). It seems probable that the eosinophilic exudate represents a type of hypersensitivity response affecting

variously the alveoli, the bronchi and the pulmonary vessels. One form of the condition known as simple pulmonary eosinophilia occurs as a hypersensitivity reaction to a wide variety of drugs, although it was originally described by Loeffler in relation to parasitic infestation due mainly to *Ascaris lumbricoides* (Loeffler's syndrome).

SIMPLE PULMONARY EOSINOPHILIA

This is usually a mild illness characterised by blood eosinophilia and transient shadows on the chest radiograph, subsiding rapidly when the offending allergen is removed. Infestation with intestinal parasites such as *Ascaris lumbricoides, Taenia saginata* and *Ancylostoma braziliense* may be responsible, but the syndrome is being increasingly described as a hypersensitivity reaction to drug therapy. The drugs include aspirin, nitrofurantoin, sodium aminosalicylate (PAS), penicillin, imipramine, chlorpropamide, mephanesin, azothioprine, sulphonamides, furazolidine, methotrexate and sulphasalazine.

The *clinical features* consist of cough, dyspnoea and a sensation of tightness in the chest without wheezing, accompanied by systemic symptoms such as malaise, fatigue and mild fever. Examination may reveal crepitations at the lung bases but no other abnormality. The chest radiograph usually shows fan-shaped opacities with ill-defined borders, sometimes occurring transiently in one part of the lungs and subsequently appearing in another, while small pleural effusions may be observed. Eosinophilia occurs in blood and sputum. The symptoms and radiological changes resolve promptly once the offending drug has been withdrawn.

Tests of pulmonary function during the acute phase of the pulmonary reaction show increased minute ventilation, hypoxaemia, hypocapnia and reduction in carbon monoxide transfer (T_L, CO).

REACTIONS TO NITROFURANTOIN

Although the antibiotic nitrofurantoin may cause simple pulmonary eosinophilia as described above, allergic pulmonary reactions to this drug may also become manifest in the following ways:

Acute Pulmonary Syndrome. In some patients, the hypersensitivity reaction to nitrofurantoin takes a very acute and alarming form with severe breathlessness, malaise, chills, fever and chest pain coming on 4 or 5 hours after ingesting the drug, associated with widespread crepitations and occasional wheezing heard on auscultation. The reaction may not occur until several days after starting treatment with nitrofurantoin, and sometimes appears only during a second or subsequent course of treatment. Cyanosis and hypotension may occur in severe cases, the condition simulating left ventricular failure

or pneumonia. Eosinophilia is sometimes observed. The reaction settles down within a few hours of discontinuing the drug, but urgent treatment with aminophylline and corticosteroid drugs may be necessary.

Progressive Pulmonary Fibrosis. This condition presents with dyspnoea of insidious onset, usually in patients on long-term or repeated courses of nitrofurantoin therapy. It is thought to be due to gradual organisation and fibrosis of alveolar and interstitial exudate and is sometimes the legacy of repeated attacks of the acute syndrome. Fine basal crepitations are heard on listening to the chest, and the chest radiograph shows bilateral basal infiltrations which, on lung biopsy, are shown to be due to interstitial fibrosis. The condition may regress slowly when nitrofurantoin is discontinued or with the administration of corticosteroid therapy.

Drug-induced Polyarteritis Nodosa

The pulmonary manifestations of polyarteritis nodosa include asthma, pneumonia, and cough and haemoptysis associated with radiological shadows, which may represent consolidation, infarction or abscess formation. Eosinophilia of the blood and sputum is a common but not invariable accompaniment. Polyarteritis nodosa is alleged to have followed therapy with a number of drugs which include sulphonamides, iodides, penicillins, organic arsenicals and mercurials, gold salts and phenothiazines.

Drug-induced Systemic Lupus Erythematosus

Among the common clinical manifestations of systemic lupus erythematosus are pleurisy and pleural effusion, pneumonia, pulmonary infarction, progressive atalectasis with shrinkage of the lungs and diffuse pulmonary fibrosis. These manifestations may also occur in the drug-related form of the disease but significant renal damage is rare and the condition as a whole is less severe than the 'spontaneous' disease. Withdrawal of the offending drug is nearly always followed by complete resolution although corticosteroid treatment is occasionally necessary.

The four drugs that most commonly induce systemic lupus erythematosus are hydrallazine, phenytoin, procainamide and isoniazid, but many others have been suspected, including antibacterial or antifungal agents (griseofulvin, penicillin, sodium aminosalicylate, streptomycin, sulphonamides, tetracycline), anticonvulsants (carbamazepine, ethosuximide, mephenytoin, primidone, troxidone), antihypertensives (methyldopa, reserpine), antithyroid drugs (thiouracils) and a miscellaneous group

(chlorpromazine, D-penicillamine, methysergide, oral contraceptive agents, phenylbutazone).

Patients receiving treatment with a drug known to be particularly liable to cause the systemic lupus erythematosus syndrome should be tested for LE cells and antinuclear antibodies at intervals during therapy, and a watch should be kept for possible manifestations of the condition.

Pulmonary Fibrosis

A number of *cytotoxic drugs* are liable to induce intra-alveolar exudation which may become chronic and lead to increased fibrosis of the alveolar walls, progressing ultimately to widespread fibrosis or honeycombing which is indistinguishable on clinical or pathological grounds from other forms of diffuse pulmonary fibrosis. Busulphan, an alkylating agent used in the treatment of chronic myeloid leukaemia, may induce this type of syndrome after three or four years of treatment, causing cough, dyspnoea and fever with typical radiological changes of interstitial and intra-alveolar fibrosis. Although corticosteroid therapy may halt the progress of the fibrosis, most patients die of advanced restrictive pulmonary disease. Similar reactions may occur with cyclophosphamide and chlorambucil, while bleomycin, a cytotoxic antibiotic, sometimes causes pulmonary fibrosis and interstitial pneumonia more acutely after a period of 6 to 12 weeks' therapy. The *ganglion-blocking antihypertensive agents* hexamethonium, pentolinium and mecamylamine may also cause pulmonary fibrosis secondary to intra-alveolar exudation.

A different type of pulmonary fibrosis occasionally complicates long-term therapy with *methysergide* for migraine. The fibrogenic effects of this drug were first observed in relation to retroperitoneal fibrosis which resulted in ureteric obstruction, but evidence of concurrent pleuropulmonary involvement has subsequently been emphasised, characterised by pleuritic pain, pleural effusion and chronic dense pleural thickening. These changes tend to advance if methysergide therapy is continued but may slowly regress when the drug is withdrawn.

Extrinsic allergic alveolitis due to a Type III immune-complex reaction occurs rarely in patients who have taken *pituitary snuff* for the treatment of diabetes insipidus. Circulating precipitins against bovine and porcine antigens are present in the patient's serum, and the clinical and pathological manifestations are characteristic of those seen in other types of extrinsic allergic alveolitis (page 227).

Pulmonary Thromboembolic Disease

Deep venous thrombosis complicated by pulmonary embolism is an

important and potentially dangerous adverse effect of therapy with oral contraceptives, the incidence of thromboembolic disorders being directly related to the oestrogen content of these agents. Medication is therefore safer using combined progestogen-oestrogen preparations with an oestrogen content not exceeding 50 micrograms.

Although the mechanism of thromboembolism induced by these drugs is not satisfactorily explained, oral contraceptives have been shown to influence blood-clotting mechanisms by causing an increase in levels of prothrombin and factors VII, IX and X, and to affect the circulation by producing peripheral venous dilatation with consequent slowing and stagnation of blood flow in the legs; both these effects would tend to promote venous thrombosis.

Opportunist Infections

Corticosteroid Drugs. It has long been recognised that among the many side-effects of corticosteroid therapy is an increased liability to bacterial, mycobacterial and fungal infections that are particularly prone to affect the respiratory tract. Two examples of current interest may be quoted: the development of *Candida* infections of the oropharynx in asthmatic patients treated with topical corticosteroid aerosol preparations, particularly when the daily dose exceeds 400 micrograms: and the recrudescence of active pulmonary tuberculosis in middle-aged or elderly patients with apparently quiescent fibrotic apical lesions, given corticosteroids for conditions such as asthma, sarcoidosis or rheumatoid arthritis. Patients with radiographic evidence of past tuberculous infection who require corticosteroid therapy for any reason should be followed with serial chest radiographs, and if the activity of the lesion is in doubt prophylactic isoniazid therapy should be given concurrently.

Immunosuppressive therapy. The administration of immuno-suppressant drugs such as azothioprine, cyclophosphamide, metho-trexate, chlorambucil and corticosteroids is becoming increasingly common in the treatment of cancers, leukaemias and Hodgkin's disease, and in the management of patients receiving organ transplants. Pulmonary infections with fungi such as *Aspergillus fumigatus, Candida albicans* and *Nocardia asteroides,* protozoa such as *Pneumocystis carinii* and viruses such as cytomegalovirus have been described.

'Transplant lung' is a descriptive name given to *Pneumocystis carinii* pneumonia which presents as a characteristic clinical syndrome in renal transplant patients, consisting of dyspnoea of insidious onset associated with an unproductive cough, fever and malaise. The chest radiograph shows a diffuse 'granular' appearance due to miliary opacities distributed initially at the lung bases and in the hilar regions,

subsequently forming a dense confluent pattern. Tests of pulmonary function show arterial hypoxaemia, an increase in the alveolar-arterial oxygen tension difference and a reduction in carbon monoxide transfer factor (T_L,CO). The organism can rarely be identified in the sputum and the diagnosis must often be presumptive, based on the clinical presentation and radiological findings. Successful treatment with pentamidine isethionate has been described.

Bibliography

The references listed in this bibliography are intended to give the reader an opportunity to widen his study of topics that are necessarily described only briefly in a short textbook. Review articles and references to medical symposia or to other textbooks have been included whenever they appear to the author to give a particularly useful or balanced account of modern views, especially in those aspects of respiratory medicine that are rapidly changing.

Clinical Symptoms and Signs

CAMPBELL, E.J.M. (1969) Physical signs of diffuse airways obstruction and lung distension. *Thorax,* **24**, 1.

FINCH, C.A. (1948) Methemoglobinemia and sulphemoglobinemia. *New Engl. J. Med.,* **239**, 470.

FISHMAN, A.P. (1958) Polycythemia. *Amer. J. Med.,* **24**, 132.

FLAVELL, G. (1956) Reversal of pulmonary hypertrophic osteoarthropathy by vagotomy. *Lancet,* **i**, 260.

FORGACS, P. (1967) Crackles and wheezes. *Lancet,* **ii**, 203.

GROSS, N.J. and HAMILTON, J.D. (1963) Correlation between the physical signs of hypercapnia and the mixed venous PCO_2. *Brit. med. J.,* **2**, 1096.

LOVELL, R.H.H. (1950) Observations on the structure of clubbed fingers. *Clin. Sci.,* **9**, 299.

MEDD, W.E., FRENCH, E.B. and WYLIE, V.M. (1959) Cyanosis as a guide to arterial oxygen saturation. *Thorax,* **14**, 247.

MENDLOWITZ, M. (1942) Clubbing and hypertrophic osteoarthropathy. *Medicine* (Baltimore), **21**, 269.

NATH, A.R. and CAPEL, L.H. (1974) Inspiratory crackles—early and late. *Thorax,* **29**, 223.

The Chest X-Ray

SIMON, G. (1973) *Principles of Chest X-ray Diagnosis,* 3rd Ed. London: Butterworth.

SUTTON, D. (1969) *Textbook of Radiology,* Ch. 11, p. 227. The normal chest: techniques. London: Livingstone.

Pulmonary Physiology and Tests of Function

BATES, D.V., MACKLEM, P.T. and CHRISTIE, R.V. (1971) *Respiratory Function in Disease,* 2nd Ed. Philadelphia: W.B. Saunders.

CAMPBELL, E.J.M. (1958) *The Respiratory Muscles and the Mechanics of Breathing.* London: Lloyd-Luke.

CAMPBELL, E.J.M. (1966) The relationship of the sensation of breathlessness to the act of breathing. In *Breathlessness,* Ed. Howell, J.B.L. and Campbell, E.J.M. Oxford: Blackwell, p. 55.

COLLINS, J.V. (1973) Closing volume—a test of small airway function? *Brit. J. Dis. Chest,* **67**, 1.

COMROE, J.H., FORSTER, R.E., DUBOIS, A.B., BRISCOE, W.A. and CARLSEN, E. (1962) *The Lung: Clinical Physiology and Pulmonary Function Tests.* 2nd Edn. Chicago: Year Book Medical Publishers Inc.

COTES, J.E. (1975) *Lung Function.* 3rd Ed. Oxford: Blackwell.

JONES, N.L. (1967) Exercise testing. *Brit. J. Dis. Chest,* **61**, 169.

MEAD, J. (1961) Mechanical properties of lungs. *Physiol. Rev.,* **41**, 281.

RAHN, H. and FAHRI, L.E. (1964) Ventilation, perfusion and gas exchange–the VA/Q concept. *Respiration,* Vol. I, Ed. Fenn, W.O. and Rahn, H. Washington: American Physiological Society, p. 735.

SCADDING, J.G. (1966) Patterns of respiratory insufficiency. *Lancet,* i, 701.

TIERNEY, D.F. (1965) Pulmonary surfactant in health and disease. *Dis. of Chest,* **47**, 247.

WEIBEL, E.R. and GOMEZ, D.M. (1962) Architecture of the human lung. *Science,* **137**, 577.

WEST, J.B. (1970) Ventilation/Blood Flow and Gas Exchange. 2nd Ed. Oxford: Blackwell.

The Pulmonary Circulation

COURTICE, F.C. (1963) Lymph flow in the lungs. *Brit. med. Bull.,* **19**, 76.

CUMMING, G., HENDERSON, R., HORSFIELD, K. and SINGHAL, S.S. (1969) The functional morphology of the pulmonary circulation. In *The Pulmonary Circulation and Interstitial Space,* Ed. Fishman, A.P. and Hecht, H.H. Chicago: University of Chicago, p. 327.

HARRIS, P. and HEATH, D. (1962) *The Human Pulmonary Circulation.* London: Livingstone.

RAPHAEL, M.J. (1970) Pulmonary angiography. *Brit. J. Hosp. Med.,* **3**, 377.

STIRLING, G.M. (1973) Current status of radioisotope investigation of the lungs: clinical aspects. In *9th Symposium on Advanced Medicine,* Ed. Walker, G. London: Pitman, p. 347.

WEST, J.B., GLAZIER, J.B., HUGHES, J.M.B. and MALONEY, J.E. (1969) Pulmonary capillary flow, diffusion ventilation and gas exchange. In *Circulatory and Respiratory Mass Transport,* Ed. Wolstenholme, G.E.W. and Knight, J. London: Churchill, p. 256.

Disordered Function in Lung Disease

ABRAHAM, A.S., COLE, R.B. and BISHOP, J.M. (1968) The effects of prolonged oxygen administration on the pulmonary hypertension of patients with chronic bronchitis. *Circulation Res.,* **23**, 147.

ARNDT, H., KING, T.K.C. and BRISCOE, W.A. (1970) Diffusing capacities and ventilation : perfusion ratios in patients with the clinical syndrome of alveolar capillary block. *J. clin. Invest.,* **49**, 408.

CAMPBELL, E.J.M. (1967) Management of acute respiratory failure in chronic bronchitis and emphysema. *Amer. Rev. resp. Dis.,* **96**, 626.

CARO, C.G. and DUBOIS, A.B. (1961) Pulmonary function in kyphoscoliosis. *Thorax,* **16**, 282.

EMERSON, P.A. (1969) The pleura and its effusions. In *Fifth Symposium on Advanced Medicine,* Ed. Williams, R. London: Pitman Medical, p. 154.

FINLEY, T.N., SWENSON, E.W. and COMROE, J.H. (1962) The cause of arterial hypoxaemia at rest in patients with 'alveolar-capillary block syndrome'. *J. clin. Invest.,* **41**, 618.

FISHMAN, A.P., TURINO, G.M. and BERGOFSKY, E.H. (1957) The syndrome of alveolar hypoventilation. *Amer. J. Med.,* **23**, 333.

GREEN, I.D. (1967) Choice of method for administration of oxygen. *Brit. med. J.,* **3**, 593.

HARRIS, P., SEGEL, N., GREEN, I. and HOUSLEY, E. (1968) The influence of the airways resistance and alveolar pressure on the pulmonary vascular resistance in chronic bronchitis. *Cardiovascular Res.,* **2**, 84.

HASLETON, P.S., HEATH, D. and BREWER, D.B. (1968) Hypertensive pulmonary vascular disease in states of chronic hypoxia. *J. Path. Bact.,* **95**, 431.

NASH, G., BLENNERHASSETT, J.B. and PONTOPPIDAN, H. (1967) Pulmonary lesions associated with oxygen therapy and artificial ventilation. *New Engl. J. Med.,* **276**, 368.

ROBIN, E.D., JULIAN, D.G., TRAVIS, B.M. and CRUMP, C.H. (1959) A physiologic approach to the diagnosis of acute pulmonary embolism. *New Engl. J. Med.,* **260**, 586.

STAUB, N.C. (1963) Alveolar-arterial oxygen tension gradient due to diffusion. *J. appl. Physiol.,* **18**, 673.

Bronchial Asthma

GELL, P.G.H. and COOMBS, R.R.A. (1968) *Clinical Aspects of Immunology.* Oxford: Blackwell, p. 580.

MAUNSELL, K., PEARSON, R.S.B. and LIVINGSTONE, J.L. (1968) Long-term corticosteroid treatment of asthma. *Brit. med. J.,* **1**, 661.

MORAN, F., BANKIER, J.D.H. and BOYD, G. (1968) Disodium cromoglycate in the treatment of allergic bronchial asthma. *Lancet,* **ii**, 137.

PEPYS, J. (1967) Hypersensitivity to inhaled organic antigens. *J. Roy. Coll. Phycns Lond.,* **2**, 42.

PEPYS, J. (1973) Immunopathology of allergic lung disease. *Clin. Allergy,* **3**, 1.

WILLIAMS, N.E. and CROOKE, J.W. (1968) The practical management of severe status asthmaticus. *Lancet,* **i**, 1081.

Chronic Bronchitis and Emphysema

BATES, D.V. (1968) Chronic bronchitis and emphysema. *New Engl. J. Med.,* **278**, 546, 600.

BURROWS, B., FLETCHER, C.M., HEARD, B.E., JONES, N.L. and WOOTLIFF, J.S. (1966) The emphysematous and bronchial types of chronic airways obstruction. *Lancet,* **i**, 830.

KUEPPERS, F. and BLACK, L.F. (1974) Alpha 1-antitrypsin and its deficiency. *Amer. Rev. resp. Dis.,* **110**, 176.

LAMBERT, P.M. and REID, D.D. (1970) Smoking, air pollution and bronchitis in Britain. *Lancet,* **i**, 853.

McNICOL, M.W. and PRIDE, N.B. (1965) Unexplained underventilation of the lungs. *Thorax,* **20,** 53.

McNICOL, M.W. (1967) The management of respiratory failure. *Hospital Med.,* **1,** 601.

Bronchiectasis

BORRIE, J. and LICHTER, I. (1965) Surgical treatment of bronchiectasis: ten year survey. *Brit. med. J.,* **2,** 908.

CROFTON, J. (1966) Diagnosis and treatment of bronchiectasis. *Brit. med. J.,* **1,** 721, 783.

SANDERSON, J.M., KENNEDY, M.C.S., JOHNSON, M.F. and MANLEY, D.C.E. (1974) Bronchiectasis: results of surgical and conservative management. *Thorax,* **29,** 407.

Cystic Fibrosis

BUSEY, J.F., FENGER, E.P.K., HEPPER, N.G., KENT, D.C., KILBURN, K.H., MATTHEWS, L.W., SIMPSON, D.G. and GRZYBOWSKI, S. (1968) The treatment of cystic fibrosis. *Amer. Rev. resp. Dis.,* **97,** 730.

GIBSON, L.E. and COOKE, R.E. (1959) A test for concentration of electrolytes in sweat in cystic fibrosis of the pancreas utilising pilocarpine by iontophoresis. *Pediatrics,* **23,** 545.

MAY, J.R., HERRICK, N.C. and THOMPSON, D. (1972) Bacterial infection in cystic fibrosis. *Arch. Dis. Childhood,* **47,** 908.

MEARNS, M.B. (1974) Cystic fibrosis. *Brit. J. Hosp. Med.,* **12,** 497.

WENTWORTH, P., GOUGH, J. and WENTWORTH, J.E. (1968) Pulmonary changes and cor pulmonale in mucoviscidosis. *Thorax,* **23,** 582.

Spontaneous Pneumothorax

KILLEN, D.A. and GOBBEL, W.G. (1968) Spontaneous Pneumothorax. London: Churchill.

LENNOX, S.C. (1970) Treatment of spontaneous pneumothorax. *Brit. J. Hosp. Med.,* **3,** 893.

LICHTER, I. (1974) Long-term follow-up of planned treatment of spontaneous pneumothorax. *Thorax,* **29,** 32.

LICHTER, I. and GWYNNE, J.F. (1971) Spontaneous pneumothorax in young subjects. *Thorax,* **26,** 409.

NORRIS, R.M., JONES, J.G. and BISHOP, J.M. (1968) Respiratory gas exchange in patients with spontaneous pneumothorax. *Thorax,* **23,** 427.

Acute Infections of the Respiratory Tract

ANDREWS, N.C., PARKER, E.F., SHAW, R.R., WILSON, N.J. and WEBB, W.R. (1962) Management of nontuberculous empyema. *Amer. Rev. resp. Dis.,* **85,** 935.

CROFTON, J. (1970) The chemotherapy of bacterial respiratory infections. *Amer. Rev. resp. Dis.,* **101,** 841.

FLAVELL, G. (1966) Lung abscess. *Brit. med. J.,* **1,** 1032.

FORSYTH, B.R. and CHANOCK, R.M. (1966) Mycoplasma pneumoniae. *Ann. Rev. Med.,* **17,** 371.

GRIST, N.R. (1968) Investigative methods. *J. clin. Path.*, **21**, Suppl. 2, 10.

HEATH, R.B. (1973) Virus infections of the respiratory tract. In *Recent Advances in Medicine*, 16th Ed. London: Churchill Livingstone, p. 181.

HOFFMAN, E. (1961) Empyema in childhood. *Thorax*, **16**, 128.

McCRACKEN, G.H., EICHENWALD, H.F. and NELSON, J.D. (1969) Antimicrobial therapy in theory and practice. *J. Pediat.*, **75**, 742, 923.

MARMION, B.P., STOKER, M.G.P., McCOY, J.H., MALLOCH, R.A. and MOORE, B. (1953) Q Fever in Great Britain. *Lancet*, i, 503.

NICKS, R. (1964) Empyema and ruptured lung abscess in adults. *Thorax*, **19**, 492.

OSWALD, N.C., SIMON, G. and SHOOTER, R.A. (1961) Pneumonia in hospital practice. *Brit. J. Dis. Chest*, **55**, 109.

STUART-HARRIS, C.H. (1965) *Influenza and Other Virus Infections of the Respiratory Tract*, 2nd Ed. London: Arnold.

Pulmonary Tuberculosis

CITRON, K.M. (1974) The chemotherapy of pulmonary tuberculosis. *Brit. J. Hosp. Med.*, **12**, 731.

CROFTON, J. (1970) The chemotherapy of bacterial respiratory infections. *Amer. Rev. resp. Dis.*, **101**, 841.

DAVIES, D. (1972) Ankylosing spondylitis and lung fibrosis. *Quart. J. Med.*, **41**, 395.

EAST AFRICAN/BRITISH MEDICAL RESEARCH COUNCILS (1974) Controlled trial of four short course (6-month) regimens of chemotherapy for treatment of pulmonary tuberculosis. *Lancet*, **ii**, 237.

JACQUES, J. and SLOAN, J.M. (1970) The changing pattern of miliary tuberculosis. *Thorax*, **25**, 237.

PROUDFOOT, A.T., AKHTAR, A.J., DOUGLAS, A.C. and HORNE, N.W. (1969) Miliary tuberculosis in adults. *Brit. med. J.*, **2**, 273.

STEAD, W.W., KERBY, G.R., SCHLUETER, D.P. and JORDAHL, C.W. (1968) The clinical spectrum of primary tuberculosis in adults. *Ann. intern. med.*, **68**, 731.

STRADLING, P. and POOLE, G.W. (1970) Twice weekly streptomycin plus isoniazid for tuberculosis. *Tubercle (London)*, **51**, 44.

Fungal Infections of the Lungs

HENDERSON, A.H., ENGLISH, M.P. and VECHT, R.J. (1968) Pulmonary aspergillosis. *Thorax*, **23**, 513.

MACLEOD, W.M., MURRAY, I.G., DAVIDSON, J. and GIBBS, D.D. (1972) Histoplasmosis. *Thorax*, **27**, 6.

MURRAY, J.F., FINEGOLD, S.M., FROMAN, S. and HILL, D.W. (1961) The changing spectrum of nocardiosis. *Amer. Rev. resp. Dis.*, **83**, 315.

SARKANY, I. (1968) Systemic Mycoses. In *Recent Advances in Medicine*, 15th Edn., Ed. Baron, D.N., Compston, N. and Dawson, A.M. London: Churchill, p. 243.

SLADE, P.R., SLESSOR, B.V. and SOUTHGATE, J. (1973) Thoracic actinomycosis. *Thorax*, **28**, 273.

Pulmonary Sarcoidosis

HOYLE, C., SMYLLIE, H.C. and LEAK, D.A. (1967) Prolonged treatment of pulmonary sarcoidosis with steroids. *Thorax*, **22,** 519.

JAMES, D.G. (1961) Erythema nodosum. *Brit. med. J.*, **1**, 853.

JONES WILLIAMS, W. (1967) The pathology of sarcoidosis. *Hospital Med.*, **2,** 21.

LONGCOPE, W.T. and FREIMAN, D.G. (1952) A study of sarcoidosis. *Medicine* (Baltimore), **31,** 1.

MARSHALL, R., SMELLIE, H., BAYLIS, J.H., HOYLE, C. and BATES, D.V. (1958) Pulmonary function in sarcoidosis. *Thorax*, **13**, 48.

SMELLIE, H. and HOYLE, C. (1960) The natural history of pulmonary sarcoidosis. *Quart. J. Med.*, **29,** 539.

Diffuse Fibrosing Alveolitis

GAENSLER, E.A., MOISTER, M.V.B. and HAM, J. (1964) Open lung biopsy in diffuse lung disease. *New Engl. J. Med.*, **270**, 1319.

HAMMAN, L. and RICH, A.R. (1944) Acute diffuse interstitial fibrosis of the lungs. *Bull. Johns Hopkins Hosp.*, **74**, 177.

LIEBOW, A.A., STEER, A. and BILLINGSLEY, J.G. (1965) Desquamative interstitial pneumonia. *Amer. J. Med.*, **39**, 369.

OSWALD, N. and PARKINSON, T. (1949) Honeycomb lungs. *Quart. J. Med.*, **18**, 1.

SCADDING, J.G. (1974) Diffuse pulmonary alveolar fibrosis. *Thorax*, **29**, 271.

STACK, B.H.R., CHOO-KANG, Y.F.J. and HEARD, B.E. (1972) The prognosis of cryptogenic fibrosing alveolitis. *Thorax*, **27**, 535.

STEEL, S.J. and WINSTANLEY, D.P. (1969) Trephine biopsy of the lung and pleura. *Thorax*, **24**, 576.

TURNER-WARWICK, M. (1974) A perspective view of widespread pulmonary fibrosis. *Brit. Med. J.*, **2**, 371.

Industrial Lung Disease

ELMES, P.C. (1971) Asbestos. In *Inhaled Particles in Clinical Practice*, Ed. Muir, D.C.F. London: Heinemann.

PARKES, W.R. (1974) *Occupational Lung Disorders*. London: Butterworth.

PEPYS, J. (1969) *Hypersensitivity Diseases of the Lungs due to Fungi and Organic Dusts*. Basel: Karger.

SEAL, R.M.E. (1967) Farmer's lung. *Hospital Med.*, **1**, 1123.

Malignant Disease of the Lungs

ABBEY SMITH, R. (1969) Bronchial carcinoid tumours. *Thorax*, **24**, 43.

ASHLEY, D.J.B. and DAVIES, H.D. (1967) Cancer of the lung. Histology and biological behaviour. *Cancer*, **20**, 165.

BAYLISS, R.I.S. (1967) Endocrine syndromes associated with bronchial carcinoma. In *Progress in Clinical Medicine*, 5th Edn., Ed. Daley, R. and Miller, H. London: Churchill, p. 86.

BIGNALL, J.R., MARTIN, M. and SMITHERS, D.W. (1967) Survival in 6086 cases of bronchial carcinoma. *Lancet*, **i**, 1067.

BRAIN, R. and HENSON, R.A. (1958) Neurological syndromes associated with carcinoma—the carcinomatous neuromyopathies. *Lancet,* **ii**, 971.

DEELEY, T.J. (1967) The treatment of carcinoma of the bronchus. *Brit. J. Radiol.,* **40**, 801.

DE VILLIERS, A.J. and WINDISH, J.P. (1964) Lung cancer in a fluorspar mining community. *Brit. J. Indust. Med.,* **21**, 94.

DOLL, R. (1955) Mortality from lung cancer in asbestos workers. *Brit. J. indust. Med.,* **12**, 81.

ELLMAN, P. and BOWDLER, A.J. (1960) Pulmonary manifestations of Hodgkin's disease. *Brit. J. Dis. Chest,* **54**, 59.

HAROLD, J.T. (1952) Lymphangitis carcinomatosa of the lungs. *Quart. J. Med.,* **21**, 353.

LENNOX, S.C., FLAVELL, G., POLLOCK, D.J., THOMPSON, V.C. and WILKINS, J.L. (1968) Results of resection for oat-cell carcinoma of the lung. *Lancet,* **ii**, 925.

Medical Research Council (1966) Comparative trial of surgery and radiotherapy for the primary treatment of small-celled or oat-celled carcinoma of the bronchus. *Lancet,* **ii**, 979.

MELMON, K.L., SJOERDSMA, A. and MASON, D.T. (1965) Distinctive clinical and therapeutic aspects of the syndrome associated with bronchial carcinoid tumours. *Amer. J. Med.,* **39**, 568.

NOHL-OSER, H.C. (1965) Mediastinoscopy. *Brit. med. J.,* **1**, 1167.

REES, G.M. (1973) Primary lymphosarcoma of the lung. *Thorax,* **28**, 429.

RICHARDSON, R.H., ZAVALA, D.C., MUKERJEE, P.K. and BEDELL, G.N. (1974) The use of fibreoptic bronchoscopy and brush biopsy in the diagnosis of suspected pulmonary malignancy. *Amer. Rev. resp. Dis.,* **109**, 63.

Royal College of Physicians of London (1971) *Smoking and Health Now.* A new report and summary on smoking and its effects on health. London: Pitman.

STRADLING, P. (1973) *Diagnostic Bronchoscopy.* 2nd Ed. London: Livingstone.

WAGNER, J.C., SLEGGS, C.A. and MARCHAND, P. (1960) Diffuse pleural mesothelioma and asbestos exposure in the North Western Cape Province. *Brit. J. indust. Med.,* **17**, 260.

WATSON, W.L. and FARPOUR, A. (1966) Terminal bronchiolar or 'alveolar' cell cancer of the lung. *Cancer,* **19**, 776.

Connective Tissue Diseases

CAPLAN, A., PAYNE, R.B. and WITHEY, J.L. (1962) A broader concept of Caplan's syndrome related to rheumatoid factor. *Thorax,* **17**, 205.

CARRINGTON, C.B. and LIEBOW, A.A. (1966) Limited forms of angiitis and granulomatosis of Wegener's type. *Amer. J. Med.,* **41**, 497.

HUGHES, G.R.V. (1974) Systemic lupus erythematosus. *Brit. J. Hosp. Med.,* **12**, 309.

ROSE, G.A. and SPENCER, H. (1957) Polyarteritis nodosa. *Quart. J. Med.,* **26**, 43.

RUBIN, E.H. (1967) Rheumatoid lung. *N.Y. St. J. Med.,* **67**, 2014.

TURNER-WARWICK, M.E. (1969) Rheumatoid arthritis, rheumatoid factors and lung disease. *Brit. J. Hosp. Med.,* **2**, 507.

WALKER, W.C. (1967) Pulmonary infections and rheumatoid arthritis. *Quart. J. Med.,* **36**, 239.

WEAVER, A.L., DIVERTIE, M.B. and TITUS, J.L. (1967) The lung in scleroderma. *Mayo Clin. Proc.,* **42**, 754.

Pulmonary Thromboembolic Disease

GOODWIN, J.F., Harrison, C.V. and WILCKEN, D.E.L. (1963) Obliterative pulmonary hypertension and thromboembolism. *Brit. med. J.,* **1**, 701, 777.

GOODWIN, J.F. (1969) The management of pulmonary thromboembolism. In *5th Symposium on Advanced Medicine,* Ed. Williams, R. London: Pitman, p. 126.

JONES, N.L. and GOODWIN, J.F. (1965) Respiratory function in pulmonary thromboembolic disorders. *Brit. med. J.,* **1**, 1089.

MILLER, G.A.H. and SUTTON, G.C. (1970) Massive pulmonary embolism. *Brit. J. Hosp. Med.,* **3**, 847.

OAKLEY, C.M. (1969) Mechanism of pulmonary embolism. In *5th Symposium on Advanced Medicine,* Ed. Williams, R. London: Pitman, p. 105.

TIBBUTT, D.A., DAVIES, J.A., ANDERSON, J.A., FLETCHER, E.W.L., HAMILL, J., HOLT, J.M., LEA THOMAS, M., LEE, G. DeJ., MILLER, G.A.H., SHARP, A.A. and SUTTON, G.C. (1974) Comparison by controlled clinical trial of streptokinase and heparin in treatment of life-threatening pulmonary embolism. *Brit. med. J.,* **1**, 343.

Drug-induced Lung Disease

D'ARCY, P.F. and GRIFFIN, J.P. (1972) *Iatrogenic Diseases.* London: Oxford University Press, p. 65.

DAVIES, P.D.B. (1969) Drug-induced lung disease. *Brit. J. Dis. Chest,* **63**, 57.

DOAK, P.B., BECROFT, D.M.O., HARRIS, E.A., HITCHCOCK, G.C., LEEMING, B.W.A., NORTH, J.D.K., MONTGOMERIE, J.Z. and WHITLOCK, R.M.L. (1973) *Pneumocystis carinii* pneumonia—transplant lung. *Quart. J. Med.,* **42**, 59.

DOLLERY, C.T. (1972) Drug interactions. In *8th Symposium on Advanced Medicine,* Ed. Neale, G. London: Pitman, p. 210.

HILL, R.B., ROWLANDS, D.J. and RIFKIND, D. (1964) Infectious pulmonary disease in patients receiving immunosuppressive therapy for organ transplantation. *New Engl. J. Med.,* **271**, 1021.

LARSSON, S., CRONBERG, S., DENNEBURG, T. and OHLSSON, N.-M. (1973) Pulmonary reaction to Nitrofurantoin. *Scand. J. resp. Dis.,* **54**, 103.

ROSENOW, E.C. (1972) The spectrum of drug-induced pulmonary disease. *Ann. intern. Med.,* **77**, 977.

SAMTER, J. and BEERS, R.F. (1968) Intolerance to aspirin. Clinical studies and consideration of its pathogenesis. *Ann. intern. Med.,* **68**, 975.

SMITH, J.W., SEIDL, L.G. and CLUFF, L.E. (1966) Studies on the epidemiology of adverse drug reactions. *Ann. intern. Med.,* **65**, 629.

Index